Medical Terminology:
A Text/Workbook

medical terminology:
a text/workbook
second edition

Alice Prendergast, R.N., M.A.
Phoenix College, Phoenix, Arizona

Addison-Wesley Publishing Company
Medical/Nursing Division
Menlo Park, California • Reading, Massachusetts
London • Amsterdam • Don Mills, Ontario • Sydney

Sponsoring Editor: Nancy Evans
Associate Editor: Tom Eoyang
Production Editor: Betty Duncan
Cover Design: Robin Ann Gold
Illustrations: Peter Hastings
          Fran Milner (Figs. 22–2, 23–1)

Copyright © 1983 by Addison-Wesley Publishing Company, Inc.
All rights reserved. No part of this publication may be reproduced,
stored in a retrieval system, or transmitted, in any form or by any
means, electronic, mechanical, photocopying, recording, or otherwise,
without the prior permission of the publisher. Printed in the
United States of America. Published simultaneously in Canada.

Library of Congress Cataloging in Publication Data

Prendergast, Alice, 1914–
    Medical terminology.

    Includes index.
    1. Medicine—Terminology—Problems, exercises, etc.
I. Title.   [DNLM: 1. Nomenclature—Examination
questions.   W 18 P926m]
[R123.P72 1982]   610'.1'4   82-16342

ISBN 0-201-05955-X
ABCDEFGHIJKL-MU-898765432

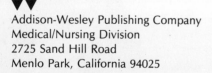

Addison-Wesley Publishing Company
Medical/Nursing Division
2725 Sand Hill Road
Menlo Park, California 94025

preface

AUDIENCE

Medical Terminology: A Text/Workbook, Second Edition is written for a one-semester allied health course, including medical records, emergency medical technology, medical reception, medical secretary, medical transcriber, medical assisting, unit clerking, and various other types of health care activities. Nursing programs at all levels found the first edition to be a valuable supplement to the basic curriculum for their students. Other professions identified a need for knowledge of medical terminology; this text can meet this need for personnel in legal, paralegal, court reporting, and medical claims work.

GOALS OF THE TEXT

When the first edition of *Medical Terminology* was published in 1977, I had been teaching the subject for 6 years and had used all the popular medical terminology texts then available. Although some were excellent books, none proved satisfactory because they simply offered too much material to cover in a one-semester course. They included more than most students in the allied health fields needed or could reasonably absorb in a short course; the result was discouragement. Judging from the response to the first edition, this text provided an answer to the problem for other instructors as well.

Instead of presenting an exhaustive list of every known medical word and forcing the student to try to memorize what is in essence a dictionary, this text helps the student learn the *basic construction* of medical terminology. Through constant practice, repetition, and simplified explanations, the student acquires a solid foundation that not only aids retention of the vocabulary learned in this text, but also facilitates understanding new vocabulary encountered in other course work and work situations.

The text accomplishes these goals by assuming no extensive knowledge of anatomy and physiology or any other previous learning that does not happen naturally in the course of daily living. The book offers concrete learning activities in the form of exercises and drills, with answers provided to allow immediate feedback and progress evaluation.

COVERAGE AND ORGANIZATION

The terms presented in *Medical Terminology* are general terms used in many medical situations. No attempt is made to include all special vocabulary pertinent to the medical specialties.

Part 1 contains 15 chapters on terminology, in which word parts, prefixes, suffixes, and root words are introduced in a logical manner. Some important medical words that are not composed of these common parts also are included. Two comprehensive chapters on abbreviations and laboratory terms are followed by a brief introduction to medications.

Part 2 contains 10 chapters, one for each body system. Each chapter offers a brief outline of anatomy and physiology, as well as information about the principal diseases that affect the system. Students will find it helpful to supplement the information on body systems with outside reading in any suitable book such as an encyclopedia, medical dictionary, health book or any of the reference books listed in Appendix E.

The sequence in which the book is studied can be altered by the instructor as desired. I use the book in this manner: one or two chapters from Part 1 together with a chapter from Part 2. For example, Chapters 1 and 2 are used with 16, Chapter 3 with 17, and so on, with a total of two or three chapters assigned at one time. This is feasible for a class that meets once a week for 3 hours. If classes meet for shorter periods two or three times a week, assignments would differ.

Tests are included in this text. Instructors, of course, may wish to use their own or combine theirs with the text to suit individual needs. More tests are provided than are needed; some may be used as additional exercises.

CHANGES IN THE SECOND EDITION

Pronunciation. The letter or letters that receive the greatest emphasis are shown in boldface type instead of italics, which did not show up well in the first edition. (This is not meant to show syllables as they are given in a dictionary but only to give the student a clue as to how to pronounce the word.)

Sequence. "Plural Endings" (Chapter 11) is brought forward and is now Chapter 7, so that these will be understood as they are encountered in subsequent chapters.

The "Nervous System" (Chapter 24) is moved forward to Chapter 23, and the "Endocrine System" (Chapter 23) is now Chapter 25. This change brings the more important "Nervous System" to a place where it will not be hurried through to complete the course.

Additions. Additional terms are introduced in every chapter, and definitions are clarified but kept as simple as possible. New headings of special interest (Chapters 17–25) include: diseases, diagnostic and surgical procedures, abbreviations in some chapters, psychiatric terms in Chapter 24, and neuromuscular disorders in Chapter 18. In all chapters, terms have been assembled in alphabetical order for easier reference.

"Abbreviations: Diagnoses and Medical Laboratory" (Chapter 14) is expanded to include SMA forms (blood chemistry profiles) and an explanation of the results. Chapter 15, "Introduction to Pharmacology," includes an assignment with the *Physicians' Desk Reference* and drug advertisements.

Most important, at least one case report is created for each body system chapter (more often several are included) to demonstrate the use of medical terminology in realistic settings. Preliminary reactions to this feature indicate that it will enhance students' comprehension of the material and their motivation to learn. The reports are not consistent in form. Some use abbreviations for headings, laboratory data, and so on; some spell out these words. *These inconsistencies have been purposely retained* so that the student can see how actual reports vary in form, completeness, and clarity.

Illustrations are added in this edition to clarify difficult concepts, and some are included that are not readily found in every text.

Two new appendices are added. These include a list of medications, with both generic and trade names; and a comprehensive list of abbreviations, with physical therapy, pulmonary function, and cancer terms listed separately.

The index is a glossary/index – comprehensive, but simple. This should be helpful for reference and enable the student to find an answer quickly.

In summary, the new edition should prove to retain its value as a text/workbook and also serve as a reference book after the course has been completed.

COURSE OBJECTIVE

At the completion of this course, the student will be able to:

1. Analyze many medical words and have a solid base on which to build a larger vocabulary.
2. Spell most medical words correctly.
3. Recognize medical words in dictation and decide whether a word makes sense in context.
4. Identify normal and abnormal functions of the human body and understand what medical terms mean in specific contexts.
5. Enjoy his or her work more because of increased understanding of medical terminology.

ACKNOWLEDGMENTS

I wish to express my gratitude to all Addison-Wesley personnel who were instrumental in the publishing of this book, with special thanks to Betty Duncan and Tom Eoyang. Their help has been invaluable.

My thanks also are extended to the instructors who reviewed the manuscript and offered suggestions for improvement; appreciation is extended to the people who gave permission for the use of illustrations and other materials.

Throughout my teaching career, I have found my students to be my greatest motivating factor. Their enthusiasm and their questions inspire me to continue learning.

Alice Prendergast

instructions for use of this workbook

Concentrate on one chapter at a time; your instructor may wish to go over new words in class, pronouncing the words so you will become familiar with their sound. As you use this book:

1. Be sure you have mastered one chapter before going on to the next, no matter in what order they are presented.
2. Practice saying the words.
3. Memorize unfamiliar word parts.
4. Learn all example words given.
5. Work and rework drill and practice sheets.
6. Continue to review as often as necessary to retain what you have learned.

PRONUNCIATION

You may not be called on to pronounce medical words often, but you will be required to recognize medical words when you hear them; you must be able to spell them correctly. Unless you have heard the words many times, you will have difficulty recognizing them; this means that to learn *useful* medical terminology, you must learn to pronounce the words as you learn them.

Knowing which letter or letters to emphasize is the most difficult part of pronunciation. In this book, bold-face type is used to assist you. For instance, electro-encephalogram looks difficult, but if you separate the word parts—electro/en**ceph**alo/gram—and if you know which letters are to be emphasized, it becomes less formidable. Dictating words for spelling practice to another student is a good way to become familiar with

pronouncing terms. (In actual practice you will find pronunciation varies considerably.)

MEDICAL DICTIONARY

A medical dictionary is essential (see Appendix C). There are a number of good ones on the market varying in price from $3.25 (paperback) to very expensive volumes. If you plan to work in medical records, you may wish to purchase a more comprehensive dictionary at the outset. For some allied health careers, an inexpensive dictionary is adequate. (Appendix E lists some dictionaries available.)

WORK OR PRACTICE SHEETS

Worksheets are provided to help you see where you are having difficulty. The "Answer Keys" are located in Appendix A. Do not refer to the answers until you have honestly tried to complete the worksheet.

Review drills are also provided to help you quickly see which word parts are causing difficulty. Make flash cards for these.

Tests for each chapter, review tests, and a final exam are included in Appendix F. These are similar in content to the worksheets, but are worded differently. These are not self-tests, and answers are not provided in the workbook; test answer keys are located in the Instructor's Manual. Your instructor will decide how these tests are to be used, or may choose to provide different tests. *Do not write on the tests until you are instructed to do so.*

Good luck in your study of this course.

contents

LIST OF FIGURES

part 1

basic medical terminology and word structure

pretests of medical words

Although pretests are not generally given in medical terminology courses (because it is presumed that the average person has no knowledge of medical terms), you will find such tests given here as an introduction to what you will find in this workbook.

pretest A

This "test" is to show you that you already have some knowledge of medical terms.

Define the following words:

1. **mi**croscope _____
2. tonsil**lec**tomy _____
3. appen**dec**tomy _____
4. **frac**ture _____
5. derma**ti**tis _____
6. in**cis**ion _____
7. **ut**erus _____
8. pre**nat**al care _____
9. pneu**mon**ia _____
10. **ster**ilized _____
11. bac**ter**ia _____
12. antibi**ot**ic _____
13. a**bor**tion _____
14. electro**car**diogram (ECG or EKG) _____
15. com**mun**icable disease _____
16. "staph" infection _____
17. "strep throat" _____
18. Spell the name of the common medication (made by Bayer) for headaches: _____
19. Spell the word for the regular monthly "period" experienced by the female: _____

If you had no difficulty with the preceding test, you have a good start on medical terms. If you found it difficult to define these words, even though you have probably used them often, see Answer Key 1.* (If you missed only two or three answers, you have scored satisfactorily.)

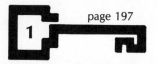

page 197

* All Answer Keys are located in Appendix A, beginning on p. 197.

-ology: the science or study of (appears at the end of a word and applies to the word that comes before it). Note that the accent is always on the **ol** syllable in **ol**ogy.

1. Define:

    a. bi**ol**ogy (bio = life or living) _____

    b. bacteri**ol**ogy _____

    c. microbi**ol**ogy _____

    d. termi**nol**ogy _____

    (Wonder why they don't just call it term**ol**ogy?)

2. What do you think these words mean?

    a. a**nat**omy _____

    b. physi**ol**ogy _____

    c. pa**thol**ogy _____

3. Name the body organs you know (an organ is a specialized body structure that performs a certain function):

    _____ _____ _____ _____

    _____ _____ _____ _____

4. Name some body systems (a system is a set of organs that work together to perform a certain function):

    _____ _____

    _____ _____

5. List several kinds of physicians (specialists), for example, urologist:

    _____

    _____

    _____

6. Name some diseases or abnormal conditions:

    _____

    _____

    _____

7. Name some kinds of operations:

    _____

    _____

    _____

Ready for Chapter 1?

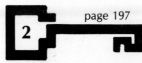
page 197
2

chapter 1
medical words
(-ectomy)

---

word parts introduction

Define:

1. prefix _____

2. suffix _____

3. root word _____

4. compound word _____

5. combining form _____

    Examples of various combinations of word parts follow. Start your new vocabulary by trying to define the indicated medical words.

Words using a prefix and root word:

Prefix	Root	Example	Define
semi-	final	semifinal	
mis-	interpret	misinterpret	
uni-	form	uniform	
pre-	mature	prema**ture**	6. _____
hyper-	active	hyper**ac**tive	7. _____

Words using a root and a suffix:

Root	Suffix	Example	Define
care	-less	careless	
violin	-ist	violinist	
psych	-ology	psy**chol**ogy	8. _____
tonsil	-ectomy	tonsil**lec**tomy	9. _____
bronch	-itis	bronch**i**tis	10. _____

Words made up of two root words (compound words):

Root	Root	Example	Define
head	ache	headache	
news	paper	newspaper	
micro	scope	**mi**croscope	11. _____
hydr/o	therapy	hydro**ther**apy	12. _____
bronch/o	pneumonia	bronchopneu**mo**nia	13. _____

Words using combining form:

14. cardio **vas**cular _____

15. gastroin **tes**tinal _____

Words using prefix and suffix only:

Prefix	Suffix	Example	Define
an-	-emia	a **ne**mia	16. _____
ex-	-cise	**ex**cise	17. _____
poly-	-uria	poly **u**ria	18. _____

Words using prefix, root, and suffix:

Prefix	Root	Suffix	Word	Define
super-	nature	-al	supernatural	
un-	lady	-like	unladylike	
peri-	card	-itis	pericar **di**tis	19. _____

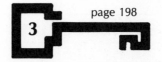

page 198

3

practice sheet

-ectomy to excise or cut out surgically. The accent is
always on the **ec** syllable in **-ec**tomy.

   With this information, write a definition for the following words. Do not worry about whether the word makes sense to you or that you have never heard of it. These are obvious.

1. tonsil **lec**tomy _excision of the tonsils_

2. appen **dec**tomy _excision of the appendix_

3. adenoid **ec**tomy _excision of the adenoids_

4. thyroi **dec**tomy _excision of the thyroids_

5. sple **nec**tomy _excision of the spleen_

These are more difficult, but they are fairly common operations.

6. hyste **rec**tomy _excision of the uterus_

7. cholecys **tec**tomy _____

8. hemorrhoi **dec**tomy _excision of the hemorrhoids_

9. gingi **vec**tomy (dental) _____

10. mas **tec**tomy _____

Less commonly performed operations. Some are quite obvious.

11. adrenal **ec**tomy _____

12. pancrea **tec**tomy _____

13. co**lec**tomy _____

14. neu**rec**tomy _____

15. duode**nec**tomy _____

16. laryn**gec**tomy _____

17. ureter**ec**tomy _____

18. gas**trec**tomy _____

19. cervi**cec**tomy _____

20. tympa**nec**tomy _____

21. oopho**rec**tomy _____

22. cys**tec**tomy _____

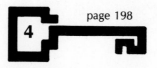

page 198

suffix -ectomy

Do not worry if you did not do well on the foregoing practice sheet. You should, however, have noticed that all -ectomy words are not formed in exactly the same way.

1. Some -ectomy words are formed by simply adding -ectomy to a familiar word (body part or organ), for example:

adenoid = adenoid**ec**tomy

2. Some -ectomy words are formed by using an unfamiliar or foreign root word, for example:

gastr- = gas**trec**tomy (stomach)
hyster- = hyste**rec**tomy (uterus)

3. Some -ectomy words have a letter added, a letter dropped, or a letter changed, for example:

tonsil**lec**tomy (tonsils)
sple**nec**tomy (spleen)
pancrea**tec**tomy (pancreas)
laryn**gec**tomy (larynx)

4. In some -ectomy words, the last syllable is dropped, for example:

colon = co**lec**tomy (large intestine)
duo**de**num = duode**nec**tomy (first part of small intestine)
ap**pen**dix = appen**dec**tomy (small appendage on cecum)

Go back to the preceding practice sheet and look at the words. Select the category that each word belongs in and write that word in the correct column of the following chart. *THEN* check your answers with the numbers given in the footnote below.*

---

* Category 1: 3, 4, 8, 11, 17, and 22; category 2: 6, 7, 9, 10, 14, 18, 21, and 22; category 3: 1, 5, 12, 16, and 19; category 4: 2, 13, 15, and 20.

Category

1 word unchanged	2 unfamiliar or foreign root	3 letter changed, added, or dropped	4 last syllable dropped

-ectomy pretest

You know what - **ec**tomy means: to excise or cut out surgically. The spelling of - **ec**tomy is always the same, and the accent is always on the **-ec** syllable.

Write a word that means:

1. Tonsils removed surgically _____ *tonsilectomy*

2. Adenoids removed surgically _____ *adenoidectomy*

3. Thyroid gland removed surgically _____ *thyroidectomy*

4. Adrenal gland removed surgically _____ *adrenectomy*

Spell: Have someone dictate these words to you from Answer Key 5.

5. _____   13. _____

6. _____   14. _____

7. _____   15. _____

8. _____   16. _____

9. _____   17. _____

10. _____   18. _____

11. _____   19. _____

12. _____   20. _____

Define:

21. ex **cis** ion _____

22. in **cis** ion _____

23. What do you think the term *body cavity* means? _____

_____

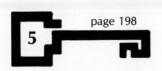

5   page 198

If your score is not 100%,
review and try again.

unfamiliar root words for body parts and organs

Figures 1–1 and 1–2 should help you to identify foreign words used to describe body parts and/or organs. Study the diagrams and **refer back to them** as often as necessary as you go on to other chapters. /o signifies combining form.

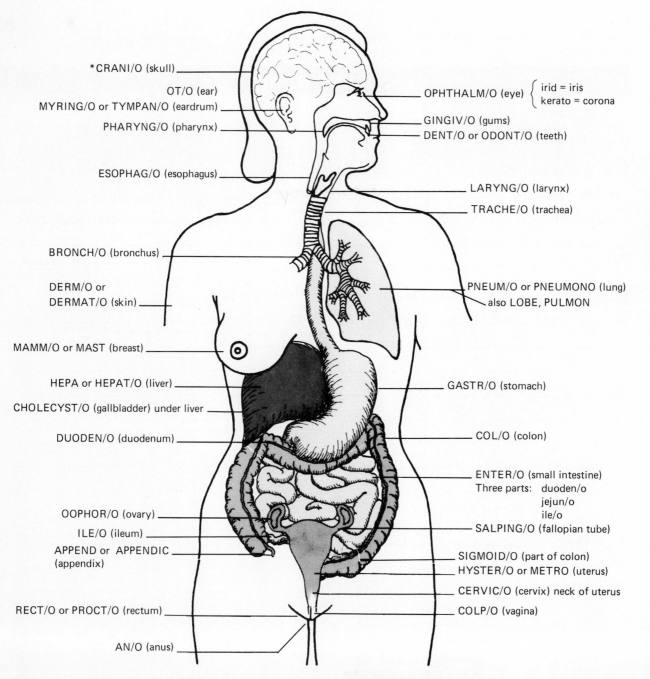

Figure 1–1. Gyne (woman). Anterior view, no bony structure shown. Showing intestinal tract, female reproductive organs, lung, and airway. Note: there is a word in this figure that refers to a part of the head (indicated by *).

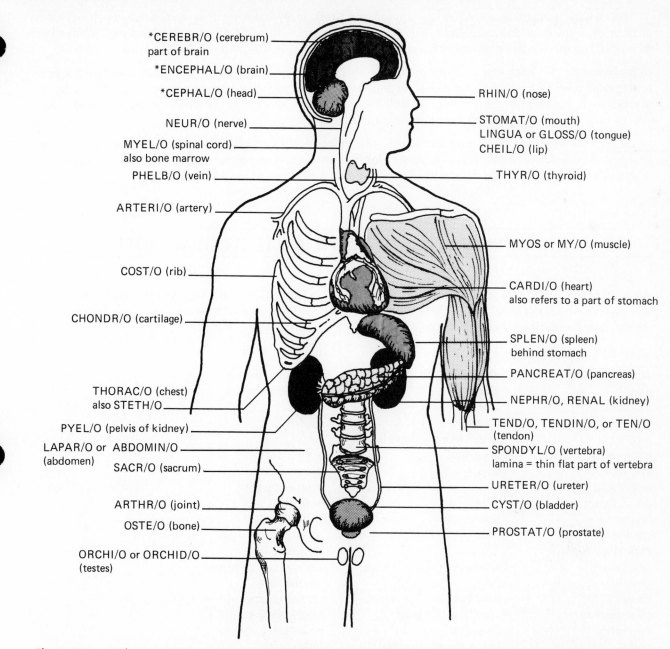

Figure 1-2. Andro (man). Anterior view, partial skeleton shown; abdominal viscera not shown. Showing male reproductive organs, urinary tract, heart, spleen, pancreas, hip joint, and some shoulder muscles. Note: there are three words in this figure that refer to parts of the head (indicated by *).

You will find that you already know some medical root words because you have heard them used in some way, for example:

derma–	(skin)	derma**tol**ogist
hepat–	(liver)	hepa**ti**tis
append–	(appendix)	appen**dec**tomy
bronch–	(bronchial tubes)	bron**chi**tis
pneum–	(lungs)	pneu**mo**nia
dent–	(teeth)	**den**tist
neur–	(nerves)	neu**ri**tis

You will be using these and other less familiar root words in the following lessons. Gradually you will learn all of them, if you continue to use them. You must review or you will forget what you have learned. Remember to pronounce the words as you write them. The accented syllable is shown in boldface type.

□ **Assignment:** Go back and study the -ectomy words on p. 5. Do not worry, at this point, if you do not fully understand what some of the root words mean. (For instance, you may not exactly know what a ureter or duodenum is, but you can still define urete**rec**tomy and duode**nec**tomy.) Work with a partner if possible. Dictate to each other for spelling and pronunciation practice.

Notice the addition of /o to most root words. This means that the o may be used in some words but may be dropped in others. In general, the o (combining form) is used when two or more root words are combined, as in gastro/enter**ol**ogy, and the o is dropped when adding a suffix, as in gas**tr/i**tis.

alphabetical list of word parts (root words)

An alphabetical listing of word parts, most of which appear in Figures 1–1 and 1–2, is given here. A few that do not appear are also given. Most of these words will have to be memorized because they are derived from foreign languages. *Cover the meaning column and see if you know some of them.*

Word part	Meaning	Example word
abdomin/o	abdomen	abdomino**pel**vic
aden/o	gland	ade**nec**tomy
an/o	anus	**a**nal
andr/o	man	**an**drogen
angi/o	vessel (lymph, blood)	**an**giogram
append	appendix	appen**dec**tomy
appendic/o	appendix	appendi**ci**tis
arteri/o	artery	arterioscle**ro**sis
arthr/o	joint	ar**thri**tis
bronch/o	bronchus	bron**chi**tis
cardi/o	heart	electro**car**diogram
cephal/o	head	ce**phal**ic
cerebr/o	cerebrum (part of brain)	**cer**ebral or ce**re**bral
cheil/o	lip	**cheil**oplasty
cholecyst/o	gallbladder	cholecys**tec**tomy
choledoch/o	common bile duct	choledo**chos**tomy
chondr/o	cartilage	chon**drec**tomy
col/o	colon (large intestine)	co**los**tomy
cost/o	rib	**cos**tal margin
crani/o	cranium (skull)	**cra**nial
cyst/o	bladder	cys**ti**tis
dent/o, odont/o	tooth	**den**tist
derm/o	skin	derma**bra**sion
dermat/o	skin	derma**tol**ogist
duoden/o	duodenum (small intestine)	duode**nec**tomy
encephal/o	brain	encepha**li**tis
esophag/o	esophagus	esopha**gi**tis
gastr/o	stomach	gas**trec**tomy
gloss/o	tongue	glos**si**tis
gyne	woman	gyne**col**ogy
hepa, hepat/o	liver	hepa**ti**tis
hyster/o	uterus	hyste**rec**tomy
ile/o	ileum (small intestine)	ile**os**tomy
irid/o	iris (eye)	iri**dec**tomy

kerat/o	cornea of eye; horny substance	**ker**atoplasty kera**to**sis
lamina	thin flat part of vertebra	lami**nec**tomy
lapar/o	abdomen	lapa**rot**omy
lingua	tongue	sub**ling**ual
lobe	lobe, as of lung	lo**bec**tomy
mast/o, mamm/o	breast	mas**tec**tomy, **mam**moplasty
my/o, myos	muscle	myo**si**tis
myel/o	bone marrow; spinal cord	osteomye**li**tis **my**elogram
myring/o	eardrum	myrin**got**omy
neur/o	nerve	neu**ri**tis
nephr/o	kidney	neph**rec**tomy
oophor/o	ovary	oopho**rec**tomy
ophthalm/o	eye	ophthal**mol**ogist
orchi/o	testicle	or**chi**tis
orchid/o	testicle	**or**chidoplasty
oste/o	bone	osteochon**dri**tis
ot/o	ear	**o**toscope
pancreat/o	pancreas	pancrea**tec**tomy
pharyng/o	pharynx	pharyn**gi**tis
phleb/o	vein	phle**bi**tis
pneum/o	lungs	pneu**mo**nia
proct/o	rectum, anus	**proc**toscope
prostat/o	prostate gland	prosta**tec**tomy
pyel/o	pelvis of kidney	pye**li**tis
rect/o	rectum	**rec**tal
ren/o	renal (kidney)	**re**nal failure
rhin/o	nose	**rhi**noplasty
sacr/o	sacrum	sacro**il**iac
salping/o	fallopian tube	salpin**gec**tomy
splen/o	spleen	sple**nec**tomy
spondyl/o	vertebra	spondy**li**tis
steth/o	chest	**stetho**scope
stomat/o	mouth	stoma**ti**tis
ten/o, tend/o, tendin/o	tendon	tendi**ni**tis, **ten**oplasty
thorac/o	thorax (chest)	tho**rac**ic
thyr/o	thyroid gland	thyroi**dec**tomy
trache/o	trachea	trache**ot**omy
tympan/o	eardrum	tympa**nec**tomy
ureter/o	ureter	urete**rec**tomy
vas/o	vessel	vasocon**stric**tion
ven/o	vein	**ve**nogram

■ **Note:** You will have noticed that more than one word may pertain to certain structures*:

Brain and head	*Kidneys*
cranio = skull only	nephro = entire kidney
cephalo = head	reno = entire kidney
cerebro = part of brain	pyelo = pelvis of kidney
encephalo = entire brain	

This also applies to words for the abdomen, rectum, eardrum, vessels, and chest.

---

* *Important:* In a few cases ONE word part can refer to two entirely different organs. Examples: myelo and kerato.

Use the preceding alphabetical listing of body parts and organs as a study guide. Cover the meaning and see if you can define the word part. Then cover the word part column and see if you know the root words.

The boldface letters show you where the accent falls. Pronounce the example words. Dictate them to a friend; write them until you are sure of the spelling.

When you think you know the -ectomy words given, proceed to the -ectomy self-test.

-ectomy self-test

Spell: Have someone dictate the words from Answer Key 6.

Define any eight:

1. _____
2. _____
3. _____
4. _____
5. _____
6. _____
7. _____
8. _____
9. _____
10. _____
11. _____
12. _____

Build a word:

13. Excision of the thyroid gland _____

14. Excision of the adrenal gland _____

15. Excision of the uterus _____

16. Excision of the tonsils _____

17. Excision of hemorrhoids _____

18. Excision of the appendix _____

Extra: What is a T & A? _____

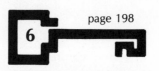
6   page 198

If your score was not 100%, review and try again.

drill: root words

Fill in the meaning of each root word. At another time, cover the first column root word and see if you can look at the meaning and write in the root word. You may not be able to use all of the roots in a word now, but you can add others as you learn more.

Root word	Meaning	Root word	Use root in a word
aden/o			
arteri/o			
appendic/o or append/			
arthr/o			
bronch/o			
cardi/o			
cerebr/o			
cholecyst/o			
col/o			
cost/o			
crani/o			
cyst/o			
derm/o, dermato			
encephal/o			
gastr/o			
hepa, hepat/o			
hyster/o			
mast/o			
my/o			
neur/o			
nephr/o			
oste/o			
ot/o			
pneum/o			
proct/o			
pyel/o			
rhin/o			
spondyl/o			
thyr/o			
trache/o			

No Answer Key

This drill should be periodically reviewed orally, working from the root and from the meanings.

chapter 2
other surgical procedures: suffixes

You have learned to use the suffix -ectomy. Here are some other surgical procedure suffixes. Many of the root words you know can be used with these endings.

Recall -ectomy: to excise or cut out surgically. The following endings have *specific meanings* other than "excising." These are other kinds of surgical procedures. Define the following example words and try to think of some others using root words you know:

Suffix	Meaning	Example	Define
-ostomy	a new permanent opening (to outside of body)	co**los**tomy	_____ _____
		trache**os**tomy	_____ _____
	(reuniting inner structures)	gastroduode**nos**tomy	_____ _____
-otomy	cutting into (making an incision)	lapa**rot**omy (or celi**ot**omy)	_____
		trache**ot**omy	_____ _____
-orrhaphy	surgical repair	herni**or**rhaphy	_____ _____
		neph**ror**rhaphy	_____ _____
-o**pex**y	fixation or suturing (a type of repair)	**neph**ropexy	_____ _____
		sal**ping**opexy	_____ _____
-o**plas**ty	plastic surgery (to improve function; to relieve pain; for cosmetic reasons)	**rhi**noplasty	_____ _____
		arthroplasty	_____ _____
		angioplasty	_____ _____

-o**trip**sy	crushing, destroying	**neur**otripsy	_____
			_____
		lithotripsy	_____
		(litho = stone)	_____
-cen**te**sis	surgical puncture to remove	abdominocen**te**sis	_____
	fluid		_____
		thoracen**te**sis or	_____
		thoracocen**te**sis	_____
		paracen**te**sis	_____
			_____
		amniocen**te**sis	_____
			_____
		arthrocen**te**sis	_____
			_____

■ **Note:** Watch the spelling of **-or**rhaphy. It is difficult but quite common in medical words. It may help if you pronounce the h (which is actually silent) when you study these words. Other words using -orrh: **hem**or-rhage, menor**rha**gia, diar**rhe**a.

The spelling of these endings is always the same, regardless of how they may sound; for example, trache**ot**omy may sometimes sound like trache**od**omy, but it is always **-ot**omy.

No Answer Key

worksheet

Define:

-ostomy

1. co**los**tomy _____
2. gas**tros**tomy _____
3. ile**os**tomy _____
4. trache**os**tomy _____
5. cys**tos**tomy _____
6. ente**ros**tomy _____
7. jeju**nos**tomy _____

-otomy

8. lapa**rot**omy _____
9. trache**ot**omy _____
10. phle**bot**omy _____
11. gas**trot**omy _____

12. cys**tot**omy _____

13. lo**bot**omy _____

The preceding words are some of the more commonly seen words with **-os**tomy and **-ot**omy endings. *Learn all of them.*

Also, study the example words given for the other surgical procedure suffixes (p. 14). Write them here. Add others as you discover them.

14. **-or**rhaphy

_____

_____

_____

_____

15. -o**pex**y

_____

_____

_____

_____

16. -o**plas**ty

_____

_____

_____

_____

17. -o**trip**sy

_____

_____

_____

18. -cen**te**sis

_____

_____

_____

Whenever you see these suffixes, you should recognize their meanings immediately. As you learn more root words, you will be able to add more words using these endings.

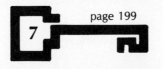

7   page 199

practice sheet

Write a specific word for:

1. Excision of the stomach _____

2. A new permanent opening into the trachea _____

3. Incision into the bladder _____

4. Plastic surgery on a joint _____

5. Fixation of a kidney _____

6. Excision of an ovary _____

7. Surgical crushing of a nerve _____

8. New permanent opening in the ileum _____

9. New permanent opening into the colon _____

10. Excision of the gallbladder _____

11. Surgical puncture (tapping) of the chest cavity _____

12. Surgical repair of a hernia _____

13. "Tapping" a joint to remove fluid _____

Spell: Have someone dictate these words to you from Answer Key 8.

Define:

14. _____   _____

15. _____   _____

16. _____   _____

17. _____   _____

18. _____   _____

19. _____   _____

20. _____   _____

21. _____   _____

22. _____   _____

23. _____   _____

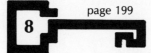 page 199

chapter 3
diseases or conditions: prefixes and suffixes

You have learned suffixes that pertain to surgical procedures. The following suffixes refer to diseases or conditions (not normal).

Define the following words. Later, starting with root words you have learned, "make up" words using **-o**sis, **-i**tis, and **-op**athy endings. Watch pronunciation of **-op**athy words (accent always on **op** syllable).

REMEMBER: The spelling of these suffixes never changes, regardless of how they may sound.

Suffix	Meaning	Examples	Define
-osis	condition of	derma**to**sis	_____
		neu**ro**sis	_____
		psy**cho**sis	_____
		scle**ro**sis (hardening)	_____
		tubercu**lo**sis (tubercle = little swelling)	_____
		diverticu**lo**sis (diverticulum = out-pouching or sac)	_____
-itis	inflammation of	appendi**ci**tis	_____
		spondy**li**tis	_____
		tonsil**li**tis	_____
		perito**ni**tis	_____
		ar**thri**tis	_____
		myo**si**tis	_____
-opathy	any disease of	hyste**rop**athy	_____
		ade**nop**athy	_____
-algia or **-o**dynia	pain	neu**ral**gia or neuro**dyn**ia	_____
		my**al**gia	_____
		coccygo**dyn**ia	_____
		den**tal**gia	_____
		o**tal**gia	_____
-cele	hernia or rupture or swelling	**cys**tocele	_____
		rectocele	_____
		me**ning**ocele	_____

-or**rha**gia	hemorrhage (blood bursting forth)	menor**rha**gia	_____
		metror**rha**gia	_____
-**ec**tasis or -ec**ta**sia	stretching or dilating	bronchi**ec**tasis	_____
		ate**lec**tasis	_____
		gastrec**ta**sia	_____

No Answer Key

■ **Notes:** Learn to spell inflam**ma**tion (but only one *m* in in**flam**ed). The cardinal signs of inflammation are redness, heat, swelling, and pain. (Inflammation can occur without infection.) Look up inflam**ma**tion and in**fec**tion in your dictionary.

Learn the word **her**nia. It is a projection of a part from its natural place and also may be called a rupture. Examples of common hernias: um**bil**ical hernia (the um**bil**icus is the navel or belly button); **ing**uinal hernia (in the groin area); hi**a**tal hernia (in the diaphragm). (See Figure 21–3 on p. 155 of direct and indirect inguinal hernias.)

Learn the words **di**late, di**la**tion, and dila**ta**tion. When something is dilated it is made larger or opened up. Dilators are instruments that may be used to dilate an opening. Dilatation can also occur spontaneously.

worksheet

Give a word for:

1. A condition of the "mind" _____

2. Inflammation of the appendix _____

3. Pain along a nerve _____

4. Hernia of the bladder _____

5. Any disease of the glands _____

6. A condition of the "nerves" _____

7. Very heavy bleeding during the menstrual period _____

8. Inflammation of the skin _____

9. A toothache (pain in a tooth) _____

10. A "condition of" acidity _____

Spell: Have someone dictate these words to you from Answer Key 9.

Define:

11. _____ _____

12. _____ _____

13. _____ _____

14. _____ _____

15. _____ _____

16. _____ _____

17. _____ _____

18. _____ _____

19. _____ _____

20. _____ _____

21. _____ _____

22. _____ _____

23. _____ _____

24. _____ _____

25. What are the symptoms of inflammation? _____

_____ _____

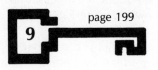

page 199

---

drill: suffixes

Fill in the first column only. At another time, cover the meaning column and see if you can remember all of the meanings. Write them in column three. This drill should be used for review as often as necessary.

Meaning	Suffix	Meaning	Suffix
excision of	_____	_____	_____
new permanent opening	_____	_____	_____
incision into	_____	_____	_____
surgical repair of	_____	_____	_____
surgical fixation	_____	_____	_____
plastic surgery	_____	_____	_____
crushing	_____	_____	_____
puncture (tapping)	_____	_____	_____
stretching (dilating)	_____	_____	_____
condition of	_____	_____	_____
inflammation of	_____	_____	_____
any disease of (general)	_____	_____	_____
pain	_____	_____	_____
hernia	_____	_____	_____
excessive bleeding	_____	_____	_____
The signs of inflammation are	_____	_____	_____

No Answer Key

introduction to prefixes

These word elements are similar in spelling and in sound, *but have different meanings*. Define the example words.

Prefix	Meaning	Examples	Give literal meaning and define. Check your dictionary.
a- an- ar-	without or not	1. a**sep**tic (septic = contaminated, dirty)	_____
		2. a**feb**rile (febrile = fever)	_____
		3. a**ne**mic	_____
		4. ar**rhyth**mic	_____
ad-	near, toward	5. ad**duc**tion	_____
		6. ad**he**sion	_____
ab-	away from	7. ab**duc**tion	_____
		8. ab**nor**mal	_____
ante-	before, forward	9. ante**flex**ion	_____
anti-	against (contra- also means against or not)	10. antibi**ot**ic	_____
		11. anti**sep**tic	_____
		12. anticon**vul**sive	_____
		13. antineo**plas**tic	_____
		14. contra**in**dicated	_____
cyto-	cell	15. cy**tom**eter	_____
cysto-	bladder	16. **cys**tocele	_____
dis-	from	17. dis**ease**	_____
dys-	painful or difficult	18. dys**u**ria (-uria = urinating)	_____
		19. dysmenor**rhe**a (meno = menses)	_____
		20. **dys**entery	_____
		21. **dysp**nea (-pnea = breathing)	_____
hemo-	blood	22. hemo**sta**sis	_____
hemi-	half (one side)	23. hemi**ple**gia (-plegia = paralysis)	_____
hyper-	too much, high	24. hyper**ten**sion	_____
		25. hy**per**trophy (-trophy = growth)	_____
hypo-	not enough, low or under	26. hypo**ac**tive	_____
		27. hypo**der**mic	_____

inter-	between	28. inter**cos**tal	_____
intra-	within	29. intra**mus**cular	_____
		30. intra**ve**nous	_____
		31. intra**the**cal	_____
		(spinal canal)	

These terms need extra study for clear understanding. (See your dictionary.) Define:

32. Sepsis _____

33. Bladder _____

34. Hernia _____

10 page 200

drill: prefixes and suffixes

As with previous drills, fill in only column one (meaning). Later, see if you can fill in the word part column and give an example of a word using the prefix or suffix. This type of review will help you to retain what you have learned.

Word part	Meaning	Word part	Example
anti-	_____	_____	_____
a- an- ar-	_____	_____	_____
ad-	_____	_____	_____
ab-	_____	_____	_____
cyto-	_____	_____	_____
cysto-	_____	_____	_____
dys-	_____	_____	_____
hemo-	_____	_____	_____
hemi-	_____	_____	_____
hyper-	_____	_____	_____
hypo-	_____	_____	_____
-ectomy	_____	_____	_____
-ostomy	_____	_____	_____
-otomy	_____	_____	_____
-osis	_____	_____	_____
-itis	_____	_____	_____
-algia	_____	_____	_____
-cele	_____	_____	_____

-**or**rhaphy _____ _____ _____

hyster- _____ _____ _____

nephro- _____ _____ _____

check your progress

You may now be given a review test on Chapters 1–3.

By this time you should be feeling a sense of accomplishment. If you scored 85 or above on the review test, proceed with Chapter 4. If you scored below 85, go back and review the material covered in Chapters 1–3. If you find that certain words are especially difficult for you, look them up in other books. Practice writing and rewriting them. Make and use flash cards. Discuss your problem with the instructor.

Your instructor may provide an alternate review test for Chapters 1–3. After you score 85 on this review, proceed with Chapter 4. (This option will depend upon your instructor.)

So far you have learned how to construct words that describe surgical procedures and disease conditions. Now you will proceed to some word parts relating to other things.

REMEMBER: Continue to review completed chapters so that you do not forget what you have learned.

chapter 4
medical instruments and machines

---
suffixes

Suffix	Meaning	Examples	Define
-oscope	instrument for looking into	**o**toscope	_____
		arthroscope	_____
		cystoscope	_____
-oscopy	procedure of using a scope	o**tos**copy	_____
		cys**tos**copy	_____
		colo**nos**copy	_____

■ **Note:** The scope instruments usually have a light at the end. The scope is inserted into an opening, and the light allows the physician to see deep into the cavity or organ. Look up the word **en**doscope. The following are exceptions:

> **Spec**ulum: instrument for looking into (and is not a scope)
> **Steth**oscope: instrument used for listening, not looking, but is called a scope
> **Fe**toscope: instrument for listening to fetal heart tones.

Suffix	Meaning	Examples	Define
-tome	instrument for cutting thin section	**der**matome	_____
		mictotome	_____
		osteotome	_____

■ **Note:** Recall that all of the suffixes that mean cutting have the letters "tom" in them: **ec**tomy, **ot**omy, **os**tomy (also a**nat**omy).

Suffix	Meaning	Examples	Define
-(o)graph	instrument (or machine) that records	electroen**ceph**alograph (EEG)	_____
		electro**car**diograph (ECG, EKG)	_____
		myograph	records muscle contractions
		radiograph	X-ray machine or picture

■ **Note:** There is not a special machine for all such procedures. An X-ray machine is used for many. (See mye**log**raphy and **my**elogram.) Look up these words in your dictionary: **an**giogram, **py**elogram, hysterosal**ping**ogram, **mam**mogram.

Suffix	Meaning	Examples	Define
-(o)graphy	procedure	electroencepha**log**raphy	_____
		electrocardi**og**raphy	_____
		my**og**raphy	_____
		mye**log**raphy (spinal cord)	_____
		ultrason**og**raphy	_____
-(o)gram	"picture" produced	electroen**ceph**alogram	_____
		electro**car**diogram	_____
		echo**car**diogram	_____
		myogram	_____
		myelogram	_____
		angiogram	_____

■ **Note:** There is a difference in accented syllables between **-o scope** and **-os**copy, and between **-o graph** and **-og**raphy.

Suffix	Meaning	Examples	Define
-(o)meter	instrument that measures or counts	ther**mom**eter	_____
		cy**tom**eter	_____
		spi**rom**eter	_____
		to**nom**eter	measures pressure in eyeball
		pel**vim**eter	_____
-ometry, **-im**etry	procedure of using the instrument	pel**vim**etry	_____
		spi**rom**etry	_____

No Answer Key

practice sheet

Which organs can the doctor look into with an instrument? Write the words and pronounce them.

	Instrument	Procedure
1. ear	_____	_____
2. stomach	_____	_____
3. sigmoid	_____	_____
4. bronchi	_____	_____
5. eye	_____	_____
6. rectum	_____	_____
7. anus	_____	_____
8. abdomen	_____	_____

Write a word for:

9. Excision of a gland _____

10. Inflammation of the appendix _____

11. Pain in the heart _____

12. Hernia of the bladder _____

13. Any disease or condition of the uterus _____

14. Instrument for looking into the ear _____

15. Instrument for cutting thin sections of skin _____

16. Condition of the "nerves" _____

17. Inflammation of the gallbladder _____

18. Instrument that records electrical impulses of the heart _____

19. X-ray picture of the spinal cord _____

20. Excision of the thyroid gland _____

21. Instrument for looking into the stomach _____

22. Inflammation of the kidney _____

23. Pain in the head _____

24. Recording or picture of brain waves _____

25. Instrument for looking into the bronchi _____

26. New permanent opening of the colon _____

27. X-ray picture of the kidney pelvis _____

28. Excision of a part or all of the stomach _____

Spell: Have someone dictate these words to you from Answer Key 11. **Define:**

29. _____ _____

30. _____ _____

31. _____ _____

32. _____ _____

33. _____ _____

34. _____ _____

35. _____ _____

36. _____ _____

37. _____ _____

38. _____ _____

39. Define speculum: _____

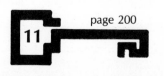

page 200

worksheet

Write a word for:

1. Instrument or device for measuring temperature _____

2. Inflammation of a gland _____

3. Pain in a nerve _____

4. Excision of the tonsils _____

5. New permanent opening into the ileum _____

6. Procedure of using a bronchoscope for an examination of the bronchi _____

7. Machine that records brain waves _____

8. Excision of the stomach _____

9. Inflammation of joints _____

10. Picture or recording of electrical impulses of the heart _____

11. Instrument for looking into the vagina _____

12. Excision of the uterus _____

13. Inflammation of the gallbladder _____

14. Incision into the abdomen _____

15. Condition of the kidney _____

True/False: Circle the number of the *true* statements only. Defend your answers. Explain what is "untrue" in the false statements.

16. A dermatome cuts a thin section of skin.

17. The physician uses an otoscope to look into the eye.

18. The electroencephalograph is a machine for recording electrical impulses of the heart.

19. A stethoscope is used to amplify sounds in the chest.

20. A bladder is a hollow organ (sac) that usually holds some fluid.

21. Sepsis is the opposite of asepsis.

22. Hemorrhage means internal bleeding.

23. Tuberculosis literally means a condition of having tubercles.

24. Hyperactive means too active.

25. ECG and EKG are both abbreviations for electrocardiogram.

Define: (See your dictionary.)

26. dilator _____

27. speculum _____

28. bougie (dilating) _____

29. sound (*Not* the sound you hear!) _____

Extra: Look up the word "radiograph." What is irregular about this word? _____

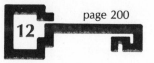

page 200

12

worksheet: review of suffixes

Without looking back, make a list of suffixes you have learned and write a word with each. Look back to the pages given after you have completed the assignment.

Cutting or surgery of some kind: (pp. 5–6, 14–15)

Suffix   *Words*

_____   _____

_____   _____

_____   _____

_____   _____

_____   _____

_____   _____

_____   _____

_____   _____

Diseases or conditions: (pp. 18–19)

Suffix   *Words*

_____   _____

_____   _____

_____   _____

_____   _____

_____   _____

Medical instruments and machines and their use: (pp. 24–25)

Suffix   *Words*

_____   _____

_____   _____

_____   _____

_____   _____

_____   _____

No Answer Key

chapter 5
medical specialties and specialists: -*ol*ogy, -*ol*ogist

You have often heard the ending **-OL**OGY. It means "the study or science of." Recall the following words:

Bi**ol**ogy	Bacteri**ol**ogy
Psy**chol**ogy	Physi**ol**ogy
Hema**tol**ogy	Termi**nol**ogy

Now you will learn the words for the persons who study these sciences: the people who practice the art or science on which the science is based. Examples include bi**ol**ogist, bacteri**ol**ogist, psy**chol**ogist, physi**ol**ogist, hema**tol**ogist, and termi**nol**ogist. These people are not all "doctors" in the common usage of the word, although they may have "doctorate" degrees. In other words, they are not necessarily physicians.

Now consider the *exceptions*. These endings also mean the same as **-ol**ogist:

-ist	in**tern**ist (internal medicine)
	ortho**pe**dist (ortho**pe**dics)
-iatrist	psy**chi**atrist (psy**chi**atry)
	po**dia**trist (po**dia**try)
-ician	pedia**tric**ian (pedi**at**rics)
	obste**tric**ian (obs**tet**rics)
	phy**si**cian
-er (**-i**tioner)	prac**ti**tioner (someone who practices, a doctor or nurse for example)

Doctors and nurses are "always practicing." It would seem that they never learn! Perhaps this is because medicine is always changing, and no one can know all there is to know.

Note the root word **iatro** in examples given here. It means "related to medicine or to physicians." Iatro**gen**ic means "any condition arising from treatment by a physician," for example: as a result of prescribed antibiotic, patient may develop a skin reaction, vaginal infection, diarrhea, or anemia.

Because the subject of specialists and specialties seems difficult for most students, a rather lengthy description and explanation follows.

education of a physician

MD (Doctor of Medicine) or DO (Doctor of Oste*op*athy)

The student must spend at least three years in undergraduate school, called premed, then four years in medical school connected with a hospital. The student receives an MD or DO degree upon graduation.

To obtain a state license to practice, the individual must have the degree plus at least one year's internship in a hospital (an intern cares for patients in the absence of the resident or attending physicians, helps out in emergencies, and assists with operations). The term "intern" is being replaced with "first-year resident."

To become a specialist (in addition to the preceding requirements).   Two to five years of residency (during which the physician is called a resident) and two years of practice are required for the physician to apply for certification. Then, if the physician passes boards (tests), he or she is board certified and is a specialist (also known as a diplomate).

License to practice.   Each state requires licensure. However, most grant reciprocity, meaning if a physician is licensed in one state, others will automatically grant a license to practice, for a certain fee. The license must be renewed yearly.

Continued education.   Once physicians are licensed, they still take postgraduate courses throughout their lives to stay current on new developments. This is becoming mandatory for renewal of license. (CEUs = continuing education units.)

General practice (GP).   General practitioner is a term applied to the nonspecialist, generally a "family doctor." Depending on the area in which he or she practices (rural or urban), this person may prescribe medications, perform surgery, deliver babies, give various treatments, and perform a variety of other services. The general practitioner usually refers complicated cases to a specialist.

Although both MD and DO practitioners may specialize, the MD is more likely to do so, and the DO is more likely to remain in general practice.

■ **Note:**   What is the difference between a medical doctor and an osteopathic doctor? They both attend school for the same amount of time, but at different and separate schools. They practice in separate hospitals (but this is gradually changing). In philosophy and treatment the osteopath places more emphasis on the interrelationship of the body's muscles, bones, and joints, but he or she treats all kinds of illnesses.

SPECIALTIES AND SPECIALISTS (MD or DO)

cardio*vas*cular diseases (cardi*ol*ogist)   a subspecialty of internal medicine; diseases of the heart and blood vessels; cardiovascular surgery.

derma*tol*ogy (derma*tol*ogist)   diseases of the skin.

endocri*nol*ogy (endocri*nol*ogist)   disorders of the ductless or endocrine glands; obesity, sterility, diabetes, and thyroid conditions, for example.

family practice specialty (family practice specialist)   similar to general practice, but has been qualified as a specialist.

gastroente*rol*ogy (gastroente*rol*ogist)   subspecialty of internal medicine; digestive tract diseases.

hema*tol*ogy (hema*tol*ogist)   disorders of the blood and blood forming organs.

internal medicine (in*tern*ist)   does many of the same things as the general practitioner, except performs no surgery or obstetrics. Often called in for consultation and diagnostic help. *Never call this person an intern!*

ob*stet*rics-gyne*col*ogy (obste*tric*ian and gyne*col*ogist)   female reproductive tract disorders; prenatal, delivery, postpartum care; gynecologic surgery; some urinary tract infections.

neu*rol*ogy or neuro*sur*gery (neu*rol*ogist or neuro*sur*geon)   diseases of the brain, spinal cord, and nerves.

ophthal*mol*ogy (pronounced ofthal-) **(ophthal*mol*ogist)**   eye diseases, eye surgery; also prescribes glasses, and does eye exams.

ortho*pe*dics (ortho*pe*dist, ortho*pe*dic surgeon or *or*thopod)   literally means "straight child" and is often confused with osteopathy; disorders of musculoskeletal system.

o*tol*ogy (o*tol*ogist)   ear surgery, hearing problems.

otorhinolaryn*gol*ogy (otorhinolaryn*gol*ogist)   (ear, nose, and throat (ENT).

pedi*at*rics (pedia*tric*ian)   disease prevention, diagnosis, and treatment of children, usually to age 16 years.

***phys*iatry (physi*at*rist)**   physical medicine and rehabilitation (PM&R).

proc*tol*ogy (proc*tol*ogist)   diseases of the rectum, sigmoid.

psy*chi*atry (psy*chi*atrist)   diagnosis and treatment of mental disorders.

radi*ol*ogy (radi*ol*ogist), also **roentge*nol*ogy (roentge*nol*ogist)**   use of radiant energy—X ray, radium, cobalt; diagnosis and treatment.

surgery (surgeon)   general surgery; also neurosurgery, orthopedic surgery, plastic surgery, and thoracic surgery, for example.

u*rol*ogy (u*rol*ogist)   urinary tract disease; male reproductive organs.

Some other medical specialties include the following:

Emergency medicine (trauma**tol**ogy)
Administrative medicine
Anesthesi**ol**ogy
Occupational medicine
Pa**thol**ogy; forensic medicine
Bariatrics
Public health
Nuclear medicine
On**col**ogy (tumors, cancer) on**col**ogists specialize in radiation, surgery, or chemotherapy.

The greatest number of specialists are in the fields of internal medicine, pediatrics, obstetrics and gynecology, surgery (general and specialized), and radiology.

Define:

Specialist _____

Intern "first-year resident" _____

Internist _____

Resident _____

Attending physician _____

other "doctors"

Some confusing terms relate to other physicians and specialists who do not hold the degree of Doctor of Medicine (MD) or Doctor of Osteopathy (DO). They are called "Doctor."

po*di*atrist   DPM, Doctor of Podiatric Medicine; specialist in care of feet, including X-ray, surgery, various therapies, and medication.

op*tom*etrist   OD, Doctor of Optometry; treats refractive errors; fits eye glasses.

***chi*roptractor**   DC, Doctor of Chiropractic; treats with manipulation only. (chiro = hand)

***na*turopath**   treats with "natural" forces or substances, such as vitamins, diets, light, heat, air, and water.

psy*chol*ogist   PhD, Doctor of Philosophy; group and individual counseling and testing; treats emotional disorders but cannot prescribe medication.

Notice the phone book listings in the Yellow Pages under "Physicians, MD" and "Physicians, DO." Look in the Yellow Pages and make a list of other specialists you find. Note that acupuncture is used by some MDs, DOs, and some DCs.

_____   _____

_____   _____

_____   _____

_____   _____
_____   _____
_____   _____
_____   _____
_____   _____

worksheet: medical specialists

Name the specialists: What kind of physicians (specialists), other than general practitioners, could treat a patient with the following health problems?

1. Upper respiratory infection (URI)   _____

2. Vaginal infection   _____

3. Urinary tract infection (UTI)   _____

4. Fractured wrist   _____

5. Deep laceration (cut)   _____

6. Hayfever, asthma   _____

7. Severe sunburn   _____

8. Ear infection   _____

9. Severe indigestion or food poisoning   _____

10. Obesity   _____

11. Object embedded in the eyeball   _____

12. Bleeding during pregnancy   _____

13. Depression   _____

14. Heart attack   _____

15. Arthritis   _____

16. Diabetes   _____

17. Cancer   _____

18. Mumps   _____

19. Epilepsy   _____

20. Blurred vision   _____

Define:

21. intern   _____

22. resident   _____

23. practitioner   _____

24. osteopath   _____

25. What does a radiologist do?   _____

_____

26. Does an internist treat children? _____

27. Who usually refers a patient to a medical specialist? _____

28. What types of practitioners do acupuncture? _____

29. Patients with leukemia are usually treated by a _____

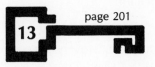

page 201

13

worksheet: medical specialties

Name ten specialists and their specialty: Define the kinds of patients or conditions each treats.

1. _____
   _____

2. _____
   _____

3. _____
   _____

4. _____
   _____

5. _____
   _____

6. _____
   _____

7. _____
   _____

8. _____
   _____

9. _____
   _____

10. _____
    _____

Name "specialists" who are _not_ MDs or DOs:

11. One who tests vision and prescribes eyeglasses _____

12. One who treats with manipulation only _____

13. One who treats _foot_ disorders only (including taking X-ray films and surgery) _____

14. One who counsels, tests, and provides therapy for emotional problems _____

True/False: Circle the number of the *true* statements only. Defend your answers. Explain what is "untrue" in the false statements.

15. Doctors, nurses, and physical therapists may all be called practitioners.

16. A resident doctor (after the first year) is working toward or at least considering specialization in one particular field of medicine.

17. An osteopath is the same as a chiropractor.

18. A family doctor is usually a general practitioner (MD or DO).

19. All doctors must renew their license to practice every year.

20. Surgeons may perform general surgery or specialize in one area such as thoracic surgery.

21. All "doctors" are physicians.

22. An intern is still a student (not yet licensed to practice).

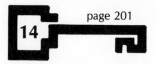

page 201

14

---

related professions

Allied health (paramedical) personnel must have some knowledge of other professionals in the health field (not all are physicians, but some may hold doctorates). All of the following *must have a license to practice:*

radiologic technologist, RT   takes X-ray films, prepares patients for X-ray films (American Registry of X-ray Technicians)

medical technologist, MT   formerly laboratory technician; performs all laboratory procedures; may specialize in one area, such as *bacteriology* (American Society of Clinical Pathologists)

public health nurse, PHN   RN with at least a BS degree, works for health departments, schools, or health agencies

registered nurse, RN   graduate nurse (from two- to four-year program); may work in hospitals, clinics, or offices; may specialize

nurse practitioner   RN with additional preparation, especially in pediatrics, obstetrics; does examinations and some treatment

physician's assistant   usually has served an internship with a physician; may also have medical corpsman experience. Does examinations, simple suturing, and so on

nurse midwife   RN with additional training. Delivers uncomplicated cases

licensed practical nurse, LPN/LVN (vocational)   graduate of a one-year program; may perform some duties similar to RN in hospitals or nursing homes, for example

registered physical therapist, RPT   performs treatments by "physical means," such as heat, cold, and exercise; accent on *gross motor* skills

occupational therapist, registered, OTR   similar to RPT but accent on *fine motor* skills, activities of daily living, and job skills

respiratory therapist or pulmonary therapist, ARRT   treats patients with breathing difficulties; uses machines to facilitate breathing; teaches breathing exercises

pharmacist   licensed to prepare and dispense drugs

general dentistry, DDS and **DMD**   (Doctor of Dental Surgery, Doctor of Medical Dentistry) usually treats all ages

ortho*don*tist   treats maloc**clu**sion (bracing)

perio*don*tist   "around" teeth; treats gum diseases (gingivitis; gingivectomy performed)

oral surgeon   extractions (especially complicated ones); maxillofacial trauma cases

prostho*don*tist   prosthesis, "false part"; dentures (artificial appliances)

pedo*don*tist   treats children only

endo*don*tist   "inside tooth"; diseases of pulp; root canal work

dental hygienist   prophylactic dental care

dental assistant   chairside assisting

The educational requirements for the preceding personnel vary considerably, from one year for LPN and dental assistant to four years or more for others (eight or more for dental specialties).

There are many other kinds of assistants and technicians with varying years of training. It is often difficult to know "who's who," and the patients are confused most of the time. Other technicians include: surgical technologist, central service aide, psychiatric aide, emergency medical technician, paramedic, cardiac technician, biomed technician, EEG technician, pharmacist assistant, nuclear medicine technician, phlebotomist, nursing assistant or aide.

review drill

Give the meaning for the following word parts: At another time, cover word part (first column) and fill in remainder.

Word part	Meaning	Word part	Example words
-oscope			
-oscopy			
-tome			
-ograph			
-ography			
-meter			
-ogram			
-ologist			
-ist			
-iatrist			
-ician			
-iatro			

Give the meaning of the following abbreviations: Later, cover the abbreviations (first column) and fill in the last column.

	Meaning		Abbreviations
MD			
DO			

DDS   _____   _____

RN   _____   _____

LPN   _____   _____

RPT   _____   _____

RT   _____   _____

MT   _____   _____

OTR   _____   _____

Fill in the blanks:

1. An internist is a specialist in   _____   _____
   (name the specialty).

2. The specialist who interprets X-ray films is a   _____

3. The specialist who treats bone injury or disease is   _____

4. The specialist who studies tissues after death as well as organs removed during surgery is a   _____
   _____

5. The "combined" specialty that treats women only is   _____

6. Define *prophy **lac**tic*   _____

7. Define *paramedical*   _____

8. Is a "technician" the same as a "technologist"?   _____

No Answer Key– if you had difficulty, review the chapter.

REVIEW EXERCISE

Refer back to Chapter 1 (p. 10–11), alphabetical listing of word parts (root words). Write the example words on a separate piece of paper and define them.

chapter 6
more medical prefixes and review

---

medical prefixes

Study the prefix and meaning, then define the examples: (Use a dictionary if needed.) Some of these have been presented earlier, and will serve as a review.

Prefix	Meaning	Examples	Define
a-, an-	without, not	a**feb**rile	1. _____
		ap**ne**a or **ap**nea	2. _____
brady-	slow	brady**car**dia	3. _____
tachy-	fast	tachy**car**dia	4. _____
de-	take away, remove	de**hy**drate	5. _____
re-	put back	re**hy**drate	6. _____
dia-	through (as in running through)	diar**rhe**a	7. _____
		diu**re**sis	8. _____
hemi-	one side, half	hemi**ple**gia	9. _____
hemo-	blood	he**mol**ysis (-olysis = destruction)	10. _____
		hemoglobin	11. _____
homo-, homeo-	likeness or resemblance	homo**sex**ual	12. _____

		homeo **sta**sis	13. _____
		(-stasis = standing still)	_____
hyper-	high; too much	hyper **ten**sion*	14. _____
			_____
		hyper **ac**tive	15. _____
			_____
hypo-	low; not enough; under	hypo **ten**sion	16. _____
			_____
		hypo **der**mic	17. _____
			_____
hydro-	water	hydro **ther**apy	18. _____
			_____
		hydro **ceph**alus	19. _____
			_____
		hydro **pho**bia	20. _____
			_____
lip-	fat	li **po**ma	21. _____
		(-oma = tumor)	_____
poly-	many, much	poly **u**ria	22. _____
			_____
		poly **cys**tic	23. _____
			_____
pre-	before	pre **op**erative	24. _____
			_____
		pre **na**tal	25. _____
			_____
pro-	preceding, coming before	prog **no**sis	26. _____
			_____
		pro **dro**mal	27. _____
		(-drome = running)	_____
post-	following, after	post **op**erative	28. _____
			_____
		post **par**tum	29. _____
		(-partus = birth)	_____

page 201

15

_____

* Does not mean "tension" in this word.

a-, an-: Remember that this little prefix completely changes the meaning of a word.

Define: *Learn* these words for future use!

1. a **feb** rile _____

2. apy **rex** ia _____

3. a **typ** ical _____

4. a **pha** sia _____

5. ap **ne** a _____

6. **at** rophy _____

7. anes **the** sia _____

8. anal **ge** sia _____

9. anaer **o** bic _____

10. ar **rhyth** mia _____

11. a **sep** sis _____

12. asympto **mat** ic _____

13. amenor **rhe** a _____

14. a **nox** ia _____

15. atrau **mat** ic _____

16. a **pha** gia _____

17. a **vas** cular _____

18. ano **rex** ia _____

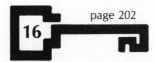

16   page 202

Make a list of words using these prefixes and define the words: Some of these words were introduced in Chapter 3. Use the dictionary if necessary.

hyper-

_____

_____

_____

_____

_____

hypo-

_____

_____

_____

_____

_____

dys-

_____

_____

_____

_____

_____

pre-

_____

_____

_____

_____

anti-

_____

_____

_____

_____

_____

post-

_____

_____

_____

_____

poly-

_____

_____

_____

_____

_____

hemo-

_____

_____

_____

_____

_____

practice sheet

True/False: If a word is misspelled, the statement is false. (Remember, one letter can change the meaning of the word.) Circle the number of the *true* statements only. Explain why the statement is false.

1. If febrile means fever, afebrile means without fever.

2. Hemoplegia means one half paralyzed.

3. Hyper- is the opposite of hypo-.

4. Dyspnea is the same as apnea.

5. Postpartum means following childbirth.

6. If esthesia means feeling, anesthesia means without feeling.

Correct spelling: Mark an **X** after the *correctly* spelled word.

7. antehistamine _____   antihistamine _____

8. hypodermic _____   hypadermic _____

9. tackycardia _____   tachycardia _____

10. prenatel _____   prenatal _____

11. hemiplegia _____   hemoplegia _____

12. anemia _____   aremia _____

Define:

13. anaer**o**bic _____

14. **at**rophy _____

15. anal**ge**sic _____

16. de**hy**drate _____

17. hyper**ten**sion _____

18. hydro**ther**apy _____

19. prog**no**sis _____

20. post**op**erative _____

21. poly**u**ria _____

22. tachy**car**dia _____

23. a**ne**mia _____

24. pro**dro**mal _____

25. he**mol**ysis _____

26. hyper**ther**mia _____

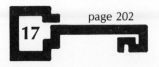

17   page 202

chapter 7
plural endings

Study the following examples. Write the plural form and define the example word:

Singular	Plural	Example	Plural form and definition
a	**ae** **(pronounced ī, ē, or ā*)**	**ver**tebra (**ver**tebrae)	_____ _____
		bursa	_____ _____
		gingiva	_____ _____
		fascia	_____ _____
		pe**te**chia (pe**te**chiae) (pinpoint hemorrhages)	_____ _____
um	**a**	memo**ran**dum (memo**ran**da)	_____ _____
		speculum	_____ _____
		diver**tic**ulum	_____ _____
		ovum	_____ _____
		datum	_____ _____
		serum	_____ _____
		medium (culture medium)	_____ _____
		bac**ter**ium	_____ _____

---

* Dictionaries do not agree on pronunciation, and many do not give *any* pronunciation for the plural form.

us	**i**	**coc**cus (cocci) (plural pronounced **cock**'seye)	_____
		ba**cil**lus	_____
		focus (foci "**fo**sigh")	_____
		nucleus	_____
		thrombus	_____
		uterus	_____
		fungus	_____
is	**es**	diag**no**sis (diag**no**ses)	_____
		uri**nal**ysis	_____
		crisis	_____
		testis	_____
ex, ix	**ices**	**a**pex (apices "**ap**iseez")	_____
		cervix	_____
		ap**pen**dix	_____
ma	**mata**	**en**ema (**enem**ata)	_____
		carci**no**ma	_____
inx	**inges**	**men**inx (men**in**ges)	_____
anx	**anges**	**pha**lanx (pha**lan**ges)	_____
ur	**ora**	**fe**mur (fe**mor**a)	_____

en   ina   lu men (lu mina)   _____

                                                    _____

No Answer Key

body openings (some confusing words)

The following words all refer to a body opening or entrance. Some are used interchangeably. You need not try to differentiate between them concerning usage. Merely become familiar with these terms so that if you hear them you will be able to recognize them. Watch the pronunciation of these terms.

Word	Pronunciation	Meaning or usage
me**a**tus	me/**ay**/tus	urinary passage or opening
orifice	**or**/ifice	any orifice, such as anal orifice
in**troi**tus	in/**troy**/tus	vaginal cavity
os	os	mouth, opening; os uteri: mouth of the uterus, or cervix
stoma	**sto**/ma	the opening established in the abdominal wall by colostomy
lumen	**lu**/men	opening within a hollow tube or organ
patent	**pay**/tent	adjective, meaning open or not plugged, as in "The tube is patent" or "That's a patent lie."
perfo**ra**tion	per/fo/**ra**/shun	a hole in something; for example, a gastric ulcer can cause perforation of the stomach wall.

Related words that often cause difficulty.

dila**ta**tion or di**la**tion   making something wider or opened up

con**stric**tion   making something smaller or narrower

Define these other terms for kinds of body openings (use a dictionary).

Aperture   _____

Fo**ra**men   _____

Cavity (oral)   _____

Canal (vaginal)   _____

Canal (ali**men**tary)   _____

Hi**a**tus   _____

Ventricle   _____

No Answer Key

practice sheet

Write the plural form:

1. vertebra _____
2. ovum _____
3. diagnosis _____
4. thrombus _____
5. apex _____

6. enema _____
7. coccus _____
8. medium _____
9. nucleus _____
10. bursa _____

Write the singular form:

11. bacteria _____
12. data _____
13. crises _____
14. prognoses _____
15. uteri _____

16. specula _____
17. carcinomata _____
18. gingivae _____
19. foci _____
20. appendices _____

Fill in the blank:

21. A catheter can be said to be _____ if its opening (_____) is not plugged up.

22. A gastric ulcer can eat through the stomach lining. This is called a _____ ulcer.

23. Three words that mean natural body opening are _____ _____ and

    _____

24. The narrowing of blood vessels is called _____

25. A patient who has a colostomy wears a bag over the _____ (opening in abdominal wall).

26. _____ (medications) cause blood vessels to become wider.

27. The medical laboratory uses many different kinds of culture _____ (on which to grow bacteria).

28. Many books have an appendix. Some large reference books have many _____

29. The os uteri is the _____

30. Tiny pinpoint hemorrhages are called _____

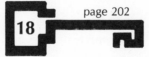

page 202

18

plural endings **45**

chapter 8
more body parts or organs: root words

Many of these root words were introduced in Chapter 1; refer back to Figures 1-1 and 1-2 in that chapter if necessary. You should be able to define most of these examples. A few of the more difficult definitions have been given for you. Later, use these pages as a drill. Cover the meaning column and see if you know the root word; then, cover the root words and see if you know the meanings. For further review write the example words. You might be able to add some more words using the suffixes you have learned previously.

Root word	Meaning	Examples	Define
carp/o	wrist	meta**car**pal (meta = after, beyond, over)	beyond wrist; bones of hand
cervic/o	neck	**cer**vical (**ver**tebra)	
		cervix (of uterus)	
chondr/o	cartilage	chon**dri**tis	
colp/o	vagina	col**pi**tis	
		colposcope	
dent/o, odont	teeth	**den**tist	
		ortho**don**tia	
		den**tal**gia	
esophag/o	esophagus	esopha**gi**tis	
lapar/o (also celi/o)	abdomen	lapa**rot**omy or celi**ot**omy	
		laparoscope	

laryng/o	larynx	laryn**gi**tis	_____
			_____
		la **ryng**oscope	_____
			_____
		la **ryng**ospasm	_____
			_____
onych/o	nail	paro **nyc**hia (par/a = around)	inflammation around a nail
			_____
oophor/o	ovary	oopho **rec**tomy	_____
			_____
		oopho **ri**tis	_____
			_____
ophthalm/o	eye	ophthal **mol**ogist	_____
			_____
		oph **thal**moscope	_____
			_____
pancreat/o	pancreas	pancrea **ti**tis	_____
			_____
pelv/i	pelvis	pel **vim**eter	_____
			_____
phleb/o	vein	phle **bi**tis	_____
			_____
pleur/o	pleura (lining membrane of chest cavity)	**pleur**isy	inflammation of pleura
			_____
pod/o	foot	po **di**atry	_____
			_____
psych/o	mind	psy **chi**atrist	_____
			_____
		psy **chol**ogy	_____
			_____
pub/o	pubes (pubic bones)	supra **pu**bic	_____
			_____
rhin/o	nose	**rhi**noplasty	_____
			_____
salping/o	fallopian tube or eustachian tube	salpin **gi**tis	_____
			_____
		salpin **gec**tomy	_____
			_____

soma	body	psychoso**mat**ic	_____
splen/o	spleen	sple**nec**tomy	_____
spondyl/o	vertebra	spondy**li**tis	_____
stomat/o	mouth	stoma**ti**tis	_____
tars/o	ankle	meta**tar**sal	_____
thorac/o	thorax (chest)	thoracocen**te**sis	_____
		tho**rac**ic vertebra	_____
tympan/o	tympanum (eardrum)	tympa**not**omy	_____
myring/o	tympanum (eardrum)	myrin**got**omy	same as tympanotomy
ureter/o	ureter (tube from kidney to bladder)	ureter**i**tis	_____
urethr/o	urethra (opening through which urine leaves body)	ure**thri**tis	_____
vas/o	vessel (artery, vein)	vasodila**ta**tion	_____
		vasocon**stric**tion	_____
		cardio**vas**cular	_____

No Answer Key

■ **Notes:** Paro**nyc**hia (pronounced "pearo**neek**ia") is another inflammation without the -itis ending. The _five_ sections of the spine (vertebral column) are

Cervical: neck region (7 vertebrae)
Thoracic or dorsal: chest region (12 vertebrae)
Lumbar: small of back (5 vertebrae)
Sacral: pelvic area (5 fused)
Coccygeal: "tail bones" (4 vertebrae)

These sections of the vertebral column are important in designating certain areas and are abbreviated in describing a certain specific region (vertebra or spinal nerve), for example:

1st thoracic vertebra is T-1 (also D-1)
2nd cervical vertebra is C-2

3rd lumbar vertebra is L-3
The sacrum is actually a single fused bone.
Coccygeal is abbrevicated Co to differentiate it from cervical.

See Chapter 18, Figure 18–7 (spinal column).

worksheet

True/False: Circle the number of the *true* statements only. Explain why statement is false. (If a word is misspelled, the statement is false.)

1. A doctor uses a pel**vim**eter to do a pelvic exam.

2. Stoma**ti**tis is inflammation of the stomach.

3. An oph**thal**moscope is used for looking into the eyes.

4. Vasocon**stric**tion is the opposite of vasodila**ta**tion.

5. Tho**rac**ic vertebrae are bones of the spine in the chest area.

6. Phle**bi**tis means inflammation of a vein.

7. Meta**car**pals are bones in the ankle.

8. Rhi**ni**tis means inflammation of the nose.

9. Pancrea**sec**tomy is excision of the pancreas.

10. A psy**chi**atrist treats diseases of the mind.

11. The u**re**thra is an opening through which urine leaves the body.

12. Bilateral salpin**gec**tomy means excision of both fallopian tubes.

13. A po**di**atrist treats diseases and deformities of the feet.

14. Den**tal**gia means toothache.

Define:

15. ortho**don**tia _____

16. **rhi**noplasty _____

17. tympa**not**omy _____

18. thoracen**te**sis (thoracocentesis) _____

19. ureter**i**tis _____

20. oopho**rec**tomy _____

21. lapa**rot**omy _____

22. **pleur**isy (pleuritis) _____

23. pel**vim**eter _____

24. supra**pu**bic _____

25. chon**dri**tis _____

Name the five sections of the vertebral column:

26. _____   29. _____

27. _____   30. _____

28. _____

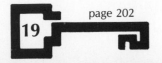

19   page 202

*If you missed any of the questions on this worksheet,
go back and review using the drill pages.*

review drill

Fill in the meaning of each word part. At another time, cover the first column and see if you can look at the meaning and write in the word part and give an example word.

Word part	Meaning	Word part	Example words
a-, an-			
anti-			
brady-			
de-			
dia-			
dys-			
hemi-			
hemo-			
hyper-			
hypo-			
hydro-			
lip-			
pre-			
pro-			
post-			
poly-			
tachy-			
-ostomy			
-itis			
-ectomy			
-otomy			
-osis			
-oscope			
-ogram			
-ography			

No Answer Key

chapter 9
more suffixes and prefixes

Study the structure of and define the following example words. Some of these should be familiar to you, as they have been used in examples in preceding lessons.

Suffix	Meaning	Examples	Define
-olysis	destruction, to separate out	he**mol**ysis	_____ _____
		oste**ol**ysis	_____ _____
		chemonucle**ol**ysis (use of an enzyme to destroy a herniated intervertebral disc)	_____ _____ _____
-oma	tumor (new growth), neoplasm, space = occupying lesion swelling	carci**no**ma or sar**co**ma	_____ _____
		hema**to**ma	_____ _____
-oid	like, similar to	**lip**oid	_____ _____
		polypoid	_____ _____
		mucoid	_____ _____
		sesamoid	_____ _____
-plasia	growth (cells)	hyper**pla**sia	_____ _____
-trophy	development	hy**per**trophy (note pronunciation)	_____ _____
-malacia	softening	osteoma**lac**ia (pronounced "ma**lash**ia")	_____ _____
		encephaloma**lac**ia	_____ _____ _____

-orrhea	flow or discharge	pyor**rhe**a (py = pus)	_____
			_____
		diar**rhe**a	_____
			_____
-pnea (also pneumo-)	breathing, air, lungs	dysp**ne**a	_____
			_____
		pneu**mon**ia or pneumo**ni**tis	_____
			_____
-plegia	paralysis	hemi**ple**gia	_____
			_____
		para**ple**gia	_____
			_____
		quadri**ple**gia, tetra**ple**gia	_____
			_____
-paresis	weakness (less than paralysis)	hemi**par**esis	_____
			_____

No Answer Key

AN IMPORTANT WORD

Genesis (remember the Bible): the origin or coming into being of something; production; birth.
   Many words are derived from this:

   gene: the unit of heredity (Greek *gennin* = to produce)

   ge**net**ics: branch of biology that deals with heredity (beginnings)

   pathogen: bacterium (or virus) that causes disease (from which disease begins)

   genitals: organs of reproduction (from which life begins)

   ho**mog**enous or homo**ge**neous: derived from like source; uniform; the same throughout, as in homog-enized milk.

Gen may come at the beginning of a word, in the middle of a word, or at the end of a word. Whenever you see it, think of genesis and see if you can figure out the meaning of the word. (*Gen* comes from the Greek; another similar word from the French means something different.)

practice sheet: -oma and -pnea (tumors & breathing words)

Define the following -oma **words:** The accent is always on **-o**ma. You will need a dictionary.

1. ade**no**ma _____

2. carci**no**ma _____

3. fi**bro**ma _____

4. gli**o**ma (glia cells = supporting tissue of brain and spinal cord) _____

5. hepa**to**ma _____

6. lym**pho**ma _____

7. granu **lo** ma _____

8. mye **lo** ma _____

9. my **o** ma _____

10. sar **co** ma _____

11. hema **to** ma _____

12. glau **co** ma (not a tumor) _____

Define the following -p*ne*a words: The accent is always on -p **ne** a. The adjective form is shown in parenthesis.

13. dysp **ne** a (dysp **ne** ic) _____

14. ap **ne** a (ap **ne** ic) _____

15. orthop **ne** a (orthop **ne** ic) _____

16. tachyp **ne** a (tachyp **ne** ic) _____

17. bradyp **ne** a (bradyp **ne** ic) _____

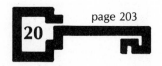

page 203

20

■ **Note**   -oma at the end of a word means a tumor or swelling. Tumors are neoplasms — new "things" formed; new growths. Tumors may be benign (innocent) or malignant (deadly, cancerous). Malignant tumors me **tas** tasize (spread to other parts of the body). A cancerous tumor that has not me **tas** tasized or infiltrated surrounding tissue is called in **si** tu (in position). An in situ tumor is a primary tumor. A secondary tumor is a meta **stat** ic tumor. Benign lesions do not me **tas** tasize, but may grow large enough to cause obstruction.

Carci **no** ma and sar **co** ma ALWAYS mean malignancy; examples: adenocarci **no** ma, lymphosar **co** ma.

■ **Note:**   -pnea words are often used in the adjectival form. For example, we usually say the patient is dysp **ne** ic (instead of the patient has dyspnea) or the patient is orthop **ne** ic (instead of the patient has orthopnea). Therefore, the spelling of the adjective is important.

worksheet

Give the correct word for the following definitions:

1. A tumor of fat _____

2. A tumor of blood (clot) _____

3. Resembling mucus _____

4. Overdeveloped (as with muscles) _____

5. Difficult breathing _____

6. Very rapid breathing _____

7. Paralysis on one side of the body _____

8. Paralysis of the lower half of body (waist down) _____

9. Flow of pus _____

10. "Running through" of stool or feces (bowel movement) _____

11. Softening of the bones _____

12. Destruction of blood (cells) _____

13. Cancerous or malignant tumor _____

14. Without breathing (adjective) _____

15. Able to breathe only when sitting upright _____

Define:

16. ho**mog**enized _____

17. quadri**ple**gic _____

18. **lip**oid _____

19. gene _____

20. hemi**par**esis _____

21. **gen**itals _____

22. ade**no**ma _____

23. pneumo**ni**tis _____

24. hyper**pla**sia _____

25. **path**ogen _____

26. Is a meta**stat**ic tumor a malignant tumor? (yes or no) _____

27. in **si**tu _____

28. secondary tumor _____

29. **ne**oplasm _____

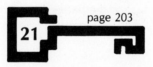

page 203

21

---

more prefixes

Define the following example words. In analyzing the example words, it will help if you separate the word parts, for example:

acro = extremities
derma = skin
itis = inflammation

Meaning: Skin on the extremities is inflamed.

Prefix	Meaning	Examples	Define
acro-	extremities, top or extreme point	acroderma**ti**tis	1. _____
		acro**ceph**aly	2. _____
aero-	air	aer**o**bic	3. _____
		anaer**o**bic	4. _____

aniso- (see iso-)	unequal	anisocy**to**sis	5. _____
dys-	bad, painful, difficult	dys**toc**ia	6. _____
		dys**pho**ria	7. _____
eu-	good, easy	eu**to**cia	8. _____
		eu**pho**ria	9. _____
		eutha**na**sia	10. _____
hetero-	different	hetero**sex**ual	11. _____
		hetero**ge**neous	12. _____
homo-	same	homo**sex**ual	13. _____
		homo**ge**neous	14. _____
iso-	equal, same	isocy**to**sis	15. _____
		iso**ton**ic	16. _____
		iso**ther**mal	17. _____
mal-	bad, poor	mal**aise**	18. _____
		maloc**clu**sion	19. _____
megalo-, -megaly	large (enlarged)	acro**meg**aly	20. _____
		megalo**car**dia or cardio**meg**aly	21. _____
meno-	menses (menstruation)	**men**opause	22. _____
		dysmenor**rhe**a	23. _____
noct-, nyct-	night	noct**u**ria, nyct**u**ria	24. _____
pan-	all, every	pan**dem**ic	25. _____
pyo-	pus	pyo**gen**ic	26. _____
		pyor**rhe**a	27. _____
syn-	going together, united	**syn**drome (Check a dictionary for specific **syn**dromes.) Make a list and define.	28. _____

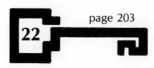

22   page 203

review drill

This review drill may be used in any manner that you find helpful in learning the material. A suggestion is to fill in the meaning for each word part, then to cover the given word part and complete the last two columns. This drill can be repeated as many times as necessary.

Word part	Meaning	Word part	Example words
-olysis			
-oma			
-oid			
-plasia			
-trophy			
-malacia			
-orrhea			
-pnea			
-plegia			
-gen-			
aero-			
hetero-			
homo-			
iso-			
mal-			
megalo-			
-megaly			
noct-			
syn-			
acro-			
pyo-			
meno-			
-itis			
-ectomy			
hemo-			
hemi-			

No Answer Key

chapter 10
bacteria, colors, and other root words

---
bacteria

Bacteria is a plural word. The singular is bacterium. Bacteriology is a study by itself. This course does not allow time for extensive coverage, but these are a few terms you should know.

The following are the two main groups of bacteria, by shape and form:

coccus   bacteria that are round in shape (plural is cocci, pronounced "cock'seye").

bacillus   bacteria that are rod shaped (plural is bacilli).

The following terms refer to the way in which bacteria grow:

strepto   twisted; bacteria that grow in twisted chains.

staphylo   bunches, like grapes; bacteria that grow in clusters.

diplo   pairs; bacteria that grow in pairs.

The two preceding sets of terms can be combined to describe certain bacteria, for example:

streptococcus   round bacteria that grow in twisted chains.

staphylococcus   round bacteria that grow in clusters.

streptobacillus   rod-shaped bacteria that grow in twisted chains.

diplococcus   round bacteria that grow in pairs.

The following are the two most important words for you to learn:

streptococcus   abbreviated "strep" infection.

staphylococcus   abbreviated "staph" infection.

The word gono**coc**cus is also important. Gono**coc**cus causes gonorrhea. Gono- is a word part that means "related to semen or seed." Gonorrhea is often abbreviated GC.

Patho**gen**ic organisms are those that cause disease. They are called **path**ogens. Bacteria, viruses, and fungi are all microorganisms that can cause disease.

□ **Assignment:**   Find a picture of kinds of bacteria in a bacteriology or microbiology book or dictionary. Make a drawing of these two kinds of bacteria.

Streptococcus   **Staphylococcus**

■ **Note:**   Bacteria can be grown on culture media in the laboratory. Studies can help in choosing the most effective antibiotic for bacterial infection.

colors and root words

Study the structure of the following examples, then define them.

Root word	Meaning	Examples	Define
chromo-	color	**chro**mosome	(soma = body) "colored bodies"
erythro-	red	e**ryth**rocyte	
leuko-	white	**leu**kocyte	abbreviated "WBC"
		leukocy**to**sis	
		leu**ke**mia	
melano-	black	mela**no**ma	
cyano-	blue	cya**no**sis	
cirrh-	orange yellow	cir**rho**sis	

No Answer Key

miscellaneous root words

Study the structure of the following examples, then define them. One of the more difficult ones has been done for you.

Root word	Meaning	Examples	Define
ankylo-	stiffening (with adhesion formation) or fusion by surgery	anky**lo**sis	
carcino-	cancer (malignancy)	carci**no**ma	
cryo-	cold	cryo**sur**gery	
		cryoex**trac**tion (of lens)	
crypt-	hidden (small, hidden sacs, especially anal)	cryp**ti**tis	
		cryp**tor**chidism	"hidden testes"—undescended
esthesia	feeling	anes**the**sia	
gravid	pregnant	primi**grav**ida	
lip-	fat	li**po**ma	

lith	stone	choleli**thi**asis*	_____
			_____
		lithotripsy	_____
			_____
necro-	dead (decayed)	ne**cro**sis	_____
			_____
par/o	to bear (children)	mul**tip**ara	_____
			_____
path-	disease	pa**thol**ogy	_____
			_____
		patho**gen**ic	_____
			_____
phago-, -phagia	eating, swallowing	phagocy**to**sis	_____
			_____
		dys**pha**gia	_____
			_____
-phasia	speech	a**pha**sia	_____
			_____
-phonia	voice	a**pho**nia	_____
			_____
schizo-	split	schizo**phre**nia (phren = mind)	_____
sclero-	hardening	arterioscle**ro**sis	_____
			_____
stasis	slowed down (sluggish)	hemo**sta**sis	_____
			_____
therapy	treatment (to cure or alleviate symptoms)	hydro**ther**apy	_____
			_____
		chemo**ther**apy	_____
			_____
		thera**peu**tic (adj)	_____
therm-, -therm	heat	**di**athermy	_____
			_____
		hyper**ther**mia	_____
			_____

_____
* -iasis means the same as -osis, but is only used in certain words.

		ther**mom**eter	_____
			_____
thrombo-	clot	throm**bo**sis	_____
			_____
trauma	injury	trau**ma**tic	_____
			_____

No Answer Key

drill

Fill in the meaning of the given root word and check your answers. After you feel you know them, cover the given root word and complete the drill using the meaning you have given. Do this as many times as necessary until you are familiar with the material.

Root word	Meaning	Root word	Example words
coccus	_____	_____	_____
bacillus	_____	_____	_____
strept/o-	_____	_____	_____
staphyl/o-	_____	_____	_____
diplo-	_____	_____	_____
gono-	_____	_____	_____
erythr/o-	_____	_____	_____
leuk/o-	_____	_____	_____
melan/o-	_____	_____	_____
cyano-	_____	_____	_____
carcin/o-	_____	_____	_____
ankyl/o-	_____	_____	_____
gravid	_____	_____	_____
par/o	_____	_____	_____
esthesia	_____	_____	_____
lith/o	_____	_____	_____
necr/o	_____	_____	_____
cryo-	_____	_____	_____
lip/o	_____	_____	_____
crypt	_____	_____	_____
path/o	_____	_____	_____
megalo-	_____	_____	_____
-megaly	_____	_____	_____
phag/o	_____	_____	_____

-phagia _____ _____ _____

phasia _____ _____ _____

schizo- _____ _____ _____

scler/o _____ _____ _____

-stasis _____ _____ _____

-therapy _____ _____ _____

therm/o _____ _____ _____

thromb/o _____ _____ _____

trauma _____ _____ _____

hemo- _____ _____ _____

uro- _____ _____ _____

hetero- _____ _____ _____

aero- _____ _____ _____

Write the word endings that pertain to surgical procedures and some words using them:

Word ending   *Example*   *Word ending*   *Example*

_____   _____   _____   _____

_____   _____   _____   _____

_____   _____   _____   _____

_____   _____   _____   _____

Write the word endings that pertain to disease conditions and some words using them:

Word ending   *Example*   *Word ending*   *Example*

_____   _____   _____   _____

_____   _____   _____   _____

_____   _____   _____   _____

No Answer Key

practice sheet

Fill in the correct word:

1. A red cell _____

2. Condition of blueness _____

3. "Black tumor" _____

4. "White blood" _____

5. Malignant tumor _____

6. Treatment with water _____

7. Fat tumor _____

8. Condition of clots or clotting _____

9. Science dealing with disease conditions _____

10. Round bacteria growing in clusters _____

11. Round bacteria growing in chain formation _____

12. Rod-shaped bacteria _____

Define:

13. pri**mip**ara _____

14. **trau**ma _____

15. arterioscle**ro**sis _____

16. hemo**sta**sis _____

17. choleli**thi**asis _____

18. ne**cro**sis _____

19. **di**athermy _____

20. anes**the**sia _____

21. hema**tol**ogy _____

22. u**re**mia _____

23. gravida III, para II _____

True/False: Circle the numbers of the *true* statements only.

24. A person who is a**pha**sic cannot speak.

25. A **leu**kocyte is a white blood cell, but the word means only white cell.

26. Schizo**phre**nia is a mental illness, commonly referred to as a split personality.

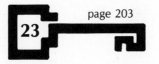

page 203

23

suffixes and some problem areas

Some of these suffixes have been used in preceding lessons in example words. This will serve as a review. Define the examples:

Suffix	Meaning	Examples	Define
-orrhexis	break open	hysteror**rhex**is	_____
		angior**rhex**is	_____
-spasm	spasm, contraction, twitching	**neu**rospasm	_____
		la**ryng**ospasm	_____
-gnos	knowledge	prog**no**sis	_____
		diag**no**sis	_____

-drome	running	**syn**drome	_____
		pro**dro**mal	_____
-opia	vision	my**o**pia*	nearsighted _____
		di**plo**pia	_____

Some word parts can be used at the beginning or at the end of a word, such as in the following examples:

Word part	Meaning	Examples	Define
megalo-, mega-, -megaly	large	acro**meg**aly	_____
		megalo**ma**nia	_____
		cardio**meg**aly	_____
		megalo**car**dia	_____
		mega**co**lon	_____
		organo**meg**aly	_____
phago-, -phagia	eat	dys**pha**gia	_____
		phagocy**to**sis	_____
therm-, -thermy	heat	ther**mom**eter	_____
		diathermy	_____

Some prefixes and suffixes that are not entirely similar have the same meaning. Note these examples. Some of the more difficult examples have been defined for you.

Meaning	Prefix	Suffix	Example	Define
urine	ur-, uro-	-uria	u**re**mia	_____
				_____
			uro**gen**ital	_____
				_____
			uri**nal**ysis	_____
				_____
			noct**u**ria	_____
				_____
			poly**u**ria	_____
				_____
			hema**tu**ria	_____
				_____
			py**u**ria	_____
				_____
			diu**re**sis	_____
				_____

---

* my/ does not mean muscle in this word.

blood   hem/o, hema, hemat/o   -emia

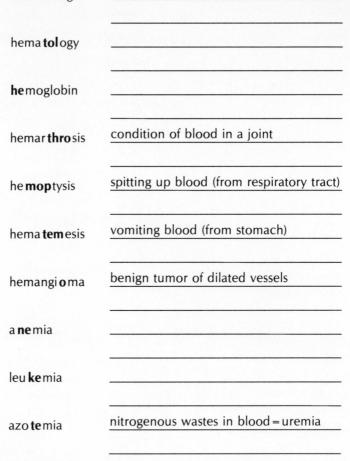

hemorrhage _____

_____

hema**tol**ogy _____

_____

hemoglobin _____

_____

hemar**thro**sis   condition of blood in a joint _____

_____

he**mop**tysis   spitting up blood (from respiratory tract) _____

_____

hema**tem**esis   vomiting blood (from stomach) _____

_____

hemangi**o**ma   benign tumor of dilated vessels _____

_____

a**ne**mia _____

_____

leu**ke**mia _____

_____

azo**te**mia   nitrogenous wastes in blood = uremia _____

_____

No Answer Key

miscellaneous practice sheet

Define:

1. **leu**kocyte _____

2. phagocy**to**sis _____

3. schizo**phre**nia _____

4. hydro**ther**apy _____

5. hemo**sta**sis _____

6. hemi**ple**gia _____

7. a**ne**mia _____

8. u**re**mia _____

9. megalo**ma**nia _____

10. hema**tol**ogy _____

11. carci**no**ma _____

12. my**o**pia _____

13. **neu**rospasm _____

14. mega **col** on _____

15. hema **tu** ria _____

Spell: Have someone dictate these words to you from Answer Key 24.

Define:

16. _____   _____
_____

17. _____   _____
_____

18. _____   _____
_____

19. _____   _____
_____

20. _____   _____
_____

21. _____   _____
_____

22. _____   _____
_____

23. _____   _____
_____

24. _____   _____
_____

25. _____   _____
_____

26. _____   _____
_____

27. _____   _____
_____

28. _____   _____
_____

29. _____   _____
_____

30. _____   _____
_____

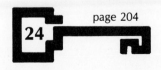

24 page 204

Fill in the blank:

1. The physician examined the boy and made a tentative _____, based on the _____, which consisted of a sore throat and fever.

2. Disease caused by a certain "round" bacteria that grow in chain formation: _____

3. The physician prescribed a medication that would retard or kill bacterial life, an _____

4. He predicted that the recovery would be complete. In other words, the _____ was good.

5. The ophthalmologist prescribed glasses for Joe Smith because he was nearsighted. The medical word for nearsightedness is _____. If a person is nearsighted, it means he can/cannot see very far. (Circle the correct word.)

6. In physical therapy many treatments are given: treatment with water is called _____; heat treatment is _____; treatment with cold is _____.

7. The laboratory technologist counted all of the *white cells* (_____) and the *red cells* (_____) in a sample of blood.

8. The abbreviation for these two procedures is _____ and _____.

9. Bacteria that cause disease are called _____. The two main kinds of bacteria (by their shape or form) are _____ and _____.

10. A woman in her first pregnancy is called a _____.

11. Gravida V, para II means _____ _____ and two _____.

12. A medication given before surgery to make the patient drowsy is called a _____ medication; one given during surgery to remove all sense of feeling is called a general _____. Medications given following surgery are called _____ medications.

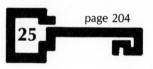

page 204

25

chapter 11
directional, positional, and numerical terms*

---

directional and positional terms

---

anterior (ventral)   toward the front, or in front of (abbreviated A).

posterior (dorsal)   toward the back, or in back of (abbreviated P), for example, AP of chest (X-ray film).

lateral   side.

bi*lat*eral   both sides.

medial (mesial)   middle.

oblique   at an angle.

superior (supra)   above; for example, superior vena cava, suprapubic.

inferior (sub) (infra)   below; for example, inferior vena cava, substernal, infraorbital.

***prox*imal**   nearest (to center). PIP = **P**roximal **i**nter**p**halangeal (joint).

distal   farthest. DIP = **D**istal **i**nter**p**halangeal (joint).

pe*riph*eral   outer edges; for example, peripheral vision.

trans-   across or through; for example, transvaginal hysterectomy; transurethral resection of prostate (TURP).

ce*phal*ic   head.

***cau*dal**   tail (base of spine), caudal anesthesia.

upright   standing.

re*cum*bent   lying down; for example, dorsal recumbent (face up).

de*cu*bitus   lying down; for example, decubitus ulcers (bed sores, sores from lying).

supine, supination   face up; palm up.

prone, pro*na*tion   face down; palm down.

ro*ta*tion (version)   turning.

eversion   turning outward, or inside out.

flexion   bending.

extension   straightening.

internal   inside.

external   outside.

sinistro   to the left, or the left, as in left eye or oculus sinister (OS).

dextro   to the right, or the right, as in right eye or oculus dexter (OD).

quadrants   "quarters" of the abdomen.

---

* See Figure 18–5 in Chapter 18; for quadrants and other areas of the abdomen, see p. 154.

TERMS THAT DESCRIBE AN EXACT POSITION   used in surgery, examination, and so on.

Tren*del*enburg   lying on back, face up, head lowered, knees bent, legs hanging over end of table.
lith*ot*omy   lying flat on back, legs in stirrups. (What does the word lithotomy mean literally?)
Sims'   lying on left side, right leg slightly forward, knees flexed.
knee-chest   kneeling, chest on table.
Fowler's   head of bed raised 1½ feet, knees elevated.
(Most medical dictionaries will list these under "positions.")

prefixes denoting direction, position, movement

Prefix	Meaning	Examples	Define
ab-	away from	1. ab**duc**tion	_____ _____
ad-	toward	2. ad**duc**tion	_____ _____
circum-	around	3. circum**ci**sion	_____ _____
contra-	opposition, against	4. contra**in**dicated	_____ _____
ecto-, exo-	outside	5. ex**og**enous	_____ _____
		6. ec**tog**enous	_____ _____
		7. ec**top**ic	_____ _____
		8. **ex**ocrine	_____ _____
endo-	within	9. **en**docrine	_____ _____
		10. en**dog**enous	_____ _____
		11. **en**doscope	_____ _____
epi-	upon, over	12. epi**gas**tric	_____ _____
extra-	outside	13. extra**u**terine	_____ _____

infra-, sub-	below, under	14. infra**ster**nal	_____
			_____
		15. sub**nor**mal	_____
			_____
ipsi-	same	16. ipsi**lat**eral	_____
			_____
meso-	middle, pertaining to mesentery	17. meso**ster**num	_____
			_____
		18. **mes**opexy	_____
			_____
meta-	after, beyond, over, change or transformation, following in a series	19. me**tas**tasis	_____
			_____
		20. me**tab**olism	_____
			_____
		21. meta**tar**sus	_____
			_____
para-	near, beside, past, beyond, opposite, abnormal, irregular, two like parts	22. para**med**ical	_____
			_____
		23. para**ty**phoid	_____
			_____
		24. para**ple**gia	_____
			_____
peri-	around, about, surrounding	25. perio**don**tal	_____
			_____
		26. peri**ton**sillar	_____
			_____
		27. peri**car**dium	_____
			_____
		28. peri**ne**um	_____
			_____
retro-	behind, backward	29. retroperito**ne**al	_____
			_____
		30. retro**ver**sion	_____
			_____
trans-	across, through	31. transu**re**thral	_____
			_____
		32. trans**vagi**nal	_____
			_____

■ **Note:** These are difficult because, in some cases, they can mean so many different things. In addition to that, some may be used interchangeably: for instance, peri**ton**sillar and para**ton**sillar are both correct and synonymous.

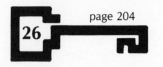

page 204

practice sheet

Define:

1. upright _____

2. flexion _____

3. decubitus _____

4. extension _____

Fill in the blank:

5. The opposite of proximal is _____. A term that means side is _____; both sides, _____

6. Recumbent, decubitus, supine, and prone are all terms that refer to the _____ position.

7. The term that refers to the "head" is _____; "tail," _____

8. The position used for a pelvic exam (with legs in stirrups) is _____

9. Internal and external mean _____ and _____

10. Interpret this X-ray order and explain what it means: AP, PA, and left lat. of chest. _____
_____

True/False: Circle the numbers of the *true* statements only. Defend your answers. Explain what is "untrue" in the false statements.

11. A transvaginal hysterectomy requires no abdominal incision.

12. A finger has three small bones—distal, medial, and proximal. The distal one is the tip of the finger.

13. Caudal anesthesia is injected into an arm vein.

14. The head is superior to the spine.

15. The abdomen is divided into quadrants to make describing an area easier and more exact.

16. An ectopic or extrauterine pregnancy is usually in the fallopian tube, but it could also be in the perineum.

17. A subnormal temperature is below 98.6 F.

18. When the gums are inflamed, we say a person has periodontal disease.

19. Paraplegia means paralysis of one side of the body.

20. Movement of the arm away from the body is called abduction. Abduction also means kidnapping (taking someone away).

21. Addiction and adduction both use the prefix ad- because they mean drawing toward something.

22. Peripheral vision means vision out to the sides.

23. The peritoneal cavity is the abdominopelvic cavity.

24. DIP refers to the joint at the far end of the finger.

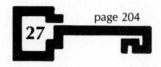

27   page 204

---
prefixes relating to numbers

Study the examples and their prefixes, then define them.

Prefix	Meaning	Examples	Define
uni-	one	uni**lat**eral	_____
bi-	two (double), twice	bi**lat**eral	_____
		bi**week**ly	(once every 2 weeks but can also mean twice a week, in which case semiweekly is the preferred term)
		bi**cus**pid	_____
tri-	three	tri**cus**pid	_____
quadri-	four	quadri**ple**gic	_____
multi-	many (more than one)	mul**tip**ara	_____
primi-	first	pri**mip**ara	_____
semi-	half (partially)	semi**co**matose	_____
hemi-	half, also one side	hemi**ple**gia	_____
ambi-	both or both sides	ambi**o**pia	double vision
		ambi**dex**trous	_____
		am**biv**alence	_____

ambly-	dull, dim, not clear	amblyopia	lazy eye _____
			_____
diplo-	double	diplopia	_____
			_____
		diplococcus	_____
			_____

UNITS OF MEASURE COMMONLY USED

diopters D, used for lenses (eye glasses).

decibels dB, used for level of sound (hearing tests).

degrees F or C, temperature, Fahrenheit or Celsius [the degree sign (°) is not used, as 98.6 F].

rads radiation dose.

units U, as TU, meaning tuberculin unit.

milligrams mg or mgm.

grams g or gm
grains gr } 1 g (gm) = 15 gr   Be careful with these abbreviations!

cubic centimeters cc or mL (milliliters, used for liquid measure; 1 cc = 1 mL).

positive + (may be 1 plus to 4 plus; 4 plus may also be written 4+ or + + + +).

negative − (written −1 or −2, for example).

review drill

Word part	Meaning	Word part	Meaning
-orrhexis	_____	infra-	_____
-spasm	_____	trans-	_____
-gnos	_____	uni-	_____
-drome	_____	primi-	_____
-opia	_____	semi-	_____
ad-	_____	hemi-	_____
ab-	_____	ambi-	_____
endo-	_____	diplo-	_____
ecto-	_____	bi-	_____
meso-	_____	tri-	_____
extra-	_____	quadri-	_____
retro-	_____	multi-	_____
peri-	_____	sinistr/o	_____
para-	_____	dextr/o	_____
epi-	_____	ipsi-	_____

Abbreviations	Meaning
AP	_____
RUQ	_____
LUQ	_____
OS	_____
cc	_____
mL (or ml)	_____
mg	_____
gr	_____
g (or gm)	_____
rad	_____

No Answer Key

worksheet

Fill in the blank:

1. To be drawn toward a habit _____

2. To move away from the midline _____

3. Arising or originating from outside of the organism (body) _____

4. Out of natural place _____ (as a tubal pregnancy)

5. Behind the peritoneum _____

6. Across (or through the urethra) _____

7. The four "areas" of the abdomen are called _____

8. Separate, conflicting emotions _____

9. A tooth or a heart valve with three cusps _____

10. Position used for pelvic exam _____ (literal meaning: surgical incision for removal of a stone)

11. Both fallopian tubes excised: _____ salpingectomy

12. Pneumonia in both lungs: _____ pneumonia.

Define:

13. semicomatose _____

14. multipara _____

15. diplopia _____

16. epigastric _____

17. endogenous _____

18. adduction _____

19. substernal _____

20. perineum _____

21. Sims' position _____

22. unilateral _____

23. periodontal _____

24. flexion _____

25. diplococcus _____

Write the abbreviation for the following:

26. right eye _____ grain _____ gram _____

27. cubic centimeter _____ positive _____ milligram _____

28. X-ray picture taken from the front of chest _____

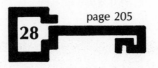

page 205

chapter 12
important words

There are many words in medicine that may or may not be made up of word parts you have learned. Their meanings are not so readily discernible, and spelling, in some cases, is difficult. Some of these have been given in previous lessons, but they are repeated here because of their importance in medicine.

drill

Define the following words: Think before you look them up. Pronounce the words as you work with them. Later rewrite each word in the third column using only the definition.

Word	Definitions	Word
1. a**bor**tion		
2. **ab**domen		
3. ab**dom**inal		
4. **ab**scess		
5. a**cute**		
6. ad**he**sion		
7. ad**nex**a		
8. auscul**ta**tion (combined with percussion)		
9. **au**toclave		
10. ax**il**la (axillary)		

11. a **nom**aly _____ _____

_____

12. **bi**opsy _____ _____

_____

13. **cat**gut _____ _____

_____

14. **cath**eter _____ _____

_____

15. **cer**vical _____ _____

_____

16. **chron**ic _____ _____

_____

17. **chro**mic _____ _____

_____

18. **coc**cyx (coccy**ge**al) _____ _____

_____

19. con **gen**ital _____ _____

_____

20. dila **ta**tion, di **la**tion _____ _____

_____

21. e **de**ma (pitting), _____ _____
    as **ci**tes, ana **sar**ca

22. **em**bolism, **em**bolus _____ _____

_____

23. **em**esis _____ _____

_____

24. **en**ema _____ _____

_____

25. ex **cre**tion _____ _____

_____

26. exacer **ba**tion _____ _____

_____

27. **fas**cia _____ _____

_____

28. **feb**rile _____ _____

_____

29. fibril **la**tion, de **fib**rillate _____ _____

_____

30. **hem**orrhage

31. **ic**terus

32. immuni**za**tion

33. in**con**tinence, in**con**tinent

34. inflam**ma**tion, in**flamed**

35. is**che**mia

36. **jaun**dice (related terms: bilirubin, Coombs')

37. me**tas**tasis, me**tas**tasized

38. **mu**cus, **mu**cous, mu**co**sa

39. o**bese**, o**bes**ity

40. **pal**pable

41. **par**alyzed, pa**ral**ysis

42. pa**ri**etal

43. per**cus**sion

44. peri**ne**um, peri**ne**al

45. perito**ne**al, perito**ne**um

46. **pleur**al

47. **pro**lapse

48. prophy**lax**is

49. **pu**rulent, pus   _____   _____

_____

50. re**mis**sion   _____   _____

_____

51. rheu**mat**ic   _____   _____

52. **se**rous   _____   _____

_____

53. **spu**tum   _____   _____

_____

54. **su**ture   _____   _____

_____

55. **vi**rus   _____   _____

56. **vis**cera   _____   _____

_____

57. void (voided)   _____   _____

_____

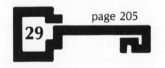

page 205

29

ROUTINE IMMUNIZATIONS

The spelling can be tricky on these terms.

> DPT (diph**ther**ia, per**tus**sis, **tet**anus) or DTP
> Rube**ol**a (hard measles)
> Ru**bel**la (German or three-day measles)
> Poliomye**li**tis
> Paro**ti**tis (mumps)
> MMR (combined measles, mumps, rubella)

IMMUNIZATIONS (NOT ROUTINE)

> Vari**o**la (smallpox), no longer required
> Typhoid, influenza, pneumonia vaccine, and so on are used only in special cases.

practice sheet

True/False: Circle the number of the _true_ statements only. Defend your answers. Explain what is "untrue" in the false statements.

1. A disease that is severe and comes on suddenly is a chronic disease.

2. A person who is afebrile has a normal temperature.

3. A congenital anomaly is one that appears late in life.

4. P & A is the abbreviation for percussion and auscultation; this means tapping and listening.

5. A person who cannot void is said to be incontinent.

6. Normal bodily excretions are urine and stool.

7. An exacerbation is an acute onset of symptoms.

8. The autoclave is one device for sterilizing medical supplies; it is used only for articles that can withstand steam under pressure.

9. Biopsy is the examination of dead tissues.

10. Mucous membranes secrete mucus.

Write a word that means:

11. vomiting _____

12. excessive fluid in body tissues _____

13. introduction of fluid into the rectum _____

14. the armpit _____

15. redness, heat, swelling, pain _____

Spell: Have someone dictate these words to you from Answer Key 30.

16. _____

17. _____

18. _____

19. _____

20. _____

Define:

21. voided _____

22. purulent _____

23. prolapse _____

24. palpable _____

25. prophylaxis _____

26. ascites _____

27. anasarca _____

Name the routine immunizations: Give the abbreviation if there is one.

28. _____

29. _____

30. _____

31. _____

32. _____

33. Name two immunizations used in special high-risk cases. _____ _____

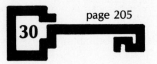

chapter 13
introduction to abbreviations (includes some diagnostic techniques)

The number of abbreviations used in medicine is overwhelming to most students. As with medical words, many abbreviations are derived from foreign words, which compounds the problem.

This chapter will introduce you to some more of the most commonly used abbreviations (Chapter 11 introduced a few abbreviations). Your need to know these will depend on your choice of a job. For instance, if you choose to work as an unit secretary, it would be important to know the abbreviations used in "physician's orders." Laboratory abbreviations and terms would be essential in this kind of job as in many other medically related jobs.

It is generally difficult to read physicians' handwriting; therefore, if you are trying to decipher scrawled handwriting and you have no idea what words or abbreviations are being used, the task of reading orders becomes almost impossible.

This chapter will only scratch the surface on abbreviations; you will gradually learn others as you are exposed to them. Along with standard abbreviations, you will find that each department or office may have their own shortcuts for writing things they use frequently. In a new situation, try to figure out what initials stand for, and if you cannot, ask! *Warning:* Abbreviations may have more than one meaning. Each must therefore be considered in context. The best "abbreviations" book I have found is *Medical Abbreviations* by Edwin B. Steen, published by the F. A. Davis Company. You will find some abbreviations listed alphabetically in medical dictionaries, and you may also find a separate section of abbreviations. An alphabetical list of abbreviations is given in Appendix h.

prescriptions and physician's orders

TIME OR NUMBER OF TIMES

qd   every day.

od   once a day.

qod   every other day.

q__h   every __ hours.

bid   twice a day.

tid   three times a day.

qid   four times a day.

hs   at bedtime.

ac   before meals.

pc   after meals.

prn   as needed.

ad lib   as desired.

UNITS OR AMOUNTS

tabs.   tablets, pills.

caps.   capsules.

supp   sup**pos**itory.

$\overline{\text{ss}}$ one-half.

mg   milligrams.

g or **gm**   grams.

gr   grains.

cc   cubic **cen**timeters or

mL or **ml**   **mil**liliters.

L   liter (1000 cc or mL [ml])

mEq   millie**quiv**alent

U   units.

gtt   drops.

℥   ounces.

ℨ   drams.

ROUTES OF ADMINISTRATION

PO by mouth.

IV intra **ve** nously.

IM intra **mus** cularly.

H hypo **der** mically

subcu, subq subcu **tan** eously.

subling sub **ling** ually.

R rec tally.

par *en* **teral administration** not by mouth.

IV 5% glu in DW (glucose in distilled water);

ns (normal saline solution). Iso **ton** ic solution.

cly **sis** fluids given by needle, under skin (not in vein).

TKO to keep open (vein).

KVO keep vein open.

ACTIVITY, TOILETING

bedrest complete bedrest. ABR (absolute).

dangle sit at edge of bed, legs over side.

ambulate walk.

OOB out of bed.

BRP bathroom privileges; may be up to BR only.

commode bedside toilet.

DIET ORDERS   (Most of these are self-explanatory):

NPO (NBM) nothing by mouth.

I & O intake and output (measured).

liq liquids only (clear, full).

fluids

lo salt, low Na

salt free

reg, full soft, bland, and so on

push fluids, force fluids (FF)

DAT diet as tolerated.

hypo hypoglycemic diet.

ADA American Dietetic Association diet.

X-RAY, LABORATORY, PULMONARY FUNCTION

AP and **Lat** routine X-ray picture of chest (front to back and side view).

up upright X-ray picture.

decub de **cu** bitus (lying).

IVP intravenous pyelogram (kidney).

BE barium enema (colon).

GI series upper (barium swallow), lower (same as BE).

GB series gallbladder X-ray picture.

RAI, RAIU radioactive iodine (uptake), thyroid function.

SCAN CT, CAT: computerized axial to **mog** raphy.*

CBC complete blood count.

Ua urinalysis.

VC vital capacity (lungs).

OTHER ROUTINE PROCEDURES

TPR temperature, pulse, respirations.

B/P blood pressure.

V/S vital signs.

ECG, EKG electrocardiogram.

EEG electroencephalogram.

SCANS

Scans can detect changes in size, shape, and position; changes in density, as happens in edema; hemorrhage; inflammation; neoplasms; clots; calcium deposits; cysts; and abscesses. CAT, CT, EMI are names of machines used.

Organs that can be "scanned" include:

Head and neck: brain, skull, ear, sinuses.

---

* Tomo **graph** ic films are serial pictures of cross sections of the body (ordinary X-ray pictures show only a flat plane). These serial pictures are "slices" of sections of the body.

Thorax: lungs, heart.

Vessels: aorta, vena cava.

Abdomen: pancreas, liver, gallbladder, adrenals, kidneys, spleen, and peritoneum.

Pelvis: reproductive organs, male and female; urinary tract.

Extremities, spinal canal, and flat bones.

Advantages of scans: more sensitive than X-ray procedures, sharper pictures are produced; therefore, earlier diagnosis is possible.

Disadvantages: relatively high cost; not useful for tiny detail (vascular).

Scans using contrast medium can have some unpleasant sensations associated with them, and some side effects; however, a scan is noninvasive and painless if no contrast is used.

ULTRASONOGRAPHY

Noninvasive technique using ultrasound is useful in obtaining "pictures" of the heart, aneurysms of the aorta, and changes in size and structure in the abdominopelvic organs; tumors, foreign bodies, and retinal detachment in the eye; fetal size and maturity in prenatal development, as well as placental placement. It is not useful for diagnosing lung cancers because ultrasound waves do not pass through structures that contain air.

MISCELLANEOUS ABBREVIATIONS

qns quantity not sufficient. (Lab requires a larger specimen.)

c̄ with.

s̄ without.

dc discontinue.

TLC tender loving care.

stat immediately. (ASAP, as soon as possible.)

EUA examination under anesthesia.

DOA dead on arrival.

OD overdose (also means right eye).

prep prepare.

pre-op preoperatively.

post-op postoperatively.

H_2O water.

O_2 oxygen.

CO_2 carbon dioxide.

CPR cardiopulmonary resuscitation.

■ Notes:

1. Abbreviations are written with or without periods. (Periods are unnecessary on most abbreviations and are required only on those that may be confusing.)
2. Roman numerals are often used: I, II, III, IV, V, VI, VII, VIII, IX, and X.
3. For any patient in the hospital, the physician's orders should always include the following:
   a. diet order (NPO, for example).
   b. activity level (BRP or OOB, for example).
   c. prn "sleep" medication and prn "pain" medication.
   d. additional orders as necessary (X-ray or lab, for example).
4. Try to read the next prescription you receive before having it filled.

worksheet

Interpret (spell out) these orders:

1. Procaine penicillin 600,000 U IM q8h _____

_____

2. Codeine 30 mg PO q4h prn for headache _____

_____

3. Seconal gr Ťss hs prn _____

4. Nembutal 100 mg PO hs _____

5. NPO after midnight _____

6. 1000 cc 5% glu in DW IV stat _____

7. BID OOB _____

8. Push fluids; I & O _____

Write the abbreviation for the following:

9. three times a day _____   15. water _____

10. grains _____   16. oxygen _____

11. grams _____   17. before meals _____

12. with _____   18. may go to bathroom only _____

13. without _____   19. gastrointestinal _____

14. discontinue _____   20. one-half _____

Identify:

21. IVP _____

22. qid _____

23. U _____

24. qns _____

25. supp _____

26. ns _____

27. TLC _____

28. IV _____

29. EKG _____

30. TPR _____

31. What are the vital signs? _____

32. What is meant by a CAT scan? _____

Extra:

What orders should always be included for a patient in hospital? _____

_____

_____

_____

_____

31 page 206

hospital or clinic departments

A & D   admitting and discharge.

CS   central service or supply.

OR   operating room, surgery (MOR, minor surgery).

RR   recovery room.

PT & OT   physical therapy and occupational therapy (May be under PM & R, physical medicine and rehabilitation).

X-ray   radiology.

lab   medical laboratory.

MR   medical records.

peds   pediatrics.

med-surg   ward for medical and surgical patients (may be combined or separate).

OB   obstetrics (includes labor and delivery rooms, postpartum ward, newborn nursery and ICN or intensive care nursery).

OPD   out-patient department.

ER   emergency room; **ED**   emergency department.

ENT   ear, nose, and throat.

GU   genitourinary.

NP   neuropsychiatric.

SS   social service.

CCU or ICU   coronary care unit or intensive care unit.

DOU   definitive observation unit (less than intensive care, but more than "floor" care).

dietary   food service.

housekeeping

pharmacy

morgue

pathology

As with the abbreviations given on pp 81–83, you will see them written in many ways. Sometimes you will see them with periods between letters and sometimes without, as in O.P.D. or OPD.

worksheet

Use abbreviations to fill in the blanks:

1. Before being admitted to the hospital as a patient, one must go through either _____ or _____.

2. After surgery in the _____, a patient usually goes to the _____ and then to the _____ unit.

3. If a fracture is suspected, the patient goes to _____ (for help in diagnosis).

4. For treatment only, not a hospital admission, a patient may go to the _____ or the _____.

5. After a severe heart attack, a patient is usually sent to the _____ or _____.

6. For delivery, a woman goes to the _____ department, _____ room. After delivery, the newborn infant is taken to the _____ and the mother is taken to the _____ unit.

7. Children are cared for in _____

8. Most reusable supplies are cleaned and sterilized for the entire hospital in _____

9. Blood and urine samples are sent to the _____ for testing.

10. After recovering from a stroke, a patient may have treatment to restore weak muscles in the _____ department.

11. After discharge from the hospital, a patient's file is sent to _____

12. After a patient dies, the body goes to the _____

13. If a patient needs help with child care or with family problems, the patient or the patient's family is referred to _____

14. Patients with psychological problems or mental illness are generally treated in _____

15. Tonsillectomies may be done in _____ or _____

16. A person who must learn a new skill because he or she is no longer able to perform on a previous job may be referred to _____

17. Intravenous fluids are generally stored in _____ and picked up or ordered from the units as needed.

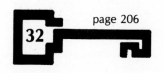

32   page 206

chapter 14
abbreviations: diagnoses and medical laboratory

---

diagnostic abbreviations

ASHD   arterioscle**rot**ic heart disease.

CA   carci**no**ma (cancer).

CBS   chronic brain syndrome.

CHD   coronary heart disease.

CHF   congestive heart failure.

COPD/COLD   chronic obstructive pulmonary (lung) disease.

CP   **cer**ebral palsy.

CVD   cardio**vas**cular disease.

CVA   cerebro**vas**cular accident (stroke).

DJD   degenerative joint disease (osteoarthritis).

FUO   fever of undetermined origin.

GC   gonorrhea.

(S)LE   (systemic) lupus erythematosus.

MD   muscular dystrophy.

MI   myo**car**dial in**farc**tion (coronary occlusion, coronary thrombosis).

MS   multiple scle**ro**sis.

PID   pelvic inflammatory disease.

RA   rheumatoid ar**thri**tis.

T & A   tonsil**lec**tomy and adenoid**ec**tomy.

TIA   transient is**che**mic attack.

URI   upper respiratory infection.

UTI   urinary tract infection.

(See the list of abbreviations in Appendix h.)

Do not let abbreviations "throw" you; recall your knowledge of terminology and use a little imagination. Often you will be able to figure out what the abbreviation stands for (in a medical history, for example) by the information given around it. In a particular work situation, you will soon learn the abbreviations pertinent to you and your job.

HISTORY-TAKING ABBREVIATIONS   abbreviations used in "history taking" are numerous. The following are just a few:

CC   chief complaint.

PI   present illness.

PH past history.

FH family history.

SR or **ROS** systemic review or review of systems.

Rx recipe, take, prescription.

Dx diagnosis.

Hx history.

Sx symptoms.

HEENT head, eyes, ears, nose, throat.

PE physical exam.

PERLA pupils equal react to light and accommodation (eyes).

SOB short of breath.

P & A percussion and auscultation.

A & P auscultation and percussion.

R/O rule out.

m murmur.

c/o complains of.

laboratory abbreviations and terms

The following material is a brief sketch of laboratory information. Although you may not understand all of it at this time, read through it; this outline contains many commonly used terms and abbreviations. Refer to lab forms on pp. 91–93 (Figures 14–1 to 14–5).

HEMATOLOGY

specimen blood; this examination includes physical properties of blood such as:

1. Numbers of cells; blood counts.
2. Size and shape: morphology.
3. Microscopic appearance.

routine tests

1. CBC: complete blood count.
2. RBC: red cell count (erythrocytes).
3. WBC: white cell count (leukocytes).
4. WBC & diff(erential) count: number of each kind of white cell: neutrophils, eosinophils, and basophils, lymphocytes, and monocytes (see "Notes" on p. 89 for further discussion of neutrophils).
5. Hb, Hgb: hemoglobin.
6. Crit, Hct: hematocrit.
7. Platelet count.
8. ESR, sed rate: erythrocyte sedimentation rate.

BIOCHEMISTRY (SMA, SMAC: chemistry profile; group of tests) See Figures 14–6 and 14–7 (pp. 94–95).

specimen blood; this examination includes tests for the following chemical elements:

1. Glucose
   FBS: fasting blood sugar.
   GTT: glucose tolerance test.
2. Sodium, potassium, chlorides, and so on.

3. BUN, BSP, NPN, SGOT, and so on. (See the explanation of blood chemistry tests, p. 96.)

specimen   urine; routine urinalysis, Ua (voided, midstream, or catheterized or cath spec) may include testing for the following:

1. Reaction (acid or alkaline, pH).
2. Albumin or glucose.
3. Specific gravity: weight as compared to water.
4. Casts, bacteria, WBCs, RBCs (microscopic exam).

SEROLOGY

specimen   blood serum; the following are blood serum tests:

1. STS (serological test for syphilis), *VDRL* (Venereal Disease Research Laboratory), Kahn, and others.
2. Pregnancy tests: Pregnosticon and UCG.
3. RA: rheumatoid arthritis.
4. Landsteiner blood types: ABO (type and crossmatch done before transfusion).
5. Rh factor.
6. Rubella.

BACTERIOLOGY

specimen   blood, sputum, spinal fluid, any excretion, feces (for presence of occult blood or parasites).

isolate and identify pathogenic bacteria

   C & S   culture and sensitivity; bacteria is grown from specimen and is subjected to various antibiotics to determine the most effective one for treatment of bacterial diseases.

common terms

   gram stain   one of the basic stains used in classifying bacteria (gram neg. or pos.).

   AFB   acid-fast bacillus (tuberculosis organism).

   hanging drop culture   placing drop on coverslip and inverting over concave slide.

HISTOLOGY AND CYTOLOGY   (study of tissues and cells)

specimen   tissues and cells; histologic and cytologic studies include the following:

1. Biopsy: examination of living tissue (tests for abnormal cells such as cancer).
2. Pap smear: cancer detection (Papanicolaou).
3. Miscellaneous tests may be done on bone marrow, gastric contents, and spinal fluid, depending on the size and scope of the lab.

■ **Notes:**   The term "neutrophil" is seldom used on lab forms. They may be called PMNs (polymorpho **nu**clear **leu**kocytes) or segs (segmented nuclei), meaning mature cells with the nucleus in segments. The terms "stabs" and "bands" refer to immature cells.

   Lab stix: Many simple lab procedures are now done with commercial *lab stix* of various kinds. For example, a treated paper stick need only be dipped into a urine sample to test for sugar. These are used in many offices and by patients who regularly test their urine at home (diabetics). Tablets are also used for simple, routine urine tests.

COMMUNICATION WITH THE LABORATORY

The laboratory is usually under the direction of a *pathologist*, with *medical technologists* performing the complicated laboratory tests and assistants the simpler tests. All hospitals and clinics have laboratories, and many lab tests can be performed in the physician's office. There are lab requisition slips for each laboratory division; every lab uses different forms, unfortunately. You will become familiar with the various laboratory forms as you use them. Figures 14–1 to 14–7, on the following pages, contain sample lab requisition forms. Some labs use color coding and code numbers.

   The following are some important points to remember in dealing with the laboratory:

1. Use care if directed to collect specimens.

2. Label specimens accurately and completely.

3. Use properly prepared containers (for example, some containers have a preservative added and some are color coded).

4. Use the right requisition form in ordering lab work.

5. Refrigerate specimens if they must be held for a specified time (unless directed otherwise).

6. If your job involves instructing patients about specimen collection, explain clearly and make sure the patient understands.

Sample lab forms   are presented in the following pages, and explanations of "SMAC" profiles are also presented.

ARIZONA MEDICAL PLAZA LABORATORY
DIVISION OF CHEMED
1728 West Glendale Avenue

DIRECTOR
CHARLES D. CONNOR, M.D.

PATIENT_____ DR._____

SPECIMEN
NO._____ DATE_____

Hemoglobin:	_____	
Hematocrit:	_____	
White Blood Count:	_____	
Red Blood Count:	_____	
Differential:	_____ Segs	
_____ Lymphs _____ Mono _____ Baso		
_____ Bands _____ Eos		
Indices: _____ MCV _____ MCH _____MCHC		
Platelet:	_____	
Sedimentation rate:	_____mm/hour	
COMMENT: _____		
_____		
_____		

URINALYSIS
Specific Gravity: _____
Ph: _____
Protein: _____
Glucose: _____
Ketones: _____
Bilirubin _____
Occult Blood: _____
MICROSCOPIC:
_____RBCs _____WBCs
_____Epithelial cells _____ casts
COMMENT: _____

CHARLES D. CONNOR, M.D.

Figure 14–1. Combined form for blood and urine testing (hematology and biochemistry). (Courtesy Arizona Medical Plaza Laboratory.)

ARIZONA MEDICAL PLAZA LAB
1728 W. GLENDALE AVENUE
PHOENIX, AZ 85021 / PHONE 995-1151

DIRECTOR: CHARLES D. CONNOR, M.D.

ID # _____
PATIENT _____
DOCTOR _____
DATE _____

COMPLETE BLOOD COUNT

	PATIENT		NORMAL
HEMOGLOBIN	gm.%	M	13 - 18 gm%
		F	11 - 16
HEMATOCRIT	%	M	40 - 54 %
		F	37 - 47
WBC	/mm³		5,000 - 10,000
RBC	/mm³	M	4.5 - 6.0
		F	4.0 - 5.5

DIFFERENTIAL

PMN	%	38 - 85%
LYMPH	%	22 - 44%
BANDS	%	2 - 5%
MONO	%	0 - 8%
EOS	%	0 - 4%
BASO	%	0 - 3%
	%	

INDICES

MCV	μ3	82 - 92 μ³
MCH	μg	27 - 32 μg
MCHC	%	32 - 40 %

PRENATAL

VDRL	R		NR	
RUBELLA	NEG		POS	1:
ABO				
RH	c̄	D		Du

		PATIENT	NORMAL
PLATELET	Est. Adeq	/mm³	150,000 - 300,000 /mm³
RETIC.		%	0 - 2 %
SEDIMENTATION		mm/hr.	M 0 - 10 mm/hr. / F 0 - 20 mm/hr.
PROTIME	CONTROL SEC.	% Activ.	% Activ.
P.T.T.		SEC.	30 - 45 SEC.
BLEEDING TIME	MIN. SEC.		LESS THAN 5 MIN.
LEE-WHITE CLOTTING	MIN. SEC.		9 - 16 MIN.

COMMENT:
_____
_____
_____

Figure 14–2. Blood test, including prenatal routine testing (*shows normal values*) (hematology and serology). (Courtesy Arizona Medical Plaza Laboratory.)

ARIZONA MEDICAL PLAZA LABORATORY
DIVISION OF CHEMED
1728 WEST GLENDALE AVENUE • PHOENIX, ARIZONA 85021

Patient: _____ Physician _____ Date _____

Specimen No.: _____ Source: _____

SMEAR	CULTURE				SENSITIVITIES			

| | | Sensitive | Resistant | | Sensitive | Resistant | |

_____ Gram Stain   _____ Routine (Culture)   _____ _____ Ampicillin   _____ _____ Erythromycin

_____ Ova, Parasites, Cysts   _____ Other   _____ _____ Chloramphenicol   _____ _____ Nitrofurantoin

_____ _____ Kanamycin   _____ _____ Penicillin G

_____ _____ Naladixic Acid   _____ _____ Streptomycin

_____ _____ Sulfonamide   _____ _____ Tetracycline

RESULTS: _____   _____ _____ Garamycin   _____ _____ Colistin

_____   _____ _____ Neomycin   _____ _____ Lincocin

_____   _____ _____ Carbenicillin   _____ _____ Methicillin

_____   _____ _____ Cephalothin

_____

_____

_____
MICROBIOLOGIST

Figure 14–3. Form used for culture and sensitivity studies (bacteriology). (Courtesy Arizona Medical Plaza Labortory.)

ARIZONA MEDICAL PLAZA LAB
1728 W. GLENDALE AVENUE
PHOENIX, AZ 85021 - PHONE 995-1151

DIRECTOR: CHARLES D. CONNOR, M.D.

ID# _____

PATIENT _____

DOCTOR _____

DATE _____

	Patient	Normals
☐ Fasting Blood Sugar	mg%	70-110
☐ 2 Hr. P.P.B.S.		
☐ Random B.S.		
☐ Glucose Tolerance	Urine	

	Blood	Sugar	Acetone
Fasting			
½ Hr.			
1 Hr.			
2 Hr.			
3 Hr.			
4 Hr.			
5 Hr.			
6 Hr.			

ENZYMES	Patient	Normals
☐ Alk. Phos.	mU/ml.	m 87-212
	child 178-556	f 68-200
☐ Acid Phos.	mU/ml.	0-11
☐ CPK	mU/ml.	0-75
☐ LDH	mU/ml.	0-74
☐ SGOT	mU/ml.	0-17
☐ SGPT	mU/ml.	0-17

CHEMISTRY

☐ B.U.N.	mg%	6-24
☐ Creatinine	mg%	0.6-1.3
☐ Cholesterol	mg%	m 141-300
		f 131-285
☐ Calcium	mg%	8.5-10.5
☐ Phosphorus	mg%	adult 2.4-4.5
		child 3.5-6.5
☐ Amylase	U.%	30-180
☐ Bilirubin Total	mg%	0.2-1.0
☐ Direct	mg%	0-0.4
☐ Indirect	mg%	0-0.6
☐ Uric Acid	mg%	m 3.4-7.0
		f 2.4-5.7
☐ Total Protein	gm%	6-8
☐ Albumin	gm%	m 3.5-4.7
		f 3.8-4.9
☐ A/G Ratio		1.48:1-2.34:1

☐ Thyroid Profile		
☐ PBI	mcg%	4-8
☐ T_3	%	25-35
☐ T_4	mcg%	3.4-11.2
☐ T_7	mcg%	0.85-3.92

☐ Lithium		mEq/L	
☐ ELECTROLYTES			
☐ Sodium	mEq/L	135-155
☐ Potassium	mEq/L	3.5-5.0
☐ Chloride	mEq/L	98-106
☐ CO_2	mmol/L	23-30

☐ Heterophil		
	Titer	1:
☐ R.A. Latex		
☐ Streptozyme		
	Titer	1:
☐ C. Reactive Protein		
☐ L.E. Slide		

☐ Pregnancy Test

MISC.

☐ _____
☐ _____
☐ _____

Chem.   COMMENTS: _____

Figure 14–4. Form used for blood chemistry, electrolytes, and other miscellaneous tests (biochemistry). (Courtesy Arizona Medical Plaza Laboratory.)

ARIZONA MEDICAL PLAZA LAB
1728 W. GLENDALE AVENUE
PHOENIX, AZ 85021 / PHONE 995-1151
DIRECTOR: CHARLES D. CONNOR, M.D.

ID # _____
PATIENT _____
DOCTOR _____
DATE _____
SOURCE _____
L.M.P. _____

CYTOLOGY

CLASSIFICATION

NEGATIVE FOR MALIGNANT CELLS	☐	CLASS I
ATYPICAL CELLS, BENIGN	☐	CLASS II
CELLS, INDETERMINATE FOR MALIGNANCY	☐	CLASS III
CELLS SUSPICIOUS FOR MALIGNANCY	☐	CLASS IV
CELLS CONCLUSIVE FOR MALIGNANCY	☐	CLASS V

ADDITIONAL FINDINGS

INFLAMMATORY EXUDATE ☐

FRESH BLOOD ☐

TRICHOMONAS PRESENT ☐

FUNGI PRESENT ☐

MATURATION INDEX

SUPERFICIAL CELLS   %

INTERMEDIATE CELLS   %

PARABASAL CELLS   %

COMMENT:

Figure 14–5.   Form used for cytology (Pap test). (Courtesy Arizona Medical Plaza Laboratory.)

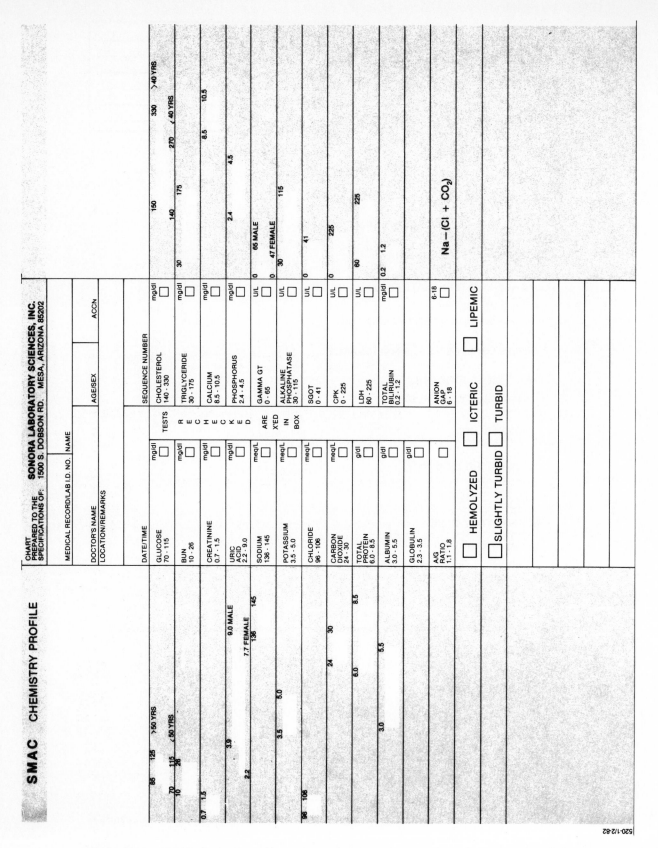

Figure 14–6. SMAC chemistry profile. (Courtesy Sonora Laboratory Sciences, Inc., Mesa, AZ.)

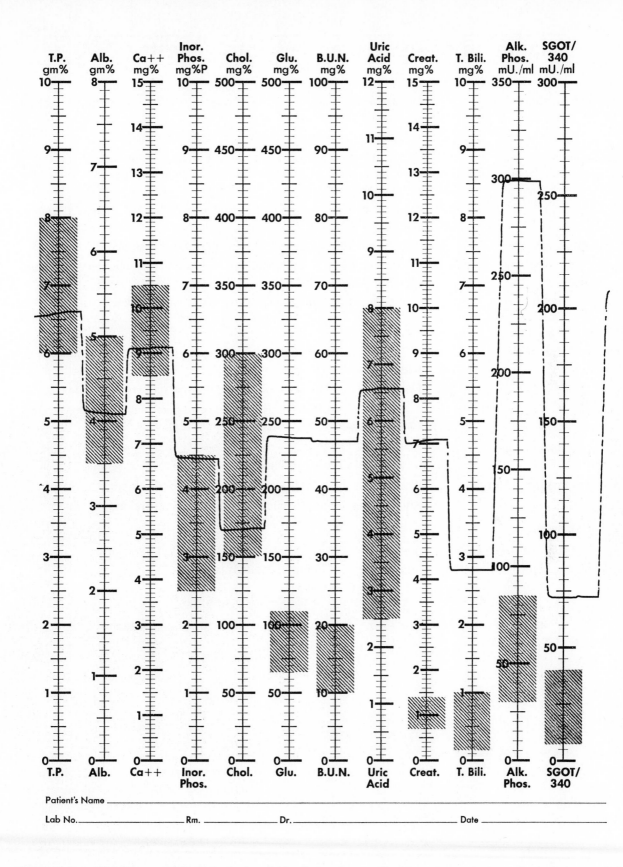

Figure 14-7. SMA (Sequential Multiple Analyzer) blood chemistry profile. Normal range is shown in shaded areas. Solid line shows patient's results. The following page explains what some of these results mean.

explanation of some blood chemistry tests (SMA)

Calcium, phosphorus
Indicative of bone function and of the parathyroid hormones that influence bone function.

Glucose
Useful test for diabetes; varies with state of fasting and age.

BUN, creatinine, BUN/creatinine ratio
Detect the presence of kidney disease but are influenced by a number of other factors; BUN may be elevated in severe dehydration and is reduced in pregnancy.

Uric acid
May be elevated in gout but levels are variable, increased during periods of stress.

Cholesterol, triglycerides (fats)
Associated with increased probability of heart disease (MI).

Total protein, albumin, globulin albumin/globulin ratio
General index of overall health and nutrition. The globulin fraction contains antibodies.

Bilirubin, direct bilirubin
Test of liver function; may be elevated because of disease of red blood cells. In circulation it indicates liver disease, hemolysis, gout, increased risk of MI.

Alkaline phosphatase
Indicates possible liver or bone disorders. Elevated in adolescence when bones are growing.

LDH
Detects cell damage of various types; not specific for any certain disease.

SGOT
May indicate possible liver disease or heart muscle damage; may also be elevated due to recent vigorous exercise.

SGPT
Test of liver function.

Iron
If low may indicate presence of anemia.

Sodium, potassium, chloride
Blood electrolytes. May be abnormal due to a number of diseases.

Magnesium
Another electrolyte, required for normal neural and muscular function.

Explanation of terms:

BUN	blood urea nitrogen.
bilirubin	orange pigment in bile (produces jaundice).
LDH	lactic dehy**drog**enase.
SGOT	serum glu**tam**ic oxaloa**ce**tic trans**am**inase.

The suffix -ase indicates an enzyme. When a tissue or organ is damaged due to disease or trauma, enzymes are released into the blood.

■ **Note:** It is important to remember that most laboratory tests are not diagnostic in themselves. Along with other findings, they do aid the physician in making a diagnosis. Blood test results are known to fluctuate from day to day, owing to changes within an individual patient and/or laboratory variation. As an interesting demonstration of this, study the two SMA forms and the chemistry form presented in this text. They all show "normal values" and all are slightly different.

Example: *Glucose* Sonora 70–115 (under age 50 years)
Other lab 65–110
(Figure 14–7)
Arizona Med. 70–110

Compare results on other items: BUN, Ca, SGOT, LDH, and so on.

blood profiles

At times, the grouping of certain blood tests gives the physician an overall picture (or profile) of the patient's status that a single test alone cannot give. The following tests are often ordered together (in part or in toto) to help the physician establish the presence of a disease, to ascertain its severity, and to aid in determining which of several possible diseases with similar symptoms is present.

Arthritis profile

Sedimentation rate (ESR)
Antinuclear antibodies (ANA)
C-reactive protein (CRP)
Rheumatoid factor (RA)
LE (lupus erythematosus) cell prep
Latex flocculation or Bentonite agglutination
ASO (antistreptolysin O) titer

Atherosclerosis profile

Triglycerides
Cholesterol
Lipids
Lipoproteins

Cardiac profile (post MI)

Serum glutamic oxaloacetic transaminase (SGOT)
Lactic dehydrogenase (LDH)
Creatine phosphokinase (CPK)
Complete blood count (CBC)
Sedimentation rate (ESR)
Prothrombin time (Pro time)

Coagulation studies

Bleeding time
Clotting time
Prothrombin time
Platelet count

Liver Profile

Serum amylase and lipase
Serum glutamic oxaloacetic transaminase (SGOT)
Serum glutamic pyruvic transaminase (SGPT)
Alkaline phosphatase
Bilirubin
Cholesterol
Protein, albumin, globulin
Thymol turbidity
Hepatitis Australia antigen (HAA)

Thyroid Profile

Thyroxine (T4)
Triiodothyronine (T3) uptake
Protein-bound iodine (PBI)

Identify:

1. CBC _____

2. WBC _____

3. RBC _____

4. Hb, Hgb _____

5. Hct, Crit _____

6. FBS _____

Complete the following:

7. Explain what diff means in "WBC and diff": _____

_____

_____

8. Name the five basic kinds of leukocytes: _____

_____

9. What are the physical properties of blood, and which lab division works in this area? _____

_____

10. Name three tests done in a routine Ua: _____

_____

_____

11. What is the difference between a voided and a catheterized urine specimen (in how it is obtained)? ____

_____

_____

Which of these would be least likely to contain contaminants? _____

_____

12. Which lab division does the VD tests? _____ Name one such test: _____

_____

13. To which lab division would a throat swab specimen be sent if strep sore throat was suspected? _____

_____

Which test would the doctor order to find out the best antibiotic to prescribe? _____

_____

14. What is a pap smear and why and how is it done? _____

_____

In which lab department? _____

15. What is a biopsy? _____

_____

_____

16. List the six important points in collection of specimens: _____

    _____

    _____

    _____

    _____

    _____

17. What is meant by a "fasting" kind of test? _____

    _____

18. What terms or abbreviations are used for neutrophils on laboratory forms (hematology)? _____

    _____

19. Which kinds of white cells (in a differential count) normally run less than (<) 1%? _____

    _____

20. An -ase suffix denotes an _____.

21. What is the normal range of hemoglobin for a woman (see lab form, hematology)? _____

page 206

33

Extra lab forms follow.   Your instructor may give you some lab results (Figures 14–8 and 14–9 on p. 100) so you can fill out these forms. You may also use results given in one of the reports included in this text. For example: C-V report in Chapter 19.

ID # _____
PATIENT _____
DOCTOR _____
DATE _____

COMPLETE BLOOD COUNT

	PATIENT	NORMAL
HEMOGLOBIN	gm.%	M 13-18 / F 11-16 gm%
HEMATOCRIT	%	M 40-54 / F 37-47 %
WBC	/mm³	5,000 - 10,000
RBC	/mm³	M 4.5-6.0 / F 4.0-5.5

DIFFERENTIAL

	PATIENT	NORMAL
PMN	%	38-85%
LYMPH	%	22-44%
BANDS	%	2-5%
MONO	%	0-8%
EOS	%	0-4%
BASO	%	0-3%
	%	

INDICES

	PATIENT	NORMAL
MCV	$\mu 3$	82-92 μ^3
MCH	μg	27-32 μg
MCHC	%	32-40%

PRENATAL

VDRL	R	NR
RUBELLA	NEG	POS 1:
ABO		
RH	c̄	D	Du

	PATIENT	NORMAL
PLATELET Est. Adeq ☐	/mm³	150,000 - 300,000 /mm³
RETIC.	%	0-2%
SEDIMENTATION	mm/hr.	M 0-10 mm/hr. F 0-20 mm/hr.
PROTIME CONTROL SEC.	% Activ.	% Activ.
P.T.T.	SEC.	30-45 SEC.
BLEEDING TIME	MIN. SEC.	LESS THAN 5 MIN.
LEE-WHITE CLOTTING	MIN. SEC.	9-16 MIN.

COMMENT: _____
_____
_____
_____

Figure 14–8. Blood test, including prenatal routine testing (shows normal values). (Courtesy Arizona Medical Plaza Laboratory.)

ID# _____
PATIENT _____
DOCTOR _____
DATE _____

	Patient	Normals
☐ Fasting Blood Sugar	mg%	70-110
☐ 2 Hr. P.P.B.S.		
☐ Random B.S.		
☐ Glucose Tolerance		Urine

	Blood	Sugar	Acetone
Fasting			
½ Hr.			
1 Hr.			
2 Hr.			
3 Hr.			
4 Hr.			
5 Hr.			
6 Hr.			

ENZYMES

	Patient	Normals
☐ Alk. Phos.	mU/ml.	m 87-212 child 178-556 f 68-200
☐ Acid Phos.	mU/ml.	0-11
☐ CPK	mU/ml.	0-75
☐ LDH	mU/ml.	0-74
☐ SGOT	mU/ml.	0-17
☐ SGPT	mU/ml.	0-17

CHEMISTRY

		Normals
☐ B.U.N.	mg%	6-24
☐ Creatinine	mg%	0.6-1.3
☐ Cholesterol	mg%	m 141-300 / f 131-285
☐ Calcium	mg%	8.5-10.5
☐ Phosphorus	mg%	adult 2.4-4.5 / child 3.5-6.5
☐ Amylase	U.%	30-180
☐ Bilirubin Total	mg%	0.2-1.0
☐ Direct	mg%	0-0.4
☐ Indirect	mg%	0-0.6
☐ Uric Acid	mg%	m 3.4-7.0 / f 2.4-5.7
☐ Total Protein	gm%	6-8
☐ Albumin	gm%	m 3.5-4.7 / f 3.8-4.9
☐ A/G Ratio		1.48:1-2.34:1
☐ Thyroid Profile		
☐ PBI	mcg%	4-8
☐ T$_3$	%	25-35
☐ T$_4$	mcg%	3.4-11.2
☐ T$_7$	mcg%	0.85-3.92

		Normals
☐ Lithium	mEq/L	
☐ ELECTROLYTES		
☐ Sodium	mEq/L	135-155
☐ Potassium	mEq/L	3.5-5.0
☐ Chloride	mEq/L	98-106
☐ CO$_2$	mmol/L	23-30
☐ Heterophil	Titer	1:
☐ R.A. Latex		
☐ Streptozyme	Titer	1:
☐ C. Reactive Protein		
☐ L.E. Slide		
☐ Pregnancy Test		

MISC.
☐
☐
☐

Chem.   COMMENTS: _____

Figure 14–9. Form used for blood chemistry, electrolytes, and other miscellaneous tests. (Courtesy Arizona Medical Plaza Laboratory.)

chapter 15
introduction to pharmacology*

In every medical situation where medications are prescribed, you will find a book called the PDR, *Physician's Desk Reference*. It is published yearly and lists all prescription drugs and information about them. During the year, a supplement is published listing new additions and new information about drugs. You will find this book helpful, especially for the spelling of drug names. Get acquainted with it. The pink section at the front of the book, "Product Name Index," is the section you will find most useful. The blue section is the "Product Category Index" (for example, analgesics). This blue section also includes a quick reference to headings and sub-headings. The yellow section is the "Generic and Chemical Name Index." Pictures of some drugs are shown in a "Product Identification Section." A Manufacturers' Index lists addresses of drug companies and the drugs they manufacture. The white pages contain information about each drug.

This introduction will give you some terms commonly used:

Rx   prescription or recipe.

OTC   over the counter (drugs), which can be obtained without prescription.

Every drug has several different names; this can be confusing to the uninitiated. Every drug has a *generic name* and a *trade* or *brand name*, for example:

Tetracycline (generic name). *Trade names:* Achro**my**cin, **Tet**racyn, My**stec**lin, Pan**my**cin, **Tet**rex, and so on.

Acetylsalicylic acid (generic name). *Trade names:* Asteric, Ecotrin, Bayer aspirin.

Acetaminophen (generic name). *Trade names:* Tylenol, Datril.

Each drug also has a chemical formula (name) with which you need not concern yourself. You do, however, need to understand about generic and trade or brand names. The recent trend seems to be for the physician to write a prescription for the drug by its generic name, so that the pharmacist may then give the patient the brand that is the best buy. If the physician writes the Rx for a specific brand name drug, the pharmacist must fill the Rx exactly, using only that particular brand name drug. This trade or brand may cost the patient more.

A *detail man* is a representative of a drug company. He, of course, thinks that his company's product is the best. He makes visits to physicians' offices and tries to convince them to use his products. He generally leaves samples, which the physician may dispense to patients.

Drugs are classified *as to the action they produce*, for example:

analgesic drugs   relieve pain (aspirin, Darvon). Includes **narcotics** (Demerol HCL, morphine).

diuretic drugs   increase urine output (Diuril).

antibiotic drugs   inhibit bacterial life (E-Mycin, Kefzol).

tranquilizers   reduce anxiety (Compazine, Valium).

decongestants   relieve congestion (Contac, Chlor-trimeton maleate).

sedatives   produce sleep (Seconal sodium, Nembutal).

Many drugs must be stored in the refrigerator, especially those used in injections. All drugs have an expiration date after which time they should not be used.

---

* See Appendix g for list of drugs.

worksheet

Define:

1. PDR _____

2. OTC _____

3. Rx _____

4. What is the action generally produced by the following drugs?

   a. a diuretic drug _____

   b. an analgesic drug _____

   c. a decongestant _____

5. Explain generic and brand names of drugs: _____

_____

_____

_____

_____

May the pharmacist substitute one for the other? Explain: _____

_____

_____

_____

6. What is a "detail man"? _____

_____

True/False: Circle the letter of the *true* statements only. Defend your answers. Explain why statement is false.

7. Some drugs must be stored in a refrigerator.

8. Drugs never "expire." They should be used up when you get sick again.

9. To learn the proper spelling of any drug, the best place to look is in the dictionary.

10. Antibiotic drugs are used to treat bacterial infections.

11. Sedatives such as Seconal sodium are given to patients who have difficulty sleeping.

12. If you have access to the PDR, look up the *brand* names of drugs and see if you can pick out ten that you have heard of. Write them here: _____

_____

_____

List five classifications (blue section of the *PDR*) not given in this text, with an example of each. _____

_____

_____

_____

_____

_____

13. The next time you receive a prescription form from your doctor, try to read it and look up the drug. You should also be able to read the abbreviations that tell how often the drug should be taken (qid or tid, for example).

14. Find a drug advertisement in a medical journal (instructor may provide these). Read through all of the information about the drug. List new words and define them, noting especially their "side effects."

_____

_____

_____

_____

_____

_____

_____

_____

_____

_____

34 page 207

part 2

terminology of body systems

A brief, simplified outline for each body system is provided in Chapters 16–25. Following each outline is a worksheet or practice test. In addition to reading the outline and learning new words contained therein, it may be helpful to do some additional reading on the system being studied. Choose any text that can be readily understood; it need not be an anatomy book (consult the Reference Material List in Appendix e). Any simple explanation will be adequate. It is better to read a book written for lay people in words that are familiar to you. Most encyclopedias and dictionaries also offer such information along with some helpful diagrams.

After you have studied the system, use the worksheets to see if you have learned the essentials for each chapter. Your instructor will be able to assist you if you need further help. Answers are provided for worksheets. Tests are included for each chapter, but no answers are provided in this workbook. DO NOT WRITE ON TESTS UNTIL DIRECTED TO DO SO. (Your instructor may choose to give tests not contained in this text).

As each body system is studied (normal anatomy and physiology), some of the abnormal (pathologic) conditions that affect each system will be presented. Only the more common diseases will be studied in this short course. Some operation reports and actual cases are included here to show use of medical terminology.

chapter 16
structure of the body

---

outline

BODY CAVITIES

*pleur*al cavity (tho*rac*ic cavity) contains lungs, **tra**chea, e**soph**agus, **thy**mus.

  mediastinum (in the middle) heart lies here.

perito*ne*al cavity (abdomino**pel**vic cavity) contains stomach, intestines, liver, gallbladder, pancreas, spleen, reproduction organs, and urinary bladder.

  The pleural and peritoneal cavities derive their names from the membranes that line them — the pleura and the perito**ne**um.

cranial cavity (skull) contains brain.

spinal cavity contains spinal cord.

  The **di**aphragm is a dome-shaped muscle that separates the pleural and perito**ne**al cavities.

STRUCTURAL UNITS OF THE BODY (from the smallest to the largest)

cells the basic unit of all living things. They are microscopic in size and vary in shape, and each cell performs functions necessary for its own life. Cells multiply by dividing. This is called mi**to**sis. The following are the *main parts of a cell:*

  *nu*cleus contains **chro**mosomes; genes (hereditary units) are in the chromosomes.

  cytoplasm protoplasm of the cell (the part outside of the nucleus).

  cell membrane holds the cell together (cell wall).

tissues groups of cells that are alike.

  epi*the*lial tissue protects, absorbs, and secretes (the skin and lining surfaces).

  connective tissue (fibrous) connects and supports and also forms blood cells (bone, tendons, and so on).

  muscle tissue contracts — **stri**ated (striped), cardiac, and smooth.

  nerve tissue conducts impulses.

organs made up of more than one kind of tissue — heart, lungs, and liver, for example.

systems groups of organs that work together. (Each system depends on the other systems of the body.)

  integu*men*tary system skin.

  musculo*skel*etal system muscles, bones, and connective tissues: ligaments, tendons, and fasciae.

  cardio*vas*cular system circulatory — heart and vessels.

  gastroin*tes*tinal system (GI) digestive organs.

  ***res*piratory system** lungs and airways.

  genito*u*rinary system (GU) reproductive and urinary organs (also called urogenital).

*en*docrine system   ductless glands.

nervous system   includes brain, spinal cord, and special senses.

ME*TAB*OLISM   the process by which foods are changed into elements the body can use for growth, energy, and repair. Metabolism includes absorption, storage, and use of foods for the maintenance of the body; combining of foods and oxygen to produce energy; and elimination of waste materials.

HOMEO*STA*SIS   the state of equilibrium or relative constancy (sameness) that the body strives to maintain — for example, body temperature, cell division rate, and so on.

BODY PLANES   imaginary lines that divide (used in anatomical diagrams).

mid*sag*ittal   a plane that divides the body, or some part of it, into equal right and left portions.

coronal (also called **frontal**)   a plane that divides the body into anterior and posterior sections (front and back).

transverse   a plane that divides the body into superior and inferior sections (top and bottom).

These terms are used as points of reference to provide clarity in diagrams; for example, a midsagittal view of the brain would show structures in the center of the brain and would divide the brain into equal right and left sides.

PATH*OL*OGY   the study of the nature and cause of disease. Diseases fall into these categories: **tu**mor, **trau**matic, meta**bol**ic, in**fec**tion, he**red**itary, **vas**cular, de**gen**erative.

worksheet

Fill in the blank:

1. Another name for the abdominopelvic cavity is _____

   Two other names for the chest cavity are _____ and _____

2. The cavity that contains the brain is _____

3. The smallest unit of living matter is _____

4. Name the main parts of a cell (3): _____

   _____

   Which part contains the genes? _____

Name the systems that include the following organs:

5. heart   _____

6. vertebra (bone)   _____

7. lungs   _____

8. stomach   _____

9. skeletal muscle   _____

10. adrenal glands   _____

11. spinal cord   _____

12. kidneys   _____

13. ovaries   _____

14. skin   _____

15. testes   _____

16. Name four kinds of tissues: _____

_____   _____   _____

17. A system is a _____ of _____ that work together to perform a certain function.

18. What are some of the processes included in metabolism? _____

_____

_____

19. Organs are made up of several kinds of _____

20. The diaphragm is a _____ that separates chest and abdominopelvic cavities.

21. Draw or describe: Use the bottom of this page to draw.

a. midsagittal plane _____

b. coronal plane _____

c. transverse plane _____

Define or describe:

22. mitosis _____

23. lower extremities _____

24. striated (muscle) _____

25. secretion _____

26. absorption _____

27. elimination _____

28. pathology _____

29. homeostasis _____

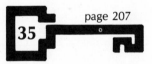

page 207

35

chapter 17
integumentary system

---

outline

SKIN   integument or external covering.

EPI*DER*MIS (cuticle)   outer layer of skin; consists of four layers: epi**the**lial tissue (see Fig. 17–1 for cross section of normal skin). Cells on the surface are dead cells.

DERMIS or **CORIUM**   deeper layer (two layers; connective tissue containing nerves, nerve endings, blood vessels, sebaceous glands (sebum = oil), and sweat glands (sudo**rif**erous).

HAIR and **NAILS**   appendages of skin.

SUBCUTANEOUS   "under the skin"; contains adipose tissue, connective tissue, vessels, and nerves.

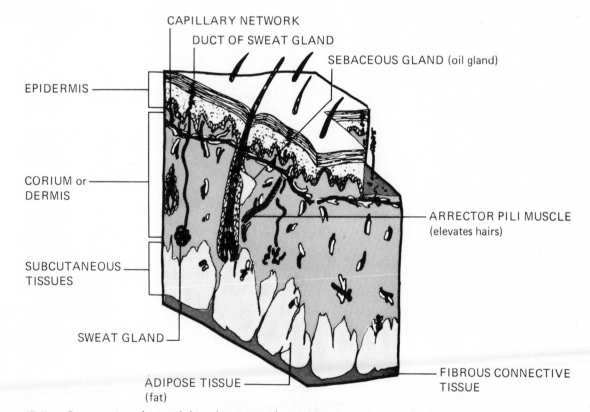

Figure 17–1.   Cross section of normal skin, showing epidermis, dermis (corium), and subcutaneous tissues. Note important structures in dermis: blood vessels, sweat glands, and sebaceous glands.

FUNCTIONS OF SKIN

protection   a waterproof overcoat that keeps body fluids in and harmful elements out (bacteria and sun, for example).

sensory organ (receptor)   for sensations of touch, pain, and temperature.

temperature regulator   for cooling and heating (perspiration and "goose flesh").

waste elimination   disposal of wastes.

BREASTS   mammary glands. Lactation is controlled by endocrine system. A *re*ola *mamma*, halo around nipple.

DERMATOLOGY   is the study of skin disorders; the dermatologist is the specialist who usually treats these, although internists often prescribe for the less complicated cases. Plastic surgeons may become involved when extensive skin damage has occurred, or for cosmetic surgery.

TREATMENT   topical (local, to surface) treatment is the most usual; various antibiotic and cortisone ointments are used. Systemic antibiotics may also be given.

DESCRIPTIVE TERMS   (see Fig. 17–2)

mac*ule   spots, not elevated (freckle, flat mole, or rash of measles, for example).

pap*ule   small, raised spots (wart, acne, mole, or pso**ri**asis, for example).

plaque   used to describe the silvery scales of pso**ri**asis.

nod*ule   larger raised lesion (cyst); can be felt more than seen.

tumor   a swelling or large nodule (may be benign or malignant); also called a neoplasm.

cyst   a type of nodule that is usually somewhat moveable; contains fluid.

wheal   elevation (individual hive) or "bleb" produced by injection of a skin test.

ves*icle   lesion containing fluid (blister).

bulla(ae)   large blister, as in burns.

pus*tule   lesion containing pus (some acne, impe**ti**go, pimple, for example); a large **pus**tule is an **ab**scess.

scales or **crusts**   flaking type of lesions (pso**ri**asis, fungus, for example).

fis*sure   crack in skin surface (anal fissure, athlete's foot lesion, for example).

e*ro*sion   "eating away," an early ulcer.

ulcer   tissue destruction, a deep lesion extending into subcutaneous tissue (**var**icose ulcer, de**cub**itus ulcer, for example).

scar   mark left by healing of a wound. **Cic**atrix (pronounced **sick**atrix) is another word for scar. A **ke**loid is an overgrowth of scar tissue.

SURGICAL TERMS

bi*opsy   excision of living tissue for examination.

cau*tery   machine or methods used to destroy tissue by electricity, freezing or chemicals.

de*bride*ment   removal of dead tissue around a wound.

derma*bra*sion   scraping off surface layers to remove scars or wrinkles.

der*matome   instrument for cutting thin sections of skin for grafts.

electrodesic*ca*tion   destruction and drying out with electricity.

eschar*ot*omy   removal of burn scar tissue.

fulgu*ra*tion   destruction of tissue with electric sparks.

grafts (skin)   tissue taken from one place to replace a defect elsewhere: au**tog**enous (from self); homograft (from another person); pig skin may be used as a temporary graft. A new type of synthetic collagen is now being used for permanent skin grafts. A skin graft may be full-thickness, split-thickness, or pedicle graft.

Hy*frecator   a type of machine for destroying tissue (high-frequency eradicator).

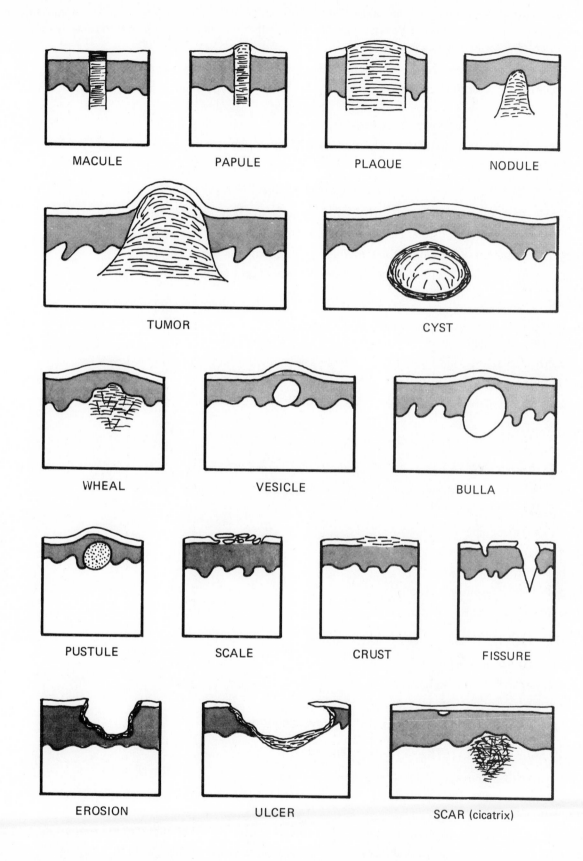

Figure 17-2. Primary and secondary lesions of the skin. Note some of these are superficial and some involve deeper tissues.

COMMON GROWTHS

carci*no*ma   skin cancer; a malignant tumor. Examples include basal cell and squamous cell carcinomas; malignant mela**no**ma or "black tumor" is the only skin cancer that me**tas**tasizes (spreads to underlying tissues or through lymphatics).

kera*to*sis   thickened, horny skin; ac**tin**ic keratosis is due to exposure to sun and X rays.

***ne*vus(i)**   mole; a discolored, flat or fleshy growth. A birthmark is a type of mole. See a medical dictionary for other types.

stea*to*ma   a wen or fatty tumor; se**ba**ceous cyst.

ver*ru*ca(ae)   wart or epi**the**lial tumor. A plantar wart is one on the sole or plantar surface of the foot. (Warts are caused by viruses.)

BACTERIAL SKIN DISEASES   (staphylo**coc**cal or strepto**coc**cal usually)

acne vul*ga*ris   inflammation of the pilose**ba**ceous glands (pilo = hair, sebum = oil).

***car*buncles** and ***fur*uncles**   pustular lesions, boils, abscesses.

cellu*li*tis   inflammation of skin and subcutaneous tissue. Ery**sip**elas is one type.

impe*ti*go   **pus**tular lesions, crusted, especially around mouth and nose. Com**mun**icable.

VIRAL SKIN DISEASES

***her*pes geni*tal*is**   blister-type lesions in genital area; may endanger infant if mother is infected at time of delivery; causes damage to child's nervous system.

***her*pes oph*thal*micus**   severe type of herpes zoster, affecting the fifth cranial nerve (eye).

***her*pes simplex**   "cold sores" or fever blisters.

***her*pes *zos*ter**   "shingles"—lesions follow the course of a nerve, usually only on one side of the trunk, pelvis, or eye.

ver*ru*ca   wart.

FUNGAL SKIN DISORDERS

***tin*ea**   ringworm—term used depends on body part involved.

> **tinea *bar*bae:**   beard.
>
> **tinea *cap*itis:**   scalp.
>
> **tinea *cor*poris:**   body.
>
> **tinea *cru*ris:**   groin ("jock itch").
>
> **tinea *pe*dis:**   foot (athlete's foot).
>
> **tinea *un*guium:**   nails.

PARASITIC DISEASES OF SKIN   cause severe itching.

pedicu*lo*sis *cap*itis   lice (head).

pedicu*lo*sis *cor*poris   lice (body).

pedicu*lo*sis *pu*bis   pubic lice or crabs.

scabies   a small parasite called a mite, which burrows under the skin.

ALLERGIC SKIN MANIFESTATIONS   due to sensitivity.

contact derma*ti*tis   caused by contact with some substance.

drug reactions   usually rash-type lesions, caused by medication and/or photosensitivity reactions when exposed to sunlight.

ec*zema   redness of skin, usually with itching, due to some substance or, possibly, food item.

insect bites, and so on   local reaction usually due to bite or sting; may become life threatening if systemic reaction follows.

neurodermatitis   usually severe itching and excoriation with unknown cause, presumed due to emotional or psychologic factors.

psoriasis   chronic, hereditary dermatosis, often associated with arthritis. Characterized by silvery flaking patches, especially on elbows and knees.

SYSTEMIC DISEASES   that may cause skin eruptions.

diabetes mellitus   various lesions and inability to heal.

erysipelas   acute febrile disease caused by "strep" infection; characterized by fiery red skin.

Hodgkin's disease   a type of cancer in which itching of the skin may occur.

lupus erythematosus   inflammatory dermatitis that may precede systemic lupus; characterized by "butterfly" lesion over nose and cheeks.

rubella   three day or German measles; characterized by rash.

rubeola   regular or hard measles; characterized by macular rash.

syphilis   cutaneous lesions in secondary stage.

varicella   chickenpox; vesicles that itch and later become scabs.

INJURIES TO THE SKIN

burns   first degree—red, tender, not blistered; second degree—blistered, dermal layer involved; third degree—subcutaneous tissue; white, charred; fat exposed; blisters often absent.

■ **Notes:**   Important factors in burn injuries are parts of body involved (hands, feet, face, genitals, joints usually most serious); percentage of body burned and depth of burn; burns complicated by fractures with extensive soft tissue damage and respiratory involvement (most critical).

lacerations   cuts; deep lacerations involve meticulous care when large nerves and blood vessels are damaged.

MISCELLANEOUS TERMS INVOLVING SKIN

actinic   pertaining to ultraviolet rays (sun).

albinism   lack of pigment; white skin and hair.

alopecia   baldness, hereditary or due to chemotherapy.

callus   localized hyperplasia caused by friction.

cicatrix   scar.

ecchymosis   bruise, black-and-blue mark due to bleeding under the skin.

eruption   any rash or "breaking out."

erythema   redness.

eschar   hard crust over a burn.

exanthem   rose-colored eruption.

excoriation   severe abrasion.

exfoliation   scaling, flaking.

gangrene   necrotic tissue (dead tissue).

hirsutism   excessive body hair, especially in women.

keloid   overgrowth of scar tissue; red, raised area that does not fade with time as usual scar does.

lesion   any kind of a "sore" is a lesion; a change in tissue structure.

nummular   having the shape of a coin; "size of a dime."

paronychia   inflammation around a nail.

pruritus   itching.

superfluous hair   excessive hair on face of women.

urticaria   hives; raised, itchy welts.

vitiligo   loss of pigment; white, patchy areas.

SKIN TESTS   These are not related to skin disease, but skin reaction determines the outcome of the test.

coccidi*oi*din (cocci)   test for valley fever (respiratory fungus disease).

histoplas*mo*sis   another fungus disease.

Mantoux or **PPD**   test for TB (bacterial disease).

If positive (red, raised area of a certain size where injection was made) person has been exposed, may now have the disease, or has had it previously.

Other skin tests include:

Dick test   for susceptibility to scarlet fever.

Schick test   for susceptibility to diph*ther*ia.

Sweat test   for presence of cystic fibrosis.

Many substances can be applied to the skin to determine if a person is allergic to them. Areas of the skin are marked off, and skin reaction is observed (redness, swelling); diagnostic for allergies.

worksheet

Fill in the blank:

1. The specialist who treats skin disorders is a _____

2. Two functions of the skin are   _____   _____

3. The outer (top) layer of skin is the   _____

4. Sweat glands are also called _____ glands.

5. Oil glands are also called _____ glands.

6. Three skin diseases are _____   _____   _____

7. The dermis is the deeper layer of skin and is also called the _____. In this layer are found

   the _____ and _____

8. Cold sores are called _____   _____

9. Three skin conditions related to allergy or sensitivity are _____

   _____   _____

10. Inflammation around the fingernail is   _____

11. Name two skin tests and their purposes:

   _____   _____

   _____   _____

True/False: Circle the number of the *true* statements only. Defend your answers. Explain why statement is false.

12. Nummular means coin shaped.

13. A biopsy is an examination of living tissue to determine malignancy.

14. A wart is a verruca.

15. The halo around the nipple of the breast is the areola mamma.

16. A vesicle is a lesion full of pus.

17. Pruritus means itching.

18. Vitiligo is an infectious disease.

Fill in the blank:

19. An instrument for cutting a thin section of skin is a _____

20. Hives are called _____

21. The plural of nevus is _____. Nevus means _____

22. A term that means redness of the skin is _____

23. Three systemic diseases that have skin symptoms are _____

_____   _____

24. Pediculosis is caused by a _____ (parasite).

25. The disease common in teenagers that produces skin lesions is called _____

26. Name some other terms not mentioned in this worksheet that describe skin lesions: _____

_____

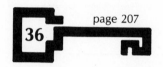

page 207

36

CASE HISTORY: DISCHARGE SUMMARY

admitting diagnosis   cellulitis of penis

discharge diagnosis   same.

This 40-year-old male reports an industrial injury to the *pubic area* by a piece of scaffolding 24 hours prior to admission. Penis was grossly *edematous* with moderate *erythema*. Admission diagnosis was *cellulitis*. Patient was treated with *intravenous* Kefzol. *Urethral* discharge cultured positive for *Staphylococcus aureus*. WBC was 26,100 with 32 *stabs*, 65 *neutrophils*; Ua 2+ blood, 0–2 white cells. *RPR nonreactive*.

    Over the next 6 days cellulitis persisted, and he began to show signs of *gangrene*. *Antibiotics* were changed to include clindamycin and minocycline during his hospital stay.

HISTORY AND PHYSICAL RECORD

CC   Swelling of the penis.

PI   This 40-year-old male apparently was struck in the mid-lower abdominal area while working on the job. He noticed considerable discomfort and pain and some swelling, which increased over a 24-hour period, and he came to the Medical Center where he was admitted.

PH   Includes episode of a kidney stone, apparently was never hospitalized for it, and it seemed to pass rather quickly. He denies any other health problems, has had no surgery or fractures.

FH   Parents *L & W*. He is married, has three children all in good health. Denies any abnormal family health history.

SH   Construction worker. Denies use of medications or excessive use of alcohol or tobacco.

ROS   Generally has been in good health. Skin normal.

skin   Dry and warm. Some *ecchymosis* and gross swelling of penis.

HEENT   *Normocephalic* male. *TMs* clear. Eyes: *EOMs* intact, good *light reflex. Funduscopic* normal. Nose and throat normal.

neck   Good *ROM*. Negative for *palpable thyroid. Carotid* pulsations normal.

chest   Clear to *A* and *P* without *rales, rhonchi* or wheezes. No history of *asthma, bronchitis* or *pneumonia*.

cardiovascular   Regular *sinus rhythm* without *murmurs, rubs* or *gallops*. Lymphatic negative.

abdomen *Scaphoid. Negative organomegaly, masses,* or *tenderness.*

genitalia Gross swelling of penis, patient in acute distress.

rectal, locomotor, extremities *Unremarkable.*

neurologic *DTRs* 2+ *bilaterally.* Cranial nerves grossly intact.

IMPRESSION Cellulitis

☐ **Assignment:** Write all of the italicized words and define them. Notice the use of the word "denies" and the word "unremarkable." These are commonly used terms. With regard to the laboratory terms, are the results within normal limits? (Refer to laboratory forms in Chapter 14 for "normals.")

_____

_____

_____

_____

_____

chapter 18
musculoskeletal system

---

outline

FUNCTIONS

1. Supports and gives shape to body.
2. Protects internal organs.
3. Makes movement possible.
4. Forms blood cells (in red bone marrow, long bones).

SKELETON   (see Fig. 18–1) the following are the main divisions:

1. **Ax**ial: skull, thorax (ribs and sternum), vertebral column.
2. Appen**dic**ular: the appendages that hang from the axial skeleton; upper and lower extremities (includes shoulder and pelvic girdle).

large bones of the body

*clav*icle   collar bone.

*ster*num   breast bone.

*hu*merus   upper arm.

*ra*dius and *ul*na   forearm.

*fe*mur   thigh.

*fib*ula and *tib*ia   lower leg.

*scap*ula   shoulder blade.

verte**bral column**   starting at the neck: cervical vertebrae (7), thoracic or dorsal (12), lumbar (5), sacral (5, fused), coccyx or tail bone (4) (see Fig. 18–2).

cranial bones

frontal   forehead (1).

pa*ri*etal   top of head (2).

*tem*poral   temples (2).

oc*cip*ital   back of head (1).

*eth*moid   upper nasal, between eyes.

*sphe*noid   behind eyes (base of skull), and laterally between parietal and temporal bones.

*man*dible   lower jaw.

max*il*la   upper jaw.

*tur*binates   cone-shaped nasal bones.

joints and **related structures**   (articulations) hold bones securely (see Figs. 18-3 and 18-4.

   ball and socket   hip and shoulder.

   hinge   elbow, knees, fingers.

   sutures   articulations in cranial bones, immovable joints.

   interverte bral disks   cartilaginous substance between vertebrae.

   aponeuro sis   flattened tendon; resembles a membrane.

   bursa(ae)   small sacs that serve to cushion joints; between tendons and bones.

   fascia   connective tissue sheath; holds muscle fibers together.

   interpha lan geal joints   fingers and toes; DIP (distal interphalangeal) and PIP (proximal interphalangeal).

   *lam*ina(ae)   the flattened part of the vertebral arch (thinnest part of a vertebra).

   *lig*ament   strong fibrous tissue connecting bone to bone.

   me nis cus(ci)   cartilage of the knee, lateral and medial, on the superior surface of the tibia (articulates with femur).

   sy no vial fluid   clear fluid present in joints (lubricates).

   tendon   fibrous tissue attaching muscle to bone.

   *the*ca   covering or sheath of a tendon.

SKELETAL DIFFERENCES   female skeleton has a wider pelvis. The infant skeleton has a larger head (for the size of its body), consists partly of cartilage so is softer than adult's, and infant skull bones have spaces between them (fontanels or soft spots).

TERMS USED TO DESCRIBE PROJECTIONS, OPENINGS, AND INDENTATIONS IN BONES

ace*tab*ulum   large socket for head of femur (hip).

fo ra men (pl. **for am ina**)   holes in a bone for large vessels and nerves to pass through, for example, fo ra men **mag**num.

fossa(ae)   depressions or hollows.

grooves   shallow linear depressions in bone (or tooth).

mal le olus   hammerlike protuberance (either side of ankle).

o lec ranon   a process on the ulnar bone (elbow).

prominences, processes, tuberosities   projections.

sinuses   air spaces in cranium that make the skull lighter and serve as resonating chambers for the voice. (Sinus has some other meanings.)

Names of the small bones of the ankle and wrist are not given in this text. Should you need these, most medical dictionaries list bones in the appendix. Taber's dictionary lists them under "skeleton." Similar lists of muscles, joints, ligaments, and so on are also usually given in the appendix of medical dictionaries.

MUSCLES   there are three kinds of muscle tissue:

1. Striated (striped): skeletal muscle (voluntary).
2. Nonstriated: smooth muscle. Called involuntary as we have no control over it. Causes peristaltic movement of stomach and intestines.
3. Cardiac muscle: heart muscle.

   Skeletal muscles are attached to two bones (origin and insertion) and are joined together by a movable joint. Skeletal muscles are attached by *tendons*. The largest tendon is the A**chil**les tendon (heel).

how muscles are named

   function   extensor carpi for extension of wrist.

   points of origin and insertion   (attachments that make movement possible) sternoclavicu **lar**is for sternum and clavicle.

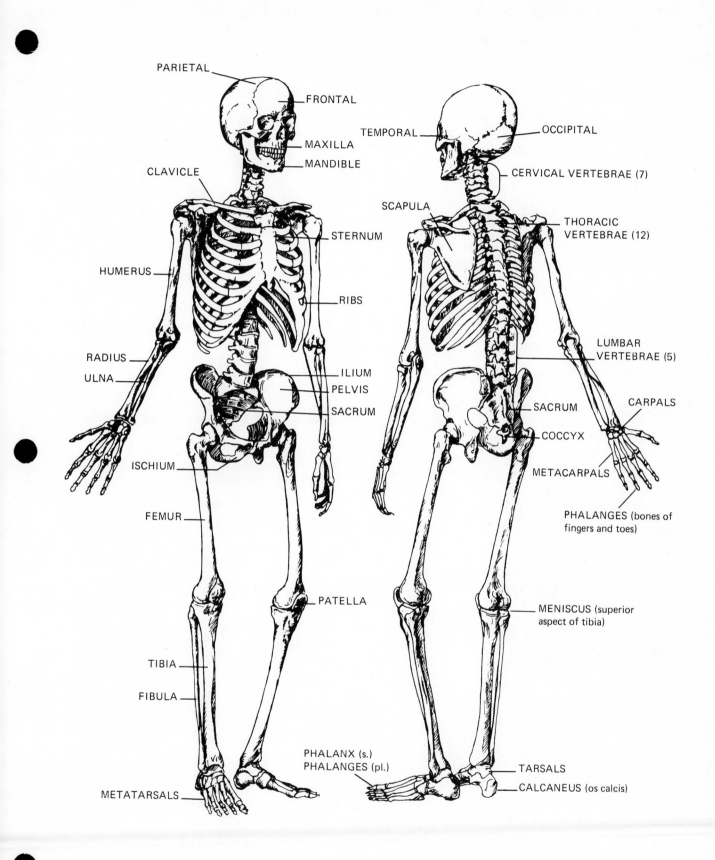

Figure 18–1. Skeleton. **Left**, Anterior view, showing large bones of the body. **Right**, Posterior view, showing large bones and sections of vertebral column.

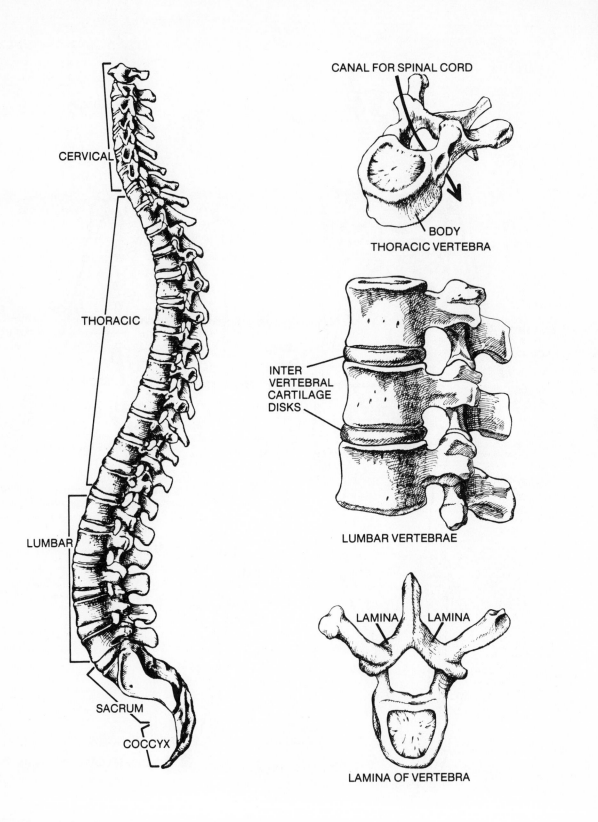

CANAL FOR SPINAL CORD

BODY
THORACIC VERTEBRA

CERVICAL

THORACIC

INTER
VERTEBRAL
CARTILAGE
DISKS

LUMBAR VERTEBRAE

LUMBAR

LAMINA   LAMINA

SACRUM

COCCYX

LAMINA OF VERTEBRA

Figure 18–2.   On the left, spinal column showing cervical, thoracic, lumbar, sacral, and coccygeal sections. On the right, individual vertebra showing spinal canal and laminae.

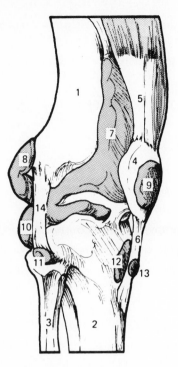

1 FEMUR

2 TIBIA

3 FIBULA

4 PATELLA

5 QUADRICEPS TENDON

6 PATELLAR TENDON

7 SUPRAPATELLAR BURSA

8 LATERAL GASTROCNEMIUS BURSA

9 PREPATELLAR BURSA

10 POPLITEUS BURSA

11 BURSA OF BICEPS TENDON

12 DEEP INFRAPATELLAR BURSA

13 SUPERFICIAL INFRAPATELLAR BURSA

14 LATERAL COLLATERAL LIGAMENT

Figure 18–3. Knee, anterolateral aspect with synovial sac and adjacent bursae. Shows large bones of the leg, some tendons and ligaments.

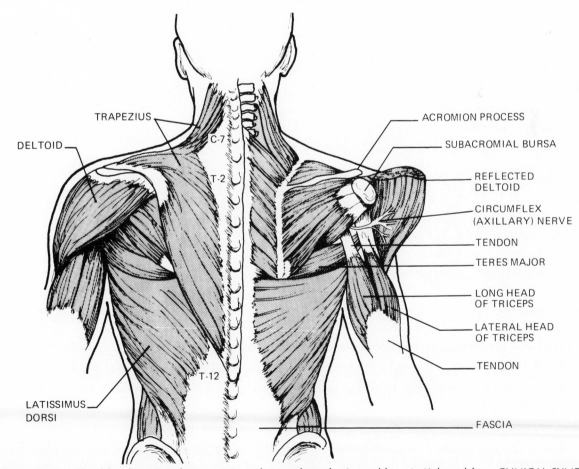

Figure 18–4. Shoulder dissection from rear (muscles, tendons, fascia, and bursa). (Adapted from CLINICAL SYMPOSIA, illustrated by Frank H. Netter, M.D. All rights reserved. Copyright © 1959 CIBA Pharmaceutical Company, Division of CIBA-GEIGY Corporation.)

form or position orbicu*lar*is *oc*uli from orbit to skin around eyes (closes eyes); pecto*ral*is minor for small chest muscle.

resemblance to an object or **for the way they are used** gastroc*ne*mius is the calf muscle shaped something like a stomach.

MUSCULOSKELETAL MOVEMENT (see Fig. 18-5)

flexion bending.

extension straightening.

adduction movement toward midline.

abduction movement away from midline.

pronation palm down (face down).

supination palm upward (face upward).

proximal nearest to midline or point of origin.

distal farthest from midline or point of origin.

MUSCULOSKELETAL TERMS

con*trac*ture permanent contraction of a muscle.

muscle *at*rophy wasting away, shrinkage; from disuse.

muscle hy*per*trophy increase in muscle size; from overuse.

muscle tone muscles partially contracted, enough to make them feel firm.

pa*ral*ysis inability to contract muscle, due to nerve damage.

pa*re*sis marked weakness, incomplete paralysis.

INJURIES

fractures see Fig. 18-6 that describes kinds of fractures.

skull fractures possible damage to brain.

"torn" ligaments, tendons, cartilage common "sports" injuries.

subluxa*tion partial dislocation (luxation = dislocation).

spondylo*lis*thesis forward displacement of a vertebra (a type of dislocation).

MUSCULOSKE*LETAL* AND NEURO*MUS*CULAR DISORDERS

ar*thri*tis inflammation of a joint; there are many kinds of arthritis. The two main types are rheumatoid, which starts at any age and causes severe deformity, and osteoarthritis (DJD, degenerative joint disease), which begins in older age groups.

bur*si*tis inflammation of a bursa.

***car*pal tunnel syndrome** pain, edema, and atrophy (thumb side of hand, due to pressure on median nerve in the wrist).

***col*lagen disease** connective tissue disease; examples include SLE (systemic lupus erythema*to*sus) and rheumatoid arthritis.

gout a type of acute arthritis, due to accumulation of uric acid crystals, especially in the great toe.

herniated nucleus pulpo*sus ruptured intervertebral disk (see surgical report, p. 127 and Fig. 18-7, p. 128).

ky*pho*sis hunchback or humpback; type of deformity of spine.

Legg-Calvé-Perthes disease osteochondr*i*tis; head of femur.

lor*do*sis convex curvature of spine ("swayback").

lupus erythematosus (systemic) collagen disease affecting connective tissues, thought to be due to abnormal immunologic response.

muscular *dys*trophy poor muscle development.

myas*the*nia gravis lack of muscle strength.

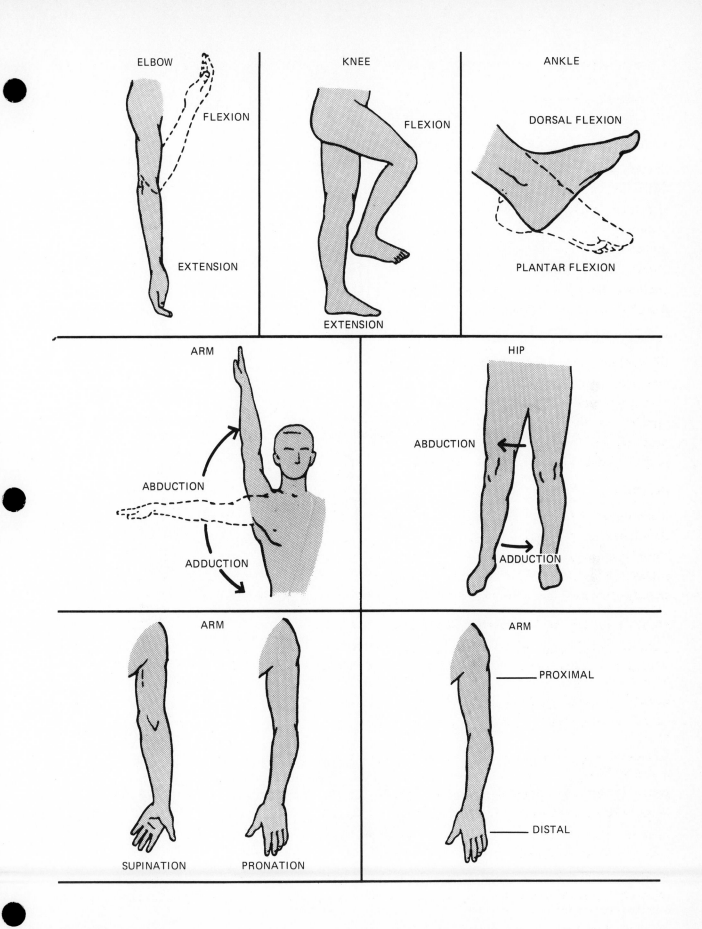

Figure 18-5. Illustration of some terms used to describe body movements and body positions.

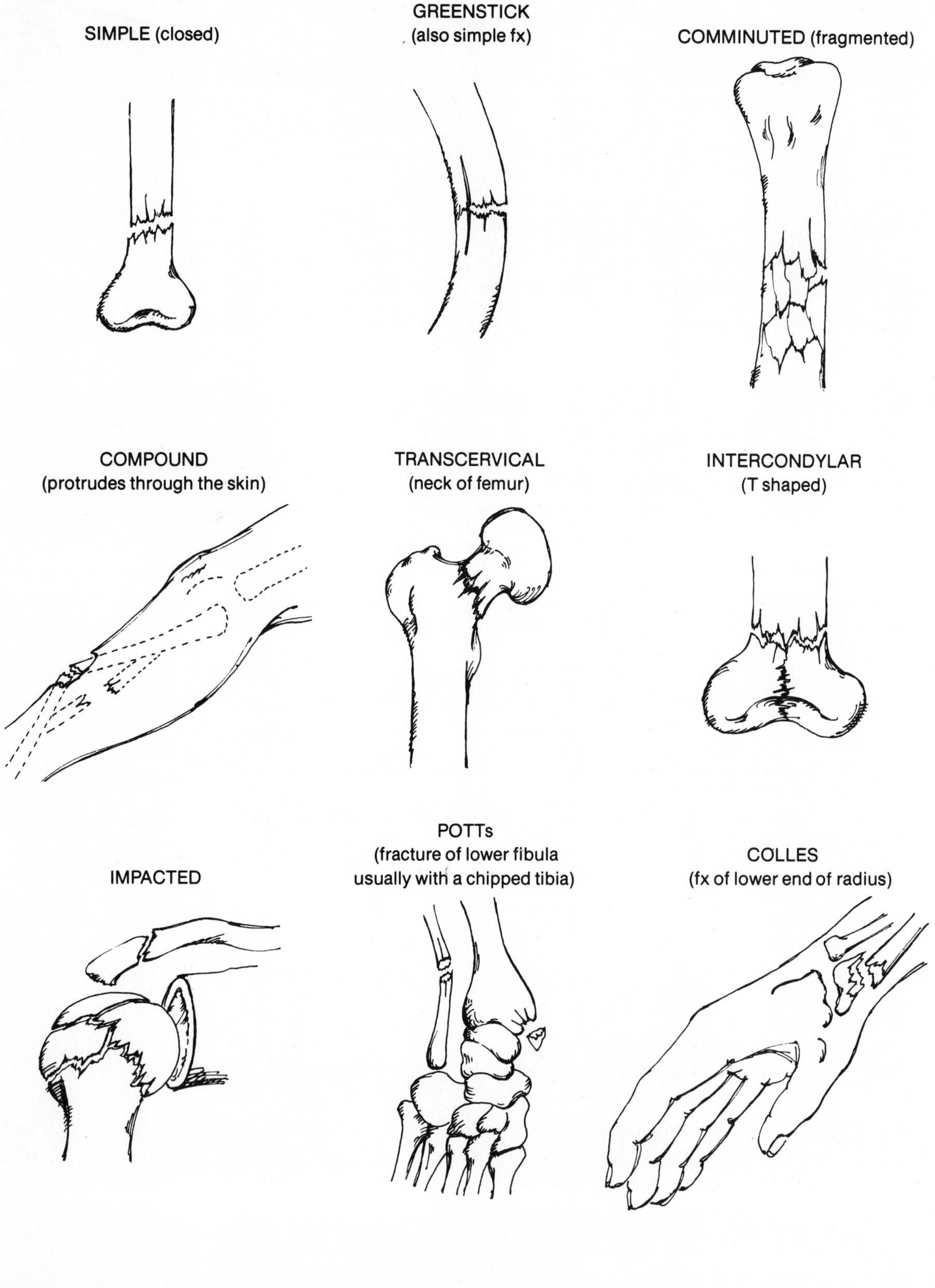

SIMPLE (closed)

GREENSTICK
(also simple fx)

COMMINUTED (fragmented)

COMPOUND
(protrudes through the skin)

TRANSCERVICAL
(neck of femur)

INTERCONDYLAR
(T shaped)

IMPACTED

POTTs
(fracture of lower fibula
usually with a chipped tibia)

COLLES
(fx of lower end of radius)

Figure 18-6. Examples of some types of fractures.

myo*si*tis   inflammation of muscle.

Osgood-Schlatter disease   osteochon**dro**sis; end of tibia (knee) in adolescents.

osteochon*dro*sis, osteochon*dri*tis   inflammation of bone and cartilage.

osteoma*la*cia   softening of bone.

osteomye*li*tis   inflammation of bone and marrow caused by bacterial invasion.

osteopo*ro*sis   porous condition of bones in old age.

rheumatism   general term for soreness and stiffness.

rickets   juvenile osteoma*la*cia, due to vitamin D deficiency.

sar*co*ma (osteogenic)   malignant bone tumor (cancer); primary tumor. Secondary (metastatic) tumors of the bone are more common than primary tumors.

scoli*o*sis   lateral curvature of spine.

spina *bif*ida   a congenital defect in spine.

spondy*li*tis (ankyl*os*ing)   inflammation of vertebrae with spontaneous fusing causing deformity.

tendi*ni*tis   inflammation of a tendon.

SURGICAL, DIAGNOSTIC, AND TREATMENT PROCEDURES

ampu*ta*tion   AK above knee, BK below knee, and so on.

arthrocen*te*sis   puncture into joint to remove fluid.

ar*thros*copy   procedure of looking into joint with scope.

ar*throt*omy   incision into a joint.

electrical stimulation   used to heal fractures more quickly.

electromy*og*raphy   making a recording of muscular contractions.

external fixation   devices used to reduce fractures, without casting.

fracture reduction   closed reduction or ORIF, open reduction with internal fixation.

lami*nec*tomy with dis*kec*tomy   surgical excision of an interver*te*bral disk (or part of it) by cutting into the lamina portion of the vertebra (see surgical report, p. 127).

meni*scec*tomy   excision of part or all of the medial or lateral me**nis**cus in the knee. Procedure is usually done for "torn cartilage in knee."

***mye*logram**   X-ray examination of spinal cord after introduction of dye into spinal cavity; often used to help diagnose herniated disk.

***my*ogram**   same as electromyogram. Do not confuse with myelogram.

replantation   of severed body part, such as hand or finger.

spondylo*syn*desis   surgical formation of ankylosis; spinal fusion.

total hip replacement   Charnley **ar**throplasty is one type, using a prosthetic head-of-femur device. Knee and other joints can also be replaced.

traction   process of drawing or pulling.

ABBREVIATIONS

ANA   laboratory serum test; antinuclear antibodies are associated with many diseases, such as LE.

DJD   degenerative joint disease (osteoarthritis).

ORIF   open reduction internal fixation.

RA   rheumatoid arthritis; RA lab test for this.

SLE (LE)   systemic lupus erythematosus.

LABORATORY ARTHRITIS PROFILE   Often ordered together to help the physician establish the presence of a disease, to determine its severity, and to help in determining which of several possible diseases with similar symptoms is present.

> sedimen**ta**tion rate (SR or ESR)
>
> antinuclear antibodies (ANA)
>
> C-reactive protein (CRP)
>
> rheumatoid (RA) factor
>
> LE (lupus erythema**to**sus) cell prep
>
> latex floccu**la**tion or bentonite aggluti**na**tion
>
> ASO (antistreptolysin O) titer

■ **Notes:**   Autoimmune antibodies are associated with many diseases, and their identification may provide diagnostic and prognostic information for management of the disease. Collagen or rheumatic diseases overlap in their clinical picture; the ANA findings support the diagnosis. *Autoimmune diseases*, a group of diseases in which the normal function of the immune system apparently becomes "mixed up," cause the body to produce antibodies against its own tissues. Normally, the immune system protects the body by producing antibodies against invaders and harmful substances.

SPECIALISTS   A great variety of practitioners treat MS and neuromuscular disorders: ortho**pe**dist, ortho**pe**dic surgeon, hand surgeon, head and neck surgeon; plastic surgeon, neurosurgeon and vascular surgeon in some cases; general practitioners, both MD and DO; **chi**ropractors, phys**i**atrists, physical therapists, and occupational therapists. In**tern**ists often treat patients with arthritis, gout, lupus, and so on.

Bonus: When you have learned the names of bones, you have also learned names of some blood vessels and nerves (for example: femur, femoral artery and nerve; tibia, tibial artery and nerve). The lobes of the brain are named the same as the cranial bones (for example, frontal, parietal, and so on).

Read the following reports, Discharge Summary and Report of Operation. It is helpful to read them aloud, and your instructor may ask you to do this in class. Look up all of the words that you do not know. Write them and write the definitions.

_____

_____

_____

_____

_____

_____

_____

_____

_____

_____

_____

CASE HISTORY ONE: DISCHARGE SUMMARY

admission diagnosis   Torn medial me**nis**cus, left knee.

discharge diagnosis   Torn medial me**nis**cus, left knee; chondroma**la**cia of the medial **fem**oral **con**dyle.

history of present illness   The patient injured her left knee on June 10, 1979, while playing tennis. She subsequently had difficulty with persistent ef**fu**sion and pain in the left knee. An **ar**throgram prior to admission revealed a tear of the medial meniscus.

physical examination   Absence of tenderness to pal**pa**tion of any of the joint structures. There was approximately 30–55 mL* of fluid within the joint. Range of motion was full (FROM).

laboratory data   Admission hemoglobin was 15.9, hematocrit 47%, white count 7400, with normal differential. Urinalysis was WNL (within normal limits). Chemistry profile showed an elevated cho**les**terol of 379 mg/dL. Chest X-ray examination was negative.

treatment and hospital course   The patient had surgery on the day of admission, at which time she underwent ar**thros**copy. This revealed a tear of the medial me**nis**cus. Ar**throt**omy was performed, with medial menis**cec**tomy. A **chon**dral fracture was noted in the medial femoral **con**dyle, measuring approximately 5 mm in greatest diameter. The edges of this were sheathed. Postoperatively, the patient's course was benign. There was no significant temperature elevation. She was ambulatory with crutches on the first postoperative day with no difficulty with straight leg raising.

disposition   Discharged to home with crutches and exercise program. To return in 1 week for suture removal.

CASE HISTORY TWO: REPORT OF OPERATION

preoperative diagnosis   **Her**niated **nu**cleus **pulp**osus, L5, S1 on the left (herniated disk).

operation performed   Lamin**ec**tomy and excision of disk.

pathologic operative findings   The disk had completely ruptured through the ligament, and the nerve root was compressed against the liga**men**tum **fla**vum.

operative procedure   Under general endo**tra**cheal anes**the**sia, with the patient in the prone position, the patient was prepped and draped in the usual manner. A linear incision extending from approximately L3 down to the sacrum was made over the spinous process through the skin and subcutaneous tissue. By means of subperi**os**teal dissection the posterior bony elements were exposed. The interspace was identified and the superior aspect of S1 and inferior aspect of L5 from the spinous processes were ron**guer**ed. By means of a cu**rette** the borders of the **lam**inae were identified and a Kerrison ronguer used to remove the superior aspect of S1 and the inferior aspect of L5.

The ligamentum flavum was cut in the midline and retracted lateralwards and removed. The nerve root was then identified, and it was markedly tight in this area. This required dissection starting superiorly to get the nerve root off the disk. After it was off the disk, the disk ruptured right into the wound, and the major fragment was removed. At this time the nerve root was held medialwards, and the remaining disk was removed from the intervertebral space.

A **cru**ciate incision was made into the **an**nulus so the pituitary ronguer could get into the interspace. After removal of the disk, the disk space was curetted, and the pituitary ronguer was used again to remove the further disk material. At this time the bleeding was controlled with gelfoam packing. The wound was copiously irrigated and closed with interrupted nylon suture for the inner spinous ligament and posterior fascia, interrupted plain suture for the subcutaneous tissue, and a continuous subcuticular nylon suture for the skin. Steri-strips were applied. Estimated blood loss was 200 mL. Blood replaced, none. All bleeders were clamped as encountered.

The patient tolerated the procedure well and returned to the recovery room in satisfactory condition.

worksheet

Fill in the blank:

1. Another word for skull is _____

2. Air spaces in the skull are called _____

3. "Cracks" in the skull are called _____

---

* A common abbreviation for milliliter is ml and cc (1 cc = 1 mL). However, preferred usage is mL.

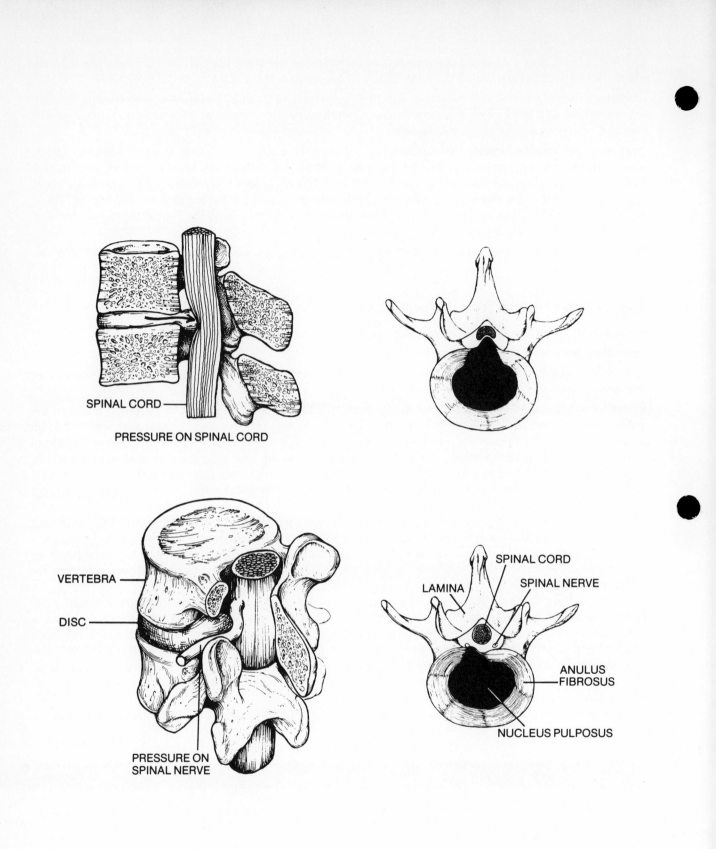

SPINAL CORD

PRESSURE ON SPINAL CORD

VERTEBRA

DISC

PRESSURE ON
SPINAL NERVE

LAMINA

SPINAL CORD

SPINAL NERVE

ANULUS
FIBROSUS

NUCLEUS PULPOSUS

Figure 18–7. Sections of spinal column showing hernia of intervertebral disk (HNP). (Adapted from Medical Times Patient Education Chart, Romaine Pierson Publishers, Inc., New York.)

4. Soft spots normally found in an infant's skull are called _____

5. Name five sections of the vertebral column (spine), in order, starting at neck: _____

   _____   _____   _____

   _____

Define:

6. adduction _____

7. ligament _____

8. tendon _____

9. bursa _____

10. Name and describe three kinds of fractures:

    _____   _____

    _____   _____

    _____   _____

11. Name three types of practitioners for bone disorders: _____   _____

    _____

12. What does "ortho" mean? _____

    Define orthopedic: _____

    _____

13. Define osteopath: _____

    _____

14. Name the common words for flexion: _____   extension: _____

15. Fixed ribs are attached anteriorly to the _____ and posteriorly to the _____

Define:

16. paralysis _____

17. atrophy (muscle) _____

18. hypertrophy _____

19. meniscus _____

20. Name three cranial bones: _____   _____   _____

21. Intercostal muscles are between the _____

22. Skeletal muscle is attached to _____

23. The dome-shaped muscle that aids breathing is called the _____

24. Name three kinds of muscle tissue: _____   _____

    _____

25. Name three diseases of the musculoskeletal system: _____   _____

    _____

26. How are muscles named? _____

    _____

27. "Foramina," "grooves," and "processes" are all terms used in relation to _____

28. The two main divisions of the skeleton are _____ and _____

29. How does the infant skeleton differ from that of the adult? _____

_____

_____

30. Diagram the skeleton and label all of the large bones.

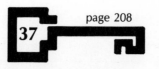

page 208

37

chapter 19
cardiovascular system

---

outline

HEART   (see Fig. 19–1). Lies in the media *sti* num (between the lungs). Has *four chambers: right and left atria* (singular, *atrium*) are receiving chambers (also called *auricles*); *right and left ventricles* are pumping chambers. The *apex* is the pointed part (bottom of the heart). The function of the heart is to pump blood, thereby maintaining circulation.

valves   keep blood from backflowing.

> **tri *cus* pid**   between right atrium and right ventricle.
>
> ***pul* monary semilunar**   between right ventricle and pulmonary artery.
>
> ***mi* tral**   between left atrium and left ventricle (also called bi **cus** pid valve).
>
> **a *or* tic**   between left ventricle and aorta.

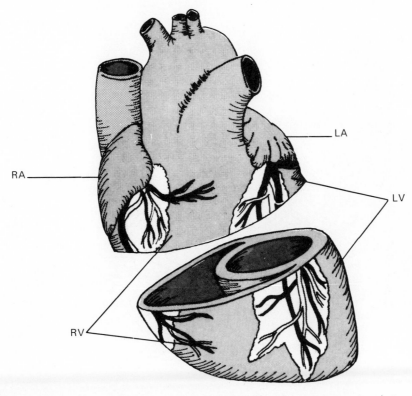

RA

LA

LV

RV

Figure 19–1.   Cross section of heart, showing coronary arteries. Also showing anatomic relationship of right ventricle, *RV*, to left ventricle, *LV*, and globular shape of left ventricle and half-moon shape of right ventricle as it drapes around left ventricle. *RA* is right auricle; *LA*, left auricle. (Adapted from Guyton, A.C.: Medical physiology, Philadelphia, 1956, W. B. Saunders Company.)

septum   divides the right and left *sides* of the heart.

muscle   myocardium is the heart muscle.

membranes   endo**car**dium lines inside of heart chambers; peri**car**dium is the outer double membranous sac; epi**car**dium (visceral layer); and outer par**i**etal layer.

conduction system

>   **sinoatrial node** or **SA node**   this is the *pacemaker* (right atrium).

>   **atrioven*tric*ular node**   in septum.

>   **bundle of His**   conducting fibers.

BLOOD VESSELS   arteries, veins, **cap**illaries (see Fig. 19–2).

arteries   always carry blood *away* from the heart (oxygenated blood except in pulmonary arteries).

veins   always carry blood *toward* the heart (deoxygenated blood except in pulmonary veins).

aorta   largest artery (ascending, aortic arch, thoracic, and abdominal sections).

vena cava   largest vein (superior and inferior venae cavae).

coronary arteries   supply the heart muscle with blood (arise from the base of the aorta). Oc**clu**sion of these causes heart attack (coronary oc**clu**sion). (See. Fig. 19–3.)

CIRCULATION   The function of circulation is to carry oxygen and nutrients to cells and to carry carbon dioxide and wastes away from the cells (see Fig. 19–4).

pulmonary circulation   right side of heart—blood returning from the body is received in the right atrium, goes to right ventricle and through the pulmonary artery to the lungs. It returns to the left atrium by way of the pulmonary veins.

systemic circulation   from left atrium, blood flows to the left ventricle and is pumped out through the aortic valve to the aorta and goes to the entire body.

portal circulation   circulation from the intestines to the liver.

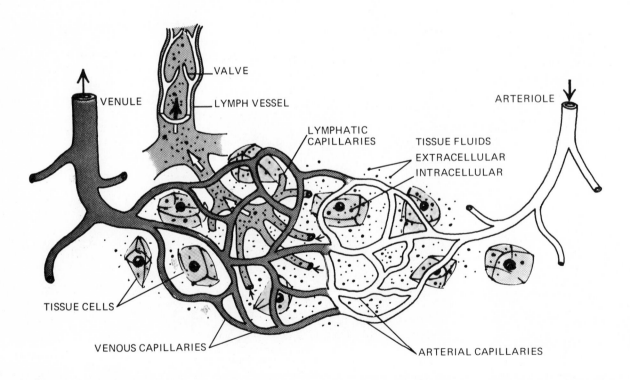

Figure 19–2.   Capillary bed, showing lymphatic vessels, and how tiny arterioles connect with tiny venules. The gaseous and nutrient exchanges take place in these capillary beds. (Adapted from Sloane, S.B.: The medical word book, Philadelphia, 1973, W. B. Saunders Company.)

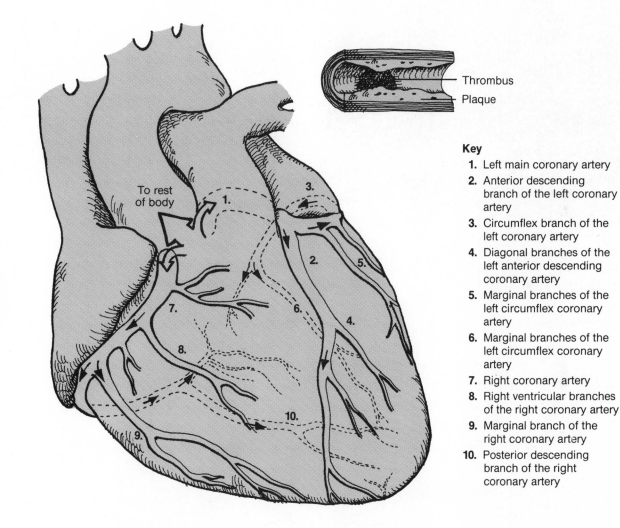

Thrombus
Plaque

Key
1. Left main coronary artery
2. Anterior descending branch of the left coronary artery
3. Circumflex branch of the left coronary artery
4. Diagonal branches of the left anterior descending coronary artery
5. Marginal branches of the left circumflex coronary artery
6. Marginal branches of the left circumflex coronary artery
7. Right coronary artery
8. Right ventricular branches of the right coronary artery
9. Marginal branch of the right coronary artery
10. Posterior descending branch of the right coronary artery

Figure 19–3. Coronary arteries, and section of artery showing thrombus and plaque formation. (Adapted from Medical Times Patient Education Charts, Romaine Pierson Publishers, Inc., New York).

LYMPHATIC VESSELS, LYMPH NODES, SPLEEN **Lymph fluid** comes from the blood; it filters out into the spaces between tissue cells, and returns to the blood via lymphatic vessels. **Lymph nodes** are numerous in certain parts of the body; nodes are palpable in the neck (cervical nodes), in the axilla (axillary nodes), and in the groin (inguinal nodes); they help filter out harmful substances such as bacteria and cancer cells. The **spleen** is the largest lymphatic organ of the body. In youth it helps build up blood cells; it also destroys old blood cells.

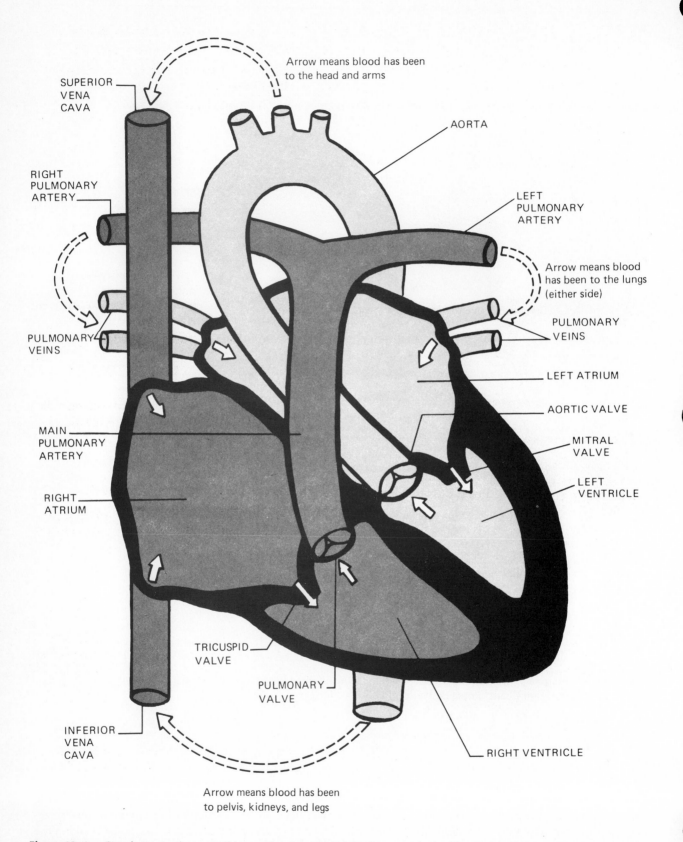

Arrow means blood has been to the head and arms

SUPERIOR VENA CAVA

AORTA

RIGHT PULMONARY ARTERY

LEFT PULMONARY ARTERY

Arrow means blood has been to the lungs (either side)

PULMONARY VEINS

PULMONARY VEINS

LEFT ATRIUM

AORTIC VALVE

MAIN PULMONARY ARTERY

MITRAL VALVE

RIGHT ATRIUM

LEFT VENTRICLE

TRICUSPID VALVE

PULMONARY VALVE

INFERIOR VENA CAVA

RIGHT VENTRICLE

Arrow means blood has been to pelvis, kidneys, and legs

Figure 19–4. Circulation in the normal heart. The right side of the heart sends the blood to the lungs (pulmonary circulation); the left side sends blood to the entire body (systemic circulation). Light areas contain oxygenated blood.

BLOOD

red blood cells (RBCs)   are called e**ryth**rocytes; they contain hemoglobin, which carries oxygen to the cells and carries carbon dioxide away from the cells.

white blood cells (WBCs)   are called **leu**kocytes. There are five basic kinds of white blood cells, numbers 1–5.

A. **Gran**ulocytes (have granules in cytoplasm) are formed in bone marrow. There are three types:

1. **Neu**trophils*: also called polymorpho**nu**clear leukocytes or PMNs because their nuclei have many shapes or forms. They defend the body by means of phagocyt**o**sis (ingesting invaders).

2. Eo**sin**ophils: are thought to be active and increased in allergic conditions.

3. **Bas**ophils: function is unclear.

B. **Agran**ulocytes (have no granules) are produced by spleen and lymph nodes. There are two types:

4. **Lymph**ocytes: produce antibodies and destroy foreign material.

5. **Mon**ocytes: perform phagocytosis and destruction of invaders.

plasma   is the liquid part of the blood, minus the cells. It is amber colored. If whole blood is allowed to stand in a container, the cells will settle to the bottom (clot), and the clear plasma will rise to the top.

serum   is plasma minus the fi**brin**ogen that promotes clotting.

platelets   are also called **throm**bocytes (clotting particles).

*re**tic**ulocyte*   immature red blood cell, in bone marrow.

■ **Note:**   An order for WBC and diff means a white blood count and differential, counting percentage of each kind of leukocyte.

BLOOD TYPES

Landsteiner types   based on type of red blood cells: A, B, AB, and O.

distribution   our population shows 3% AB, 10% B, 40% to 44% A, and 40% to 44% O. When incompatible bloods are mixed, clumping of cells occurs. Example: Type A red cells that are dropped into type B blood cause clumping or sticking together. These clumps could cause fatal injury as they pass through the heart or brain.

universal donor   group O.

universal recipient   group AB.

type and crossmatch (x-match)   before a transfusion is given, this is done to determine compatibility. Cells from the donor and serum from the recipient are mixed to see if clumping occurs. A second test is done using the cells of the recipient and the serum of the donor. If no clumping occurs, it can be assumed that the two bloods are of the same type.

Rh FACTOR   so named because it was first found in the blood of the Rhesus monkey.

> 85% of population have this factor, called Rh+.
> 15% *do not have this factor*; they are Rh−.

The Rh factor acts like a foreign substance to anyone who is negative. If an Rh-negative person receives Rh-positive blood, that person's own blood will make a substance called an antibody, which will act against the Rh-positive blood. If an Rh-negative woman mates with an Rh-positive man, their child may inherit the Rh factor from his father. The mother's blood may produce so many antibodies against it that the baby may die before or shortly after birth. This does not usually affect the first child of these parents because not enough antibodies are present, but will affect subsequent pregnancies.

Antibody titers (tests) done during pregnancy aid the doctor in determining when intervention is necessary. If the titer rises rapidly, the pregnancy can be terminated early or preparation for exchange transfusion at time of delivery can be made. *RhoGAM* can be given to the Rh-negative mother following her first delivery. This prevents Rh antibodies from forming.

---

* Neutrophils are generally not called neutrophils on laboratory forms. They may be called "segs" because of their segmented nuclei, or they may be called polys or PMNs. Immature forms are often called "bands" or "stabs" or "juvs." (See laboratory forms, p. 91.) "-phil" as in neutrophil may also be spelled "-phile."

DISORDERS OF THE HEART, VESSELS, AND BLOOD

anemias   a group of diseases characterized by insufficient red blood cells; may be due to iron deficiency, some life-threatening condition (such as aplastic anemia, sickle cell anemia), a bone marrow defect, or heredity.

an*eu*rysm   a weak, ballooned area in a vessel.

an*gi*na *pec*toris   pains in the chest due to spasm of coronary arteries.

ar*rhyth*mia   irregular heart beat; often occurs after MI.

arterioscle*ro*sis   thickening, hardening, and loss of elasticity of the walls of blood vessels, causing the lumen to become narrowed.

a*sys*tole   cardiac standstill.

atheroscle*ro*sis   a form of arteriosclerosis due to buildup of fatty material (plaque) in arteries.

cardiac arrest   heart action ceased (CPR indicated).

coarc*ta*tion   compression or narrowing of the walls of a vessel, especially the aorta.

congenital defects   septal defects (ASD, VSD), **pa**tent **duc**tus arteri**o**sus, tet**ral**ogy of Fal**lot**.

congestive heart failure (CHF)   inability to pump blood effectively throughout the body.

coronary oc*clu*sion and **coronary throm*bo*sis**   see heart attack.

CVA   see stroke.

em*bolus, *em*bolism   a thrombus that has broken loose and been carried along in the circulation until it blocks a vessel (air and fat globues may also cause this).

endocar*di*tis   inflammation of the endocardium.

fibril*la*tion   quivering or trembling type of contraction caused by injury to heart, as in MI, or by certain drugs; a heart in fibrillation cannot maintain circulation. Treatment is defibrillation.

heart attack   a clot in a coronary artery, cutting off circulation to the heart muscle; also called coronary oc**clu**sion, coronary throm**bo**sis, myo**car**dial in**farc**tion or **in**farct, MI (see Fig. 19–3).

heart block   a type of ar**rhyth**mia; conduction of impulses from atrium to ventricle disturbed; pacemaker may be inserted.

heart murmur   a soft, blowing sound heard on ausculta tion, indicating the valve may be incompetent and does not close properly.

hemo*phil*ia   congenital lack of clotting factor in blood.

Hodgkin's disease   (and other malignant lymphomas) malignant tumors of the lymph nodes and spleen.

hyper*ten*sion   *essential* hypertension (cause unknown) is high blood pressure (see p. 139).

is*che*mia   insufficient blood supply to a part.

leu*ke*mias   a group of diseases of the blood-forming organs and white blood cells; acute or chronic.

MI   see heart attack.

myocar*di*tis   inflammation of the heart muscle.

pericar*di*tis   inflammation of the double membranes on outside of the heart.

rheumatic heart disease   a form of myocarditis with mitral valve insufficiency; occurs as a se**que**la to rheumatic fever. Beta strepto**coc**cus is the causative organism.

stroke   cerebro**vas**cular accident (CVA); damage to the cerebrum due to ruptured vessel or clot.

thrombophle*bi*tis   inflammation in a vein with clot formation.

transient ischemic attack (TIA)   brief period of inadequate blood supply to brain, sometimes referred to as "small strokes."

varicose veins   dilated veins caused by defective valves; heredity is a factor; also called varices. Surgical stripping removes varicosities.

DIAGNOSTIC, SURGICAL, TREATMENT, AND RELATED CV TERMS

angi*og*raphy   X-ray examination of vessels.

angioplasty   see PTCA.

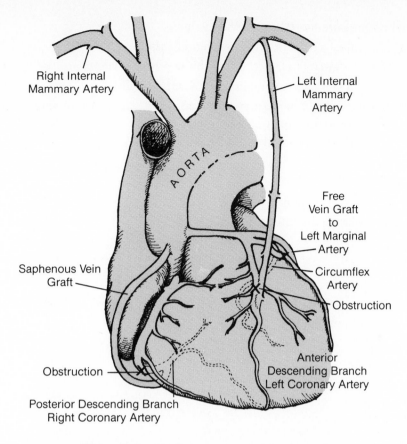

Right Internal Mammary Artery

Left Internal Mammary Artery

AORTA

Free Vein Graft to Left Marginal Artery

Saphenous Vein Graft

Circumflex Artery

Obstruction

Obstruction

Anterior Descending Branch Left Coronary Artery

Posterior Descending Branch Right Coronary Artery

Figure 19–5. Triple coronary artery bypass graft.

anticoagulant   medication to delay clotting (blood thinner).

antihypertensive drugs   relax artery walls or neutralize a hormone that causes arterial spasm.

bradycardia   slow heart rate, less than 60.

bypass   see coronary artery bypass graft.

cardiac catheterization   catheter passed into heart through a vein in the arm to detect abnormal flow in coronary arteries.

collateral circulation   "new" expanded small vessels that try to accommodate ischemic area when primary circulation has been blocked.

commissurotomy   cutting heart valve that is defective to improve flow of blood.

coronary artery bypass graft   substituting a vein from the leg to bypass the occluded artery in MI patients (see Fig. 19–5); ileofemoral bypass is similar, to supply blood to ischemic lower extremities.

digitalized   subjection of the patient to digitalis drug in a quantity sufficient to maintain heart contraction force without side effects (digitalization).

diuretic   a type of medication, often called a "water pill," that lowers blood pressure by reducing blood volume.

Doppler   ultrasonic probe that checks blood flow in artery under it.

dyscrasia (blood)   any abnormal condition.

electrocardiogram   ECG, EKG; picture of electrical impulses of the heart; also echocardioography using ultrasound.

endarterectomy   "boring out" the inner lining of artery to increase size of the lumen.

hemoglobin   iron-containing pigment in red blood cells, essential for transport of oxygen.

heparin   an anticoagulant in the blood; also given as a medication.

Holter monitor   portable ECG.

low-salt diet   lowers blood pressure by reducing blood volume.

*lu*men   the opening within a tubal structure, such as a blood vessel.

pacemaker   a battery-powered device implanted under the skin to regulate heart rate.

phle*bot*omy   a "cut down" to a vein when **ve**nipuncture is unsuccessful.

PTCA   percu**ta**neous trans**lu**minal coronary **an**gioplasty; an alternative to bypass surgery in selected cases; balloon-type catheter exerts pressure on area of plaque, thus "opening" the blocked area.

sinus rhythm   normal cardiac rhythm initiated by SA node.

tachy*car*dia   rapid heart rate.

vasodilator   agent that causes dilatation.

vasopressor   agent that causes constriction.

***ve*nipuncture**   puncturing a vein for any purpose.

ABBREVIATIONS

ALL   acute lympho**cyt**ic leukemia.

AML   acute myelo**blas**tic (myelomonocytic) leukemia (**my**eloblast is a primitive bone marrow WBC).

ASD   atrial septal defect (often referred to as a "hole in the heart").

baso   basophil (kind of WBC).

B/P   blood pressure.

CABG   coronary artery bypass graft.

CBC   complete blood count.

CCU   coronary care unit.

CHF   congestive heart failure.

CO_2   carbon dioxide (a colorless gas).

CPR   cardiopulmonary resuscitation.

CVA   cerebro**vas**cular accident (a stroke); cva (lower case letters) also means costovertebral angle.

ECG, EKG   electro**car**diogram.

Eos   eo**sin**ophil (type of WBC).

Lymph   **lym**phocyte (type of WBC).

MI   myo**car**dial **in**farct (heart attack).

Mono   **mon**ocyte (type of WBC); mono can also mean mononucleosis.

O_2   oxygen (a colorless gas); essential for life.

PMI   point of maximal impulse (of heart on chest wall).

PMN   polymorpho**nu**clear (leukocyte).

PTCA   percu**ta**neous trans**lu**minal coronary **an**gioplasty.

PVC   premature ven**tric**ular contractions.

RBC   red blood cell; red blood count.

Segs   white blood cells with segmented nuclei.

TIA   **tran**sient is**chem**ic attack.

VSD   ven**tric**ular septal defect.

WBC   white blood cell; white blood count.

BLOOD PRESSURE   the amount of pressure on the walls of blood vessels as blood passes through.

hyper*ten*sion   high blood pressure. *Essential hypertension* is high blood pressure with no apparent cause.

sphygmoman*om*eter   B/P cuff (mercury and aneroid types).

sys*tol*ic pressure   Top number in B/P reading. The greatest force exerted on the walls of the artery by the ventricles contracting.

*di*astolic pressure   Bottom number in B/P reading. The least amount of force exerted on the walls of the artery when the ventricles relax.

normal B/P   Pressure up to about 140/90 is usually considered "within normal range." Anything above this bears watching.

■ Notes: One B/P reading that is above normal does not constitute high blood pressure. Several readings, at intervals, are taken over a period of several weeks before a diagnosis of hypertension is made.

Factors that affect blood pressure include
1. The volume or amount of blood.
2. The force or strength of the heart beat.
3. The condition of the arteries; if narrowed by disease, pressure will be higher.
4. Thickness or viscosity of the blood.

Blood pressure may also vary with exercise or lack of it; eating, smoking, or fasting; taking stimulants or other drugs; strong emotions, fever, fatigue, hemorrhage, or shock.

Treatment of essential hypertension: lose weight, if overweight; eliminate salt from diet; exercise. If this does not lower the B/P sufficiently, a diuretic medication is given. If further treatment is needed, antihypertensive drugs may be prescribed. These medications must be taken regularly and usually for a life time. This is the problem in treating hypertensives; they do not feel ill and often do not take the medication as prescribed.

SPECIALISTS   cardiologist, internist, cardiovascular surgeon, hematologist, oncologist; pediatric cardiologist and hematologist.

TREATMENT   varies from encouraging patients to change their lifestyle (lose weight, exercise, stop smoking, and so on) to prescribing a great variety of drugs and surgical correction of various heart and vessel disorders. Biofeedback may also be used.

READ THE FOLLOWING REPORT. WRITE NEW WORDS AND DEFINE THEM.   Using the laboratory data given, consult laboratory forms (Chapter 14). Which results are out of normal range (if any)?

CASE HISTORY

final diagnosis   1. Recurrent episode of chest pain, probably on an ischemic basis.
2. History of an inferior wall MI, August 1978, with cardiac arrest, which was apparently not due to atherosclerosis.
3. Hiatal hernia by history.
4. Type IV hyperlipoproteinemia

The patient is a 48-year-old white male admitted to this hospital for evaluation of an episode of chest pain on the morning of admission. He has a history of undergoing cardiac catheterization and coronary angiography in January 1977 because of persistent PVCs and atypical chest pain. This catheterization gave completely normal results with normal left ventricular function and completely normal coronary arteries. He subsequently sustained an acute transmural inferior wall myocardial infarction with secondary cardiac arrest in August 1978, for which he was hospitalized. Repeat cardiac catheterization and coronary angiography performed subsequent to his MI showed total occlusion of his right coronary artery but no other abnormalities aside from markedly abnormal left ventricular function secondary to his infarct.

He has been maintained on no cardiac medications. A stress test was apparently performed approximately one month prior to his admission and, according to the patient, gave normal results.

He was in his usual state of health until breakfast time on the morning of admission when he noted the gradual onset of crampy type discomfort between the shoulder blades and a substernal heaviness with radiation into his jaw, accompanied by chills and slight nausea. These symptoms lasted a total of approximately 20 minutes. He describes the back and chest discomfort as being more severe than that which occurred with his prior MI. He denies any other accompanying symptoms. He came to the ER for evaluation where an ECG was obtained, which showed a normal sinus rhythm with changes consistent with an old inferior wall MI without other definite acute changes except for some frequent unifocal PVCs. He was given a bolus of lidocaine and started on a lidocaine drip. Because of his past and present history he was admitted for further evaluation and treatment.

physical examination   Well-nourished, well-developed, alert, cooperative, responsive white male resting comfortably in no apparent distress.

Pertinent diagnostic data: Admission CBC—hemoglobin 15.3 g, hematocrit 45.8%, WBC 6900 with a normal differential; RPR nonreactive; prothrombin time and PTT WNL; Ua normal; electrolytes—sodium 143, potassium 4.2, chloride 102, CO_2 28; blood glucose 97; BUN 18; cholesterol 279; uric acid 7.6; phosphorus 2.8; calcium 9.8; total bilirubin 0.4; total protein 8.2; albumin 5.0; SGOT 18; LDH 109; alkaline phosphatase 79; CPK 60; serial cardiac isoenzymes completely WNL; lipid profile shows a pattern consistent with type IV abnormality; HDL level is not recorded; serial ECGs show a normal sinus rhythm with changes of an old transmural inferior wall MI and some vacillating ST-T wave changes consistent with new inferolateral wall ischemia; chest X-ray examination WNL.

A recurrent acute MI was essentially ruled out with negative enzymes and ECGs. He was initially started on nitroglycerine ointment but did not tolerate this in any dose, developing severe headaches. His hospital course was totally uneventful except for the presence of some unifocal PVCs on admission, which responded to intravenous lidocaine and oral Norpace. He had no recurrent anginal symptoms whatsoever. At the time of discharge he was feeling well and was fully ambulatory. He will be followed as an outpatient.

Therapy on discharge: Low-saturated-fat diet and Norpace 150 mg po qid.

worksheet

Fill in the blank:

1. Define cardiovascular disease _____
   _____

2. What is a CVA or stroke? _____
   _____

3. There are two phases to circulation of blood in the body. In one, deoxygenated blood is sent to the lungs, this is _____ circulation. In the other, the oxygenated blood is sent to the rest of the body, this is _____ circulation.

4. Blood from the right ventricle passes through the pulmonary valve and goes to the _____ (vessel) and _____ (organ); it returns to the (chamber) _____ of the heart, through the _____ (vessel).

5. Blood from the left ventricle goes to the entire body, leaving the left ventricle through the _____ valve to the _____ (artery).

6. The heart valves between the atria and ventricles are the _____ (right side) and the _____ (left side).

7. The largest veins in the body, which return blood to the heart from the upper and lower parts of the body, are the _____ _____ _____ and the _____ _____ _____.

8. The function of valves in the heart and in the veins is to _____
   _____

9. Arteries, veins, arterioles, venules, and capillaries are all _____ _____

10. Circulation that takes over when regular circulation is cut off or blocked is called _____ circulation.

11. The blood carries _____ (gas) and _____ to all tissues of the body and carries away _____ (gas) and _____ for excretion.

Define:

12. septum (heart) _____

13. systole _____

14. diastole _____

15. myocardium _____

16. type and x-match _____

17. hematology _____

18. deoxygenated _____

19. varicose _____

20. coronary arteries _____

Fill in the blank:

21. The four main blood types (Landsteiner) are _____

22. a. Red blood cells (RBCs) are called _____

    b. White blood cells (WBCs) are called _____

    c. Cells that aid clotting are _____

    d. Name five kinds of white blood cells: _____ _____

    _____ _____ _____

23. If a person does not have the Rh factor in his blood, he is said to be _____

24. The sinoatrial node is called the _____

25. Name the specialist who diagnoses and treats circulatory disorders: _____

    "blood" diseases (diseases of bone marrow) _____

26. Give three names for a heart attack: _____

    _____ _____

27. The outer and inner membranes of the heart (in order) are _____ and _____

28. Identify: ECG _____

    CCU _____

29. Factors that can affect B/P (give three): _____

    _____

    _____

30. Give root words for heart _____ vein _____ artery _____

    (blood) vessels _____ blood clot _____ circulating clot _____

31. The universal donor is type _____

32. RhoGAM is given following delivery (of Rh-negative mother). What does it do? _____

_____

_____

33. Name three disorders of the heart, vessels, or blood not mentioned in this worksheet: _____

_____   _____

34. Identify: a. MI   _____

           b. CHF   _____

           c. CVA   _____

           d. ASD   _____ (congenital)

           e. TIA   _____

35. What is the usual treatment for essential hypertension?

     a. _____

     b. _____

     c. _____

38 page 208

chapter 20
respiratory system

---
outline

RESPIRATORY SYSTEM FUNCTION   to provide the body tissues with oxygen and to remove carbon dioxide.

ORGANS   (airways) (See Fig. 20–1.)

nasal cavity   nose; nares (naris is singular); nasal septum divides cavity.

*phar*ynx   throat (through which air and food pass).

*lar*ynx   voice box; vocal cords.

*tra*chea   windpipe.

*bron*chi **(bronchus)**   one to each lung; lined with cilia (hairlike projections).

*bron*chioles   smaller divisions of bronchi.

al*ve*oli **(al***ve*olus)   tiny air sacs at the ends of bronchioles that comprise lung tissue. In the alveoli, the gaseous exchanges take place (oxygen picked up, carbon dioxide dropped off).

lungs   right, three lobes; left, two lobes. *Apex* (**a**pices is plural) is the top of the lung; the *base* is the bottom. They lie in the *pleural cavity* (thoracic cavity).

RESPIRA*TION*   breathing; consists of *inspiration* and *expiration*. Air enters the nasal cavity and oral cavity and travels through the preceding organs.

*DI*APHRAGM   dome-shaped muscle that separates the pleural cavity from the abdominopelvic cavity. It *moves downward* on inspiration, creating suction in the chest to draw in air, expand lungs.

ACCESSORY STRUCTURES

eu*sta*chian **tubes**   tubes from pharynx to middle ear, they equalize pressure (see Fig. 24–3, p. 186).

epi*glott*tis   flap that covers entrance to trachea; it closes during swallowing to prevent aspiration of food.

inter*cos*tal **muscles**   muscles between ribs.

paranasal *sin*uses   air spaces in cranium, connected to nasal cavity (frontal, maxillary, ethmoid, sphenoid).

pleura   double mucous membrane that covers the lungs (**vis**ceral layer) and lines the thoracic cavity (par**i**etal layer).

tonsils and **adenoids**   part of the lymphatic system; act as filters (see Fig. 20–1).

*uv*ula   muscle tissue that hangs down from the soft palate; it guards the opening from the nasal cavity, preventing food from entering; staphyl/o = rootword for uvula; for example, **staph**yloplasty.

RESPIRATORY DISEASES AND DISORDERS

abscess (lung)   accumulation of pus (many causes).

ARDS   adult (acute) respiratory distress syndrome, "shock lung"; impaired gaseous exchange from any cause (aspiration, trauma, and so on).

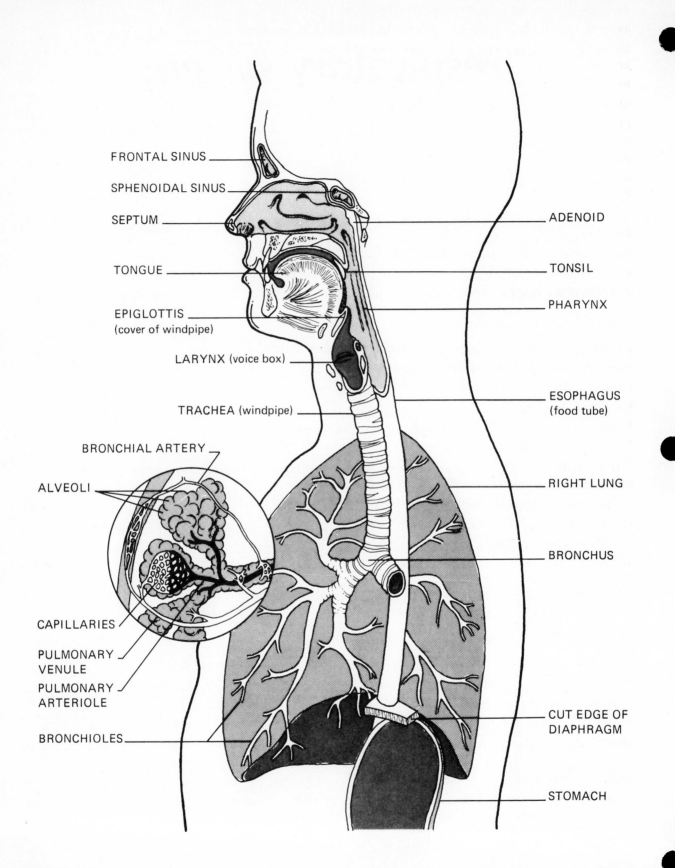

FRONTAL SINUS

SPHENOIDAL SINUS

SEPTUM

TONGUE

EPIGLOTTIS
(cover of windpipe)

LARYNX (voice box)

TRACHEA (windpipe)

BRONCHIAL ARTERY

ALVEOLI

CAPILLARIES

PULMONARY
VENULE

PULMONARY
ARTERIOLE

BRONCHIOLES

ADENOID

TONSIL

PHARYNX

ESOPHAGUS
(food tube)

RIGHT LUNG

BRONCHUS

CUT EDGE OF
DIAPHRAGM

STOMACH

Figure 20–1. Lungs and airways, showing the structures through which air passes on its way to the lungs. Inset shows alveoli and capillaries.

asphyxia*tion*   suffocation due to interference with breathing.

***asth*ma**   usually due to allergy; dyspnea and wheezing due to spasm and swelling of airways.

ate*lec*tasis   "incomplete dilatation" or collapsed lung; due to trauma, obstruction, or as a complication in lung disease.

bronchi*ec*tasis   "dilated bronchi" usually secondary to repeated early infections; foul pus discharge.

bron*chi*tis   inflammation of bronchi; acute or chronic.

carci*no*ma   broncho*gen*ic carcinoma, originating in bronchi; squamous, adenocarcinoma, oat cell are types; meta*stat*ic carci*no*ma of lung also occurs.

coccidioidomy*co*sis   "valley fever," caused by fungus that lies dormant in spore form in hot, dusty climates; produces symptoms similar to pneumonia.

COPD (COLD)   chronic obstructive pulmonary (lung) disease, especially emphysema, chronic bronchitis, and asthma.

cor pulmon*a*le   heart failure due to pulmonary disease.

co*ry*za   the common cold; caused by viruses.

cystic fi*bro*sis   mucovisci*do*sis; disorder of mucous glands leading to pancreatic insufficiency.

deviated septum   defect in wall between nostrils that can cause partial or complete obstruction.

diph*ther*ia   acute bacterial disease (immunization available).

ef*fus*ion   "flowing out" of liquid (see pleurisy).

emphy*se*ma   the functioning tissue of lungs (alveoli) become distended or ruptured; irreversible; characterized by severe dyspnea, especially exertional. Related to cigarette smoking. One form of COPD.

empy*e*ma   pus in pleural cavity (abscess).

fi*bro*sis   abnormal formation of fibrous tissue (scar tissue in lungs) usually due to previous infections; may be referred to as idio*path*ic (cause unknown).

flail chest   erratic movement of chest due to multiple injuries of ribs or sternum.

"flu"   a term that has come to mean almost anything (used by laymen).

hay fever   allergic coryza, pollin*o*sis.

hemo*thor*ax   blood in thoracic cavity.

hia*tal hernia   diaphrag*mat*ic hernia; opening in diaphragm allows part of the stomach to move up into chest; usually treated conservatively with diet, antacids, and elevation of head when lying down.

hiccough, hiccup   spasm of diaphragm due to many things; may involve phrenic nerve; also called sin**gul**tus.

histoplas*mo*sis   fungus disease of lungs; lesions resemble TB.

***hy*aline membrane disease**   poorly developed alveoli leading to collapse of lungs; disease of premature infants. Leading cause of neonatal deaths.

influ*en*za   "la grippe"; group of virus-caused acute febrile pulmonary diseases, most serious in the very young or very old.

laryn*gi*tis   inflammation of larynx (loss of voice or hoarseness).

laryngotracheobron*chi*tis   "croup"; so named because of croupy cough with air hunger (in young children).

per*tus*sis   acute febrile disease (whooping cough) caused by bacterial infection; immunization available in DPT.

pharyn*gi*tis   "sore throat."

***pleur*isy**   fluid discharged by inflamed pleural membranes (effusion), causing severe pain and dyspnea.

pneu*mon*ias   many causes and types; bacterial or viral lung infections; also aspiration and hypostatic pneumonia; may involve a lobe, a lung, or bronchial tubes.

pneumoconi*o*sis   any of the pulmonary disorders caused by irritating dusts, such as in asbes**to**sis and sili*co*sis, and other irritants (including chemicals) used in industry.

rhi*ni*tis, rhinor*rhe*a   inflammation of nose; "runny nose."

sinu*si*tis   inflammation of paranasal sinuses; acute or chronic.

SID   sudden infant death syndrome; cause unknown but may be due to lung disorder.

streptococcal sore throat   "strep throat"; due to specific organism; if not adequately treated with antibiotics may result in rheumatic fever as a sequela and even to rheumatic heart disease (all caused by streptococci).

tonsillitis   inflammation of tonsils with "crypts" of pus formation (usually); treated with antibiotics. T & A may be indicated but is not as routine as it used to be.

tuberculosis   infectious disease that produces "tubercles" in the lung (sometimes elsewhere also); caused by specific organism; treated with INH (isoniazid), PAS, and other drugs; patient need not be isolated if under treatment.

URI   upper respiratory infection; general term for colds or what people call the "flu."

valley fever   see coccidioidomycosis.

whooping cough   see pertussis.

RESPIRATORY TERMS   (diagnostic, surgical, miscellaneous)

aerosols   medications in spray form for relief of asthma symptoms.

anoxia (hypoxia)   insufficient oxygen.

apnea (apnea)   temporary periods of not breathing.

blood gases   oxygen (O_2) and carbon dioxide (CO_2) quantities in arterial blood (laboratory test).

bifurcation   separation into two branches as with the bronchus.

bronchodilators   medications to dilate bronchi.

bronchoscope   lighted instrument for viewing bronchi.

bronchoscopy   use of the above instrument.

bronchospasm   contraction causing bronchi to constrict.

Cheyne Stokes   ("chain stoks") irregular breathing; slow and shallow, increasing in rate and depth, then decreasing until breathing stops for 10–20 seconds; cycle repeats.

CO_2   carbon dioxide; gas expired in expiration.

consolidation   solidification of lung tissue (in pneumonia).

CPR   cardiopulmonary resuscitation; method of restoring circulation and breathing.

cyanosis   condition of blueness due to insufficient oxygen, especially seen in nailbeds and skin.

dysphonia   impaired voice.

dyspnea (dyspnea)   difficulty breathing; may be paroxysmal nocturnal (PND) (sudden, severe) or exertional (with exertion).

ET tube   endotracheal tube; intubation used during surgery and for temporary airway in emergency situations.

expectorants   medications that loosen secretions.

hemoptysis   expectoration of blood from lungs (frothy).

hiatus   an opening, especially in diaphragm.

hilus   root of lung where vessels, nerves, and bronchi enter.

hypercapnia   increased CO_2 in blood.

hyperventilation   hyperpnea; increased rate and/or depth of respirations; seen in anxiety states.

hyposensitization   type of treatment sometimes used in allergic states; increasing doses of the offending substance given to patient in an effort to build up his tolerance.

IPPB   intermittent positive pressure breathing (used as treatment with ventilators).

Kussmaul breathing   deep, gasping type of breathing.

laryngectomy   excision of larynx, making it necessary for person to use esophageal speech or a prosthetic larynx.

laryngoscopy   procedure of using laryngoscope to view larynx.

lavage of sinuses   washing out or irrigating sinuses.

lobectomy   excision of lobe of lung.

Mantoux ("mantoe")   TB skin test.

O₂   oxygen, gas inhaled and carried in the blood; administered as therapy by mask or cannulae.

orthopnea (orthopnea)   able to breathe only in sitting position.

parenchyma (lung)   the "working part" of any organ is the parenchyma; in the lung the alveoli are the structures where gases are exchanged.

perfusion   supplying organ with nutrients and oxygen.

P and A   percussion and auscultation; tapping and listening to chest; also A and P.

pneumothorax   introduction of air into thoracic cavity as a therapeutic measure or spontaneously as the result of an injury (puncture).

pulmonary function   various tests used to evaluate ventilation.

postural drainage   "postures" assumed by the patient to facilitate loosening and expectoration of secretions to improve ventilation.

PPD   purified protein derivative (TB test).

productive cough   a cough that produces sputum.

rales, rhonchi   sounds in the chest indicating pathology.

rarefaction   term used to describe decreased density in X-ray films.

residual air   air remaining in lungs after expiration; there is always some, but it is increased in some lung diseases.

respirators (ventilators)   mechanical assistance in breathing; Bird Mark 7, Bennett, and so on.

rhinoplasty   plastic surgery on nose; cosmetic and/or to improve breathing.

scan (lung, pleura)   use of radioactive isotopes to produce a "picture."

SOB   short of breath.

spirometer, spirometry   instrument and its use in pulmonary function tests.

sputum   secretions from bronchi.

SMR   submucous resection (for deviated septum); surgical procedure to correct defect.

tachypnea (tachypnea)   rapid breathing.

thoracentesis or **thoracocentesis**   "tapping" of chest to remove fluid.

thoracoplasty   multiple rib resection to collapse diseased area of lung.

Tine test   TB test.

tracheotomy   incision into trachea when airway is obstructed.

tracheostomy   new permanent opening into trachea.

ventilators   see respirators.

vital capacity   amount of air that can be forcibly expelled from lungs after deep inspiration (pulmonary function test).

X-ray examination   routine, of chest; AP and lat (anteroposterior and side view).

SPECIALISTS   internist (pulmonary diseases), ENT (otolaryngologist), oncologist, thoracic surgeon, head and neck surgeon, radiologist.

TREATMENT   Much of the treatment in respiratory disease is medication; frequently prescribed drugs include antibiotics, antihistamines, corticosteroids. Surgery is indicated in some cases.

CASE REPORTS   The following reports are presented so that you experience the use of medical terminology in practice. Sometimes you will be able to understand a word you do not know simply because it becomes clear in context. Read the reports and write the words you are not familiar with. Define them.

CASE HISTORY ONE: X-RAY REPORT

posteroanterior, lateral chest   There is opacity of the lower portion of the right hemithorax, apparently resulting from a large amount of fluid. The cardiac size is difficult to evaluate, but the heart may be somewhat enlarged, and the appearance of the visualized lung fields suggests passive congestion. The possibility of underlying fibrotic process in the right base cannot be excluded. There is calcification in the arch of the aorta.

CASE HISTORY TWO: MEDICAL REPORT

admitting diagnosis   bronchitis.

subjective data   A 34-year-old male admitted to the hospital because of a cough. He stated he was in his normal state of health until 1 week prior to admission when he began to experience a hacking cough that became extremely severe and was associated with malaise and sweating the night prior to admission.

objective data   CBC showed a leukocytosis of 19,000. Electrolytes, urinalysis, RPR were all WNL. Sputum for C & S grew out the usual upper respiratory tract flora. Noted on this rotochem was an elevated blood glucose; however, blood glucoses obtained after that showed the glucose to be within normal limits. Urine and blood cultures also were performed and revealed no growth. Alkaline phosphatase is 79, SGOT 38, SGPT 35, LDH 109, and a Gamma GT of 87. All of these are minimally elevated. ECG was totally WNL. Chest X-ray films were not helpful.

hospital course   The patient was admitted and treated with multiple antibiotic agents, mainly Keflex 500 mg qid; for his breathing Brethine 2.5 mg tid was used; however, he developed a drug reaction from Keflex and was changed to gentamicin sulfate 80 mg IV q12h, with Keflin 1 g q4h. Patient apparently did well on this medical regimen and after 10 days with medication was discharged from the hospital to be followed in the office in approximately 10 days.

CASE HISTORY THREE: REPORT OF OPERATION

preoperative diagnosis   bronchogenic carcinoma arising from the left upper lobe bronchus.

operation   bronchoscopy; radical left upper lobectomy.

With the patient under satisfactory anesthesia, in the supine position and connected to the ECG monitor, a bronchoscopy was performed by introduction of 7×40 bronchoscope into the trachea. Epiglottis, vocal cords, trachea, right and left main bronchi were normal. There was a tumor originating 5 to 8 mm from the orifice of the left upper lobe with partial obstruction of the bronchus. A sample of bronchial washing was taken for C & S, and the bronchoscope was withdrawn.

The patient was then put in the thoracotomy position with the left side of the chest elevated and was connected to the ECG monitor. The skin of the chest wall was prepped with Betadine (pronounced **bay**tadine), and patient was draped and exposed. A costolateral thoracotomy incision was made. Muscle layers were transected with electrocautery. Chest was entered through the fifth intercostal space. Posterior thoracotomy was made through the fourth and fifth ribs to facilitate exposure. There was adhesion from the left upper lobe on the chest, which was lysed. The left superior hilum was reached. There was marked chronic inflammatory fibrosis of the pulmonary arteries and in the hilum, but, overall, there was no nodal involvement in this area. With considerable difficulty the branch of the pulmonary artery coming into the left upper lobe was dissected, ligating continuously, and transected. The superior segment of the left lower lobe was detached from the left upper lobe using a stapler. The superior pulmonary vein was dissected also, ligating continuously, and transected. All of the nodes were dissected towards the specimen, and the bronchus was dissected free of the adjacent structure. The bronchial artery was clipped.

At this point using the stapler and the transected upper lobe, cancer was noted in the stapler line. Again 2-0 stay sutures were placed over the main bronchus, and the remainder of the bronchus, which was about 8 mm in length, was cut flush with the left main bronchus. Bronchial closure was done using interrupted sutures of 4-0 silk. This closure was airtight. The second bronchial margin was negative for cancer.

After complete hemostasis two chest tubes were inserted in the chest, exteriorized through the lower interspaces. The wound was then closed in layers, using interrupted sutures of No. 2 chromic, muscular layers with No. 1 chromic. The rest of the incision was closed in layers.

The patient tolerated the procedure well and was sent to the recovery room in satisfactory condition. Estimated blood loss was 4 units. The patient was transfused accordingly to keep up with the blood loss.

Fill in the blank:

1. Cavity in which lungs are located (chest): _____ or _____

2. Name the organs, *in order*, through which inspired air travels:

   _____   _____   _____

   _____   _____   _____   _____

3. The muscle that separates the heart and lungs from the abdominal organs is the _____
   When it contracts, it moves up/down (circle correct word), which makes more/less (circle correct word)
   room in chest cavity. It contracts during inspiration/expiration (circle correct word).

4. The _____ keeps food from entering the larynx.

5. Where are the tonsils located? _____ Where are the eustachian tubes? _____
   _____ What do they do? _____

6. Define alveoli: _____

7. When the membrane that covers the lungs is inflamed, you have _____

8. Respiration includes the exchange of two gases. Name them and give the abbreviations: _____

   _____

9. The medical term for nostrils is _____ What is the dividing cartilage in the nose?

   _____

10. The top part of the lung is the _____ What is the plural form?   What

    is the bottom or lower portion of lung? _____

11. Air spaces in the cranium are called   _____

12. The trachea is in front of/in back of (circle correct phrase) the esophagus.

13. The physician who interprets X-ray films: _____

14. The physician who performs tonsillectomies: _____

15. _____ is a new permanent opening into the trachea.

16. A hiatal hernia is a hernia in the   _____

17. A collapsed lung is called _____ Mantoux and tine tests are tests for

    _____

18. What is meant by vital capacity?   _____

    _____

19. COPD and COLD refer to chronic obstructive pulmonary disease. Name one such disease: _____

    _____

20. Difficult or labored breathing is called   _____

21. _____ means able to breathe only when sitting upright.

22. A temporary cessation of breathing is called   _____

23. Write all of the -itis words you can using the organs in the respiratory system: _____

    _____

    _____

Give the meaning of the following:

24. URI _____

25. SOB _____

26. IPPB _____

27. AP and lat (chest) _____

28. In treatment of respiratory disorders several general kinds of medications are used. Name one designed to

    loosen secretions: _____   Name a mist type: _____

29. Unusual chest sounds are also called _____

30. Name a malignant lung disease _____

Define:

31. tachypnea _____

32. sputum _____

33. asthma _____

34. productive cough _____

35. spirometer _____

36. bronchoscope _____

37. inspiration _____

38. thoracocentesis _____

39. bilateral pneumonia _____

40. The plural of bronchus is _____

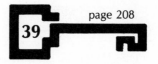

page 208

39

chapter 21
gastrointestinal system

---
outline

GASTROINTESTINAL SYSTEM FUNCTIONS   ingestion, digestion, and absorption of food or nutritive elements. The gastrointestinal (GI) system is also called the digestive system (review Fig. 1–1 in Chapter 1 and see Fig. 21–1).

ORGANS THROUGH WHICH FOOD PASSES   alimentary canal.

mouth

***phar*ynx**   throat.

e*soph*agus   tube to stomach, *behind* the trachea.

stomach   cardiac sphincter at entrance; pyloric sphincter at exit (greater and lesser curvatures – large and small outer walls of stomach).

duo*de*num, je*ju*num, *il*eum   small intestine, three parts; *ileocecal valve* prevents contents of large bowel from reentering small intestine.

***ce*cum**   appendix attached; first part of large intestine.

ascending colon   large intestine. Hepatic flexure where ascending colon turns into

transverse colon   large intestine. Splenic flexure where transverse colon turns into

descending colon   large intestine.

***sig*moid colon**   large intestine.

***rec*tum**   large intestine.

***a*nus**   anal sphincter (sphincter muscle is circular, like a purse string).

ACCESSORY ORGANS

teeth   incisors (central and lateral); cuspids or canines; bicuspids or premolars; and molars (first and second); third are "wisdom" teeth.

tongue   muscular organ, covered with mucous membrane; taste buds are present on surfaces of papillae.

***sal*ivary glands**   three pairs: pa**rot**id, sub**ling**ual, and subman**dib**ular.

***pan*creas**   behind stomach; excretes pancreatic juice to duodenum (papilla of Vater); also secretes the hormone *insulin* into blood (function of endocrine system).

liver   largest gland (RUQ); responsible for hundreds of chemical reactions.

1. Stores fats and sugars; makes proteins (albumin, globulins).
2. Secretes bile (essential for digestion of fats).
3. Regulates blood sugar.
4. Removes wastes from blood; detoxifies substances.

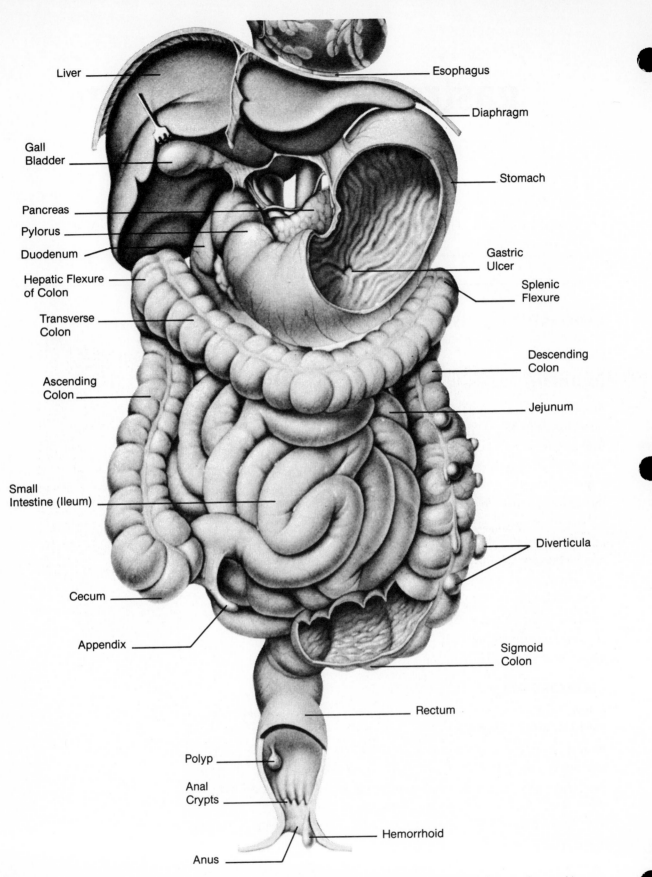

Figure 21-1. Gastrointestinal organs showing some pathologic conditions: peptic ulcer, diverticulosis, polyp, and hemorrhoid. (Adapted from Reed and Carnrick chart, copyright by Robert J. Demarest, Columbia Presbyterian Medical Center, New York.)

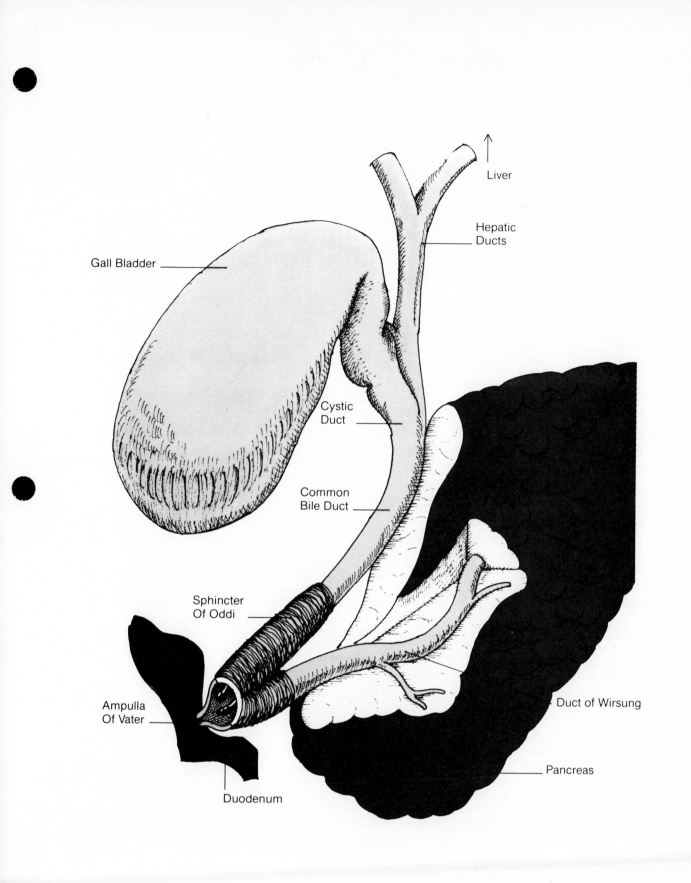

Gall Bladder

Liver

Hepatic Ducts

Cystic Duct

Common Bile Duct

Sphincter Of Oddi

Ampulla Of Vater

Duodenum

Duct of Wirsung

Pancreas

Figure 21–2. The gallbaldder and its ducts and their relationship to the pancreas and duodenum.

gallbladder   behind liver; stores and concentrates bile. *Hepatic ducts* drain bile from liver; *cystic duct* by which bile enters and leaves gallbladder; *common bile duct*, union of these two, into duodenum (by way of ampulla of Vater at sphincter of Oddi). The common bile duct and pancreatic duct meet to enter the duodenum (see Fig. 21–2).

AREAS OF ABDOMEN

***quad*rants**   four divisions: RUQ, RLQ, LUQ, and LLQ.

divisions   nine sections.

RUQ	LUQ
RLQ	LLQ

1. Right and left hypo**chon**dria.
2. Right and left lumbar.
3. Right and left **ing**uinal or **il**iac.
4. Epi**gas**tric.
5. Um**bil**ical.
6. Supra**pu**bic or hypo**gas**tric.

1	4	1
2	5	2
3	6	3

DIGESTION

mechanical process   food is broken up, mixed with digestive juices. It is moved along by peri**stal**sis (rhythmic contraction of the intestines).

chemical process   food reacts with enzymes. Large molecules are broken down so they can pass through the mucous membrane into the blood and from there to the cells.

absorption   takes place in the small intestines. **Vil**li, which are tiny projections lining intestines, provide large surface area through which nutrients can be absorbed.

elimination   of solid wastes in the form of feces. Also called fecal matter, stool, and bowel movement.

metabolism   the sum of all physical and chemical changes that take place within the body and all energy and transformations that occur within cells; change of food to mechanical energy or heat.

nutrients   food; proteins, fats, carbohydrates, plus vitamins and essential minerals. Proteins and carbohydrates (CHO) contain 4 calories per gram; fats contain 9. Protein is essential for growth and repair of tissue. Fats and carbohydrates provide heat and energy.

    Essential vitamins: A, B_1 (thiamine), B_2 (riboflavin), niacin, B_6 (pyridoxine), B_{12} (cyanocobalamin), C (ascorbic acid), D, folic acid, and K.

    Essential minerals: calcium, iron, iodine, zinc, copper, magnesium, potassium, phosphorus, sodium.

GI DISEASES AND DISORDERS

ad*he*sions   abnormal bands or fibers that bind one organ to another (especially intestines); can result from abdominal surgery or infection; surgical treatment is adhesi**ol**ysis, adhesi**ot**omy.

***al*coholism**   addiction to alcohol, leading to malnutrition and liver damage (also brain damage and sociologic problems).

ano*rex*ia nervosa   an aversion toward food ("hysterical").

appendi*ci*tis   inflammation of the appendix; ruptured appendix can lead to peritonitis.

***bot*ulism**   a severe type of food poisoning caused by anaerobic bacteria, leading to GI, eye, and neurologic symptoms; can be fatal.

carci*no*ma   malignant tumor (may involve any GI organ).

choleli*thi*asis   condition of gallstones.

cir*rho*sis   replacement of liver cells by fibrous tissue; occurs frequently in alcoholics.

cleft lip/palate   congenital anomaly; failure of lip and/or palate to fuse; treatment is surgical cheiloplasty.

co*li*tis (ulcerative, spastic)   inflammation of colon.

cryp*ti*tis   inflammation of "crypts," especially those in anus and penis.

diverticu*li*tis, diverticu*lo*sis   inflammation or condition of having diverticula that are "pouches," especially in the sigmoid colon (see Fig. 21–1).

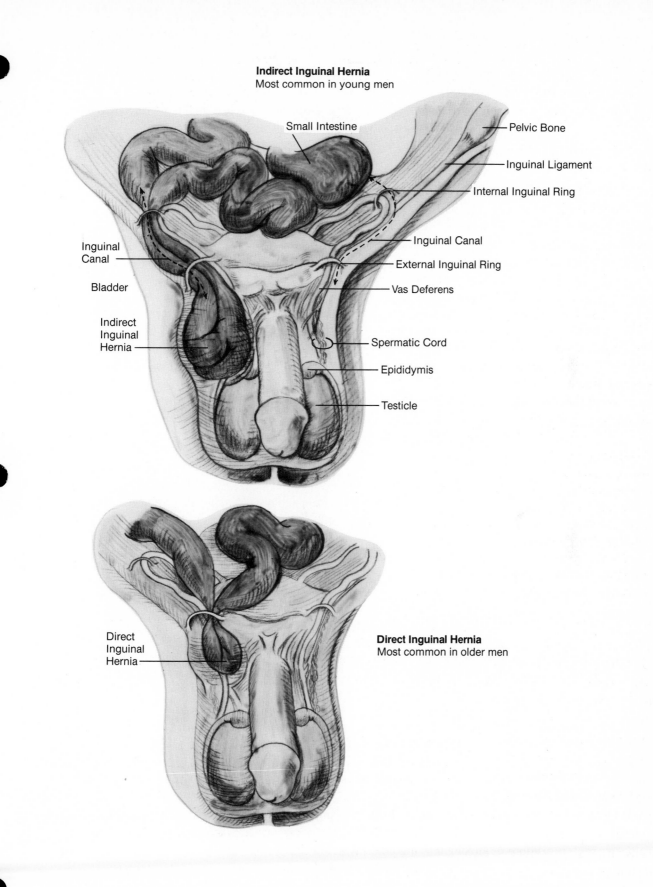

Indirect Inguinal Hernia
Most common in young men

Small Intestine

Pelvic Bone

Inguinal Ligament

Internal Inguinal Ring

Inguinal Canal

External Inguinal Ring

Vas Deferens

Spermatic Cord

Epididymis

Testicle

Inguinal Canal

Bladder

Indirect Inguinal Hernia

Direct Inguinal Hernia

Direct Inguinal Hernia
Most common in older men

Figure 21–3. Inguinal hernias, indirect and direct. (Adapted from Medical Times Patient Education Charts, Romaine Pierson Publishers, Inc., New York).

dys entery   severe dehydrating diarrhea; types include amebiasis, shigellosis, salmonella; slang term: Montezuma's revenge.

esophagitis   inflammation of the esophagus (food tube).

esophageal atresia   esophagus ends in a blind end instead of opening into the stomach.

esophageal varices   enlarged, incompetent veins in distal esophagus due to portal hypertension in cirrhosis.

flexure   a "turning" or angle, as the hepatic flexure of the colon (near the liver).

food poisoning (gastroenteritis)   acute nausea and vomiting, cramps, and diarrhea due to a variety of ingested toxins or bacteria.

gastric ulcers (peptic or duodenal)   inflamed area with destruction of tissue; may cause bleeding and pain and may perforate.

gastritis   gastroenteritis; inflammation of stomach or entire GI tract; common in alcoholism.

glossitis   inflammation of the tongue.

hepatitis   inflammation of the liver; type A, formerly called "infectious," and type B, formerly called "serum"; also nonA and nonB type. A vaccine is now available for hepatitis B high risk groups.

hernia   many types; hiatal, inguinal (Fig. 21–3), umbilical, femoral; protrusion of a part out of its natural place. Hiatal indicates that the stomach is pushed up through diaphragm into thoracic cavity; other types involve intestines and may cause bowel obstruction (strangulated hernia).

impaction (fecal)   hard stool impacted in rectum that usually must be removed manually; this condition is a problem in elderly populations (especially in nursing homes) and is due to many factors, especially inactivity and low roughage intake.

intussusception   telescoping of intestine (slides into itself).

nausea and vomiting   N and V; common symptoms in many GI disorders.

obesity   overweight 20%–30% above normal.

pancreatitis   inflammation of the pancreas.

peritonitis   inflammation of the peritoneal cavity, usually due to rupture of an organ (appendix, for example).

polyposis   condition of having polyps (growths that hang from a thin stalk); familial and a precursor to cancer.

PKU   phenylketonuria is a congenital inability to metabolize phenylalanine, which leads to mental retardation; treated with special diet.

pyloric stenosis   congenital condition; outlet of stomach is narrow and will not allow food to pass into duodenum, causing projectile vomiting.

rectocele   hernia of rectum.

sialolith   stone in salivary duct.

ulcers   see "gastric."

■ **Note:**   Treatment for many of the above conditions is surgery. Conservative treatment is often the treatment of choice in ulcers, colitis, diverticulosis, and hiatal hernia.

DIAGNOSTIC PROCEDURES

biopsy   examination of living tissue; tissue may be taken from any of the GI organs, and this can be done through an endoscope usually. Needle biopsy may be done on liver.

blood chemistry (laboratory work)   tests for liver function; frequent tests done are bilirubin, alkaline phosphatase, SGOT and SGPT (enzymes); other helpful lab tests are gastric analysis, stool specimen examination for occult blood and parasites, and so on.

cholangiography   X-ray examination of the bile ducts using contrast medium (IV or, if during surgery, directly into ducts).

colonoscopy   procedure of looking into the colon with a flexible, fiberoptic scope.

digital examination   insertion of the gloved finger into the rectum.

esophagogastroduodenoscopy (EGD)   using scope to examine these structures.

flat plate of abdomen   X-ray film of abdomen.

gallbladder series (GBS) X-ray film is taken after patient has been given a dye that will outline gallbladder; a second set of X-ray films is then taken after the patient has eaten a "fatty" meal.

gastrointestinal series (GI series) UGI (upper GI) or barium swallow; lower GI or barium enema (BE); an opaque substance called barium is given by mouth/enema and X-ray films are taken.

gas*tros*copy examining the stomach with a gastroscope.

proc*tos*copy examining the rectum, sigmoid, with scope.

scan using a special device, CAT (computerized axial tomography), to produce a "picture" of any organ.

stool specimen sent to laboratory for occult blood (guaiac) or for parasites, such as worms, amoebas.

ultrason*og*raphy using ultrasound method to obtain a "picture" of any organ.

■ **Note:** Preparation may be very vigorous for some of the above procedures, for example NPO (nothing by mouth) at least 12 hours prior to test, laxatives and enemas until clear. Without such preparation the endoscopic and GI tests cannot be useful in diagnosis. Printed instructions are usually given to the patient.

SURGICAL PROCEDURES

anasto*mo*sis joining together two parts of intestine or common bile duct when portion has been removed.

appen*dec*tomy excision of appendix.

***bi*opsy** of any organ (diagnostic).

bypass removal of large portion of small intestine in cases of morbid obesity.

***chei*loplasty** especially for cleft lip (cheilo = lip).

cholecys*tec*tomy excision of the gallbladder.

choledochoduoden*os*tomy new permanent opening between the common bile duct (choledoch/o) and duodenum.

co*los*tomy new permanent opening of colon to surface of abdomen with a stoma.

gas*trec*tomy usually subtotal removal of stomach; Billroth I and II techniques, anastomosis between stomach and duodenum or jejunum.

herni*or*rhaphy surgical repair of a hernia.

ile*os*tomy new permanent opening into ileum; continent type holds contents until released by inserting tube.

lapa*rot*omy incision into abdomen, usually "exploratory."

portacaval shunt portal vein stitched to inferior vena cava to bypass the obstructed cirrhotic liver.

stomach stapling staples across stomach to allow only very small amounts of food to be eaten; used in cases of intractable obesity.

va*got*omy cutting vagus nerve; a procedure sometimes used to treat ulcers.

RELATED TERMS

ana*sar*ca severe, generalized edema.

a*sci*tes edema, collection of fluid in peritoneal cavity.

buccal ("buckle") pertaining to the cheek.

ca*chex*ia ("ka*kex*ia") severe malnutrition and wasting; emaci*a*tion.

***cal*orie** unit of heat; energy value of food.

CBD common bile duct; union of hepatic and cystic ducts; choledoch/o = common bile duct; the CBD enters the duodenum through the ampulla of Vater.

cho*les*terol a chemical component of oils and fats (it is believed that cholesterol contributes to plaque formation in arteries).

deglu*ti*tion swallowing.

enema introduction of fluid into the rectum for cleansing and/or for diagnostic purposes in preparation for barium enema, in which cases "enemas until clear" are ordered.

enzymes   more than 650 complex proteins manufactured by living tissue; they stimulate specific chemical changes, such as breakdown of starches to sugars (amylase enzyme), so that they can be absorbed by the intestines; most enzyme names end in -ase (exceptions are rennin, pepsin, and so on).

fistula   abnormal opening between two organs (rectovaginal) or to surface of skin.

Fleet's (enema)   prepackaged, disposable type of enema.

gamma globulin   substance containing antibodies; used to provide passive (temporary) immunity in people who have been exposed to an infectious disease (infectious hepatitis, for example).

gavage   feeding by tube (especially premature infants).

glossal   pertaining to the tongue.

hyperalimentation   TPN (total parenteral nutrition) with a subclavian catheter.

lavage   to wash out, especially the stomach after ingestion of a poisonous substance.

lingual   pertaining to the tongue; sublingual means "under the tongue."

NG tube   nasogastric tube; a soft, flexible tube introduced through the nose into the stomach for gavage, lavage, or suction.

NPO   "nothing by mouth" in preparation for tests and before and after surgery (until peristalsis is established again).

parotid   "near the ear"; parotitis or mumps results when the salivary glands near the ear become inflamed.

peritoneum   membrane lining the abdominal cavity. The mesentery is part of the peritoneum; it attaches intestines to the posterior body wall. The greater and lesser omentum are also part of the peritoneum; they connect abdominal viscera with the stomach.

stoma   "mouth"; the artifically created opening in colostomy and ileostomy on the surface of the abdomen.

viscera   internal organs; eviscerate means internal organs coming out, as when a wound opens.

SPECIALISTS   GI disorders may be treated by an internist (gastroenterologist), family practice specialist, general surgeon, oncologist, proctologist. Public health physicians are involved in cases of infectious hepatitis, food poisoning, and so on.

TREATMENT   Treatment is often "surgical." Diet is often an important part of treatment in GI disorders. Bland diets and soft diets may still be used in some cases, but the trend recently has been toward more roughage in diets. Drugs that are important in treatment include antispasmodics, antacids, antinauseants, antiobesity anorexics (including amphetamines), antidiarrheals, laxatives, stool-softening drugs, as well as various antibiotics in the acute inflammatory disorders.

Read the following reports. Define the italicized words.

CASE HISTORY ONE

Miller, John
Joseph Kantor, MD
Admitted: 7–10–80

present illness   This is the third hospital admission for this 69-year-old man with a past medical history of *essential hypertension*, *ischemic* heart disease with *angina*, *osteoarthritis* of the *lumbar* spine, and known *diverticulosis* with irritability of the *descending* and *sigmoid colon*. He was seen in my office with approximately a 4-day history of lower abdominal crampy pain, two or three bowel movements daily, which were soft in nature, *anorexia*, and some *dysuria*. He had noted an episode of *hematospermia* in June, which has continued until the present time. He denied, however, having mucus in the bowel movements. There were no complaints of *nausea*, temperature elevation, or food intolerances. Because of the amount of pain it was felt that hospitalization for investigation and treatment was warranted.

past history   Has been well reviewed in patient's old chart of 1972. It should be noted that recently the patient has been treated by J. Russell, MD for his ischemic heart disease and hypertension.

review of systems   See old chart.

personal and social history   patient's current medications include Apresoline, 25 mg *tid*; Inderal, 20 mg *tid* ac, plus hs; Esidrix, 50 mg *bid*; and Nitrostat, 0.4 mg *prn*. He states that in spite of his medications his *B/P* on his most recent visits to Dr. Russell has been running in the area of 200/100.

physical examination   At the time of admission reveals a fellow of his stated age with a stoic appearance and complaints of lower abdominal pain. Temperature 98.6, pulse 72, respirations 18, B/P 184/88.

skin   Warm and dry with no evidence of rashes or eruptions.

HEENT   No evidence of recent cranial trauma. *Tympanic membranes* are grossly intact. *Conjunctivae* clear. Extraocular movements grossly intact. *Fundi* unremarkable. Nose and throat unremarkable. No notable lymph nodes in the usual areas. Thyroid does not appear to be enlarged.

thorax   There are equal and full respiratory excursions bilaterally. No spinal or *cva* tenderness noted.

lungs   All lung fields are clear to *A & P.*

heart   Regular sinus rhythm with no murmurs or rubs. No apparent *cardiomegaly.*

abdomen   No abdominal *organomegaly* nor abdominal masses noted. Bowel sounds are normally active. Patient exhibits some right lower quadrant, suprapubic, and left lower quadrant *guarding* with no masses felt, along with moderate tenderness in these areas. No *rebound tenderness* referred to these areas however.

rectal   Patient expresses a moderate amount of tenderness on rectal exam; prostate moderately enlarged, soft, tender and nonnodular.

genitals   *WNL.*

neurologic   WNL.

impression   Abdominal pain, probably secondary to *diverticulitis.*

CASE HISTORY TWO

barium enema   There has been a history of surgical intervention in the large bowel. On the filled film there are *diverticula* present in the distal descending and sigmoid regions, as well as in the ascending colon. There is overlapping of bowel in the transverse colon, and whether this represents redundancy or a side-to-side *anastomosis* could not be determined either fluoroscopically or radiographically. On the evacuation film there is noted *contrast media* extending outside the bowel wall in the region of the sigmoid diverticula, and the possibility that these represent abscesses resulting from diverticulitis must be considered. The terminal *ileum* is visualized. No filling defects are seen.

CASE HISTORY THREE

cholecystectomy   Under spinal anesthesia the patient was prepared and draped in the supine position. A right *subcostal* Kocher incision was made. The skin was incised and the incision carried down through the anterior rectus sheath, rectus muscle, posterior sheath, and *peritoneum.* Bleeders were clamped and ligated with 000 chromic suture.

The gallbladder was found to be markedly *edematous,* thickened, and *hyperemic.* It measured approximately 15 cm in length and 4 cm in diameter. There were numerous *adhesions* around the gallbladder, which were *lysed* by blunt dissection.

Exploration of the abdominal contents was normal. The finger could be inserted into the *foramen* of Winslow. The common duct was free of stones.

The gallbladder was removed using clamps to grasp the *fundus* and Hartmann's pouch. The cystic duct was then clamped, divided, and doubly ligated with 000 cotton. The cystic artery was likewise clamped, divided, and ligated with 00 cotton and the gallbladder removed. The gallbladder bed was oversewn with continuous locking 00 chromic. A medium-sized Penrose drain was placed into the foramen of Winslow and brought out through a separate stab wound in the abdomen. The peritoneum was closed using chromic. The fascia was closed in layers with cotton, the skin with Dermalon.

worksheet

Fill in the blank:

1. Another name for the GI system is _____ The name of the cavity in which the GI viscera are contained is _____ or _____

2. Name an organ in the RUQ: _____ RLQ: _____

3. The six accessory GI organs that aid in the digestive process are _____

   _____

   _____

4. Name three sections of the small intestine, *in order*: _____ _____

   _____

5. The tube from the pharynx through which food passes to the stomach is the _____

   Food passage is assisted by muscular contraction called _____

6. Name all of the sections of the large intestine (in order): _____

   _____

   _____

   _____

   _____

7. The _____ is the opening to the outside of the body for solid wastes.

8. _____ and _____ are other words for bowel movement.

9. Three X-ray procedures used in diagnosing GI disorders are _____ _____

   _____. Name three other procedures (not X-ray) _____

   _____ _____

10. Where is bile produced? _____ Stored? _____ What does it do?

    _____ Name the three ducts connected to the gallbladder: _____

    _____ _____

11. Give the root word for common bile duct: _____ gallbladder: _____

    Procedure of X-raying common bile duct _____

Define:

12. enema _____

13. villi _____

14. sphincter muscle _____

15. proctoscope _____

16. The three main food groups are _____ _____ _____

    How many calories do each of these contain (per gram)? _____ _____

    _____

17. Of these, which is important for growth and repair of tissue? _____

18. Draw and label the nine regions of the abdomen.

19. The mesentery is actually a part of the _____ membrane. The omentum
    is attached to the stomach – to the _____ and _____ curvatures.

20. Gavage means _____

21. Lavage means _____

Define:

22. stomatitis _____

23. glossitis _____

24. cholecystectomy _____

25. colostomy _____

26. hepatitis _____

27. cholelithiasis _____

28. anorexia _____

29. WNL _____

Complete these sentences:

30. Nutrients are largely absorbed in the _____ intestine, which is lined with projections
    called _____ that increase the surface area.

31. Three surgical procedures on the GI tract not mentioned in this paper: _____
    _____ _____

32. Name three diseases of this system, not already mentioned: _____
    _____ _____

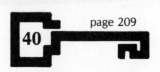
40 page 209

chapter 22
genitourinary system
(reproductive and urinary)

---

outline

URINARY ORGANS AND STRUCTURE   (see Fig. 22–1)

kidneys   two, lie behind the abdominal organs against muscles of the back (retroperitoneal) and are held in place by fat. The parts of the kidney include the following:

   *cor*tex   outer layer.

me*dul*la   inner portion.

***neph*rons**   kidney cells and capillaries. The *glomerulus, Bowman's capsule,* and *renal collecting tubule* are all parts of the nephrons. The nephrons are the pa**ren**chyma (functioning parts) of the kidney.

renal pelvis   the wide, upper end of the ureter (lies inside kidney).

u*re*ters   narrow tubes lined with mucous membrane. Urine passes from the kidneys, through the renal pelvis, and is moved through the ureters by peri**stal**sis.

urinary bladder   lined with mucous membrane; urine collects here, and bladder expands to hold urine.

u*re*thra   in female—narrow short tube from bladder to exterior; in male—narrow long tube, carries urine and seminal fluid to exterior.

urinary me*a*tus   opening of the urethra to exterior.

FUNCTION OF THE SYSTEM   to filter the blood. Urine is formed by the nephrons.

   1. Water and substances in solution are removed from blood.

   2. Essential water and substances are reabsorbed.

   3. Some water and dissolved substances are excreted to regulate reaction of the blood. Reaction of blood (pH) normally is slightly alkaline: 7.38 to 7.44 (1 to 7 is acidic; 7 to 14 is alkaline).

URINARY DISEASES, DISORDERS, AND SURGICAL PROCEDURES

*cal*culus **(renal)**   kidney stones; cause blockage with severe, colicky pain.

cys*ti*tis   inflammation of bladder; if not treated, will travel upward through ureters.

di*al*ysis   filtering blood with artificial kidney.

"floating kidney"   displaced and moveable; nephropexy may be done.

glomerulone*phri*tis   a form of nephritis involving glomeruli.

hydrone*phro*sis   collection of urine in pelvis of kidney due to obstruction of outflow.

nephroli*thi*asis   see calculus (lith=stone), treatment is nephrolithotomy.

nephrop*to*sis   prolapse or downward displacement of kidney, treatment is nephropexy.

neph*ror*rhaphy   surgical repair of kidney.

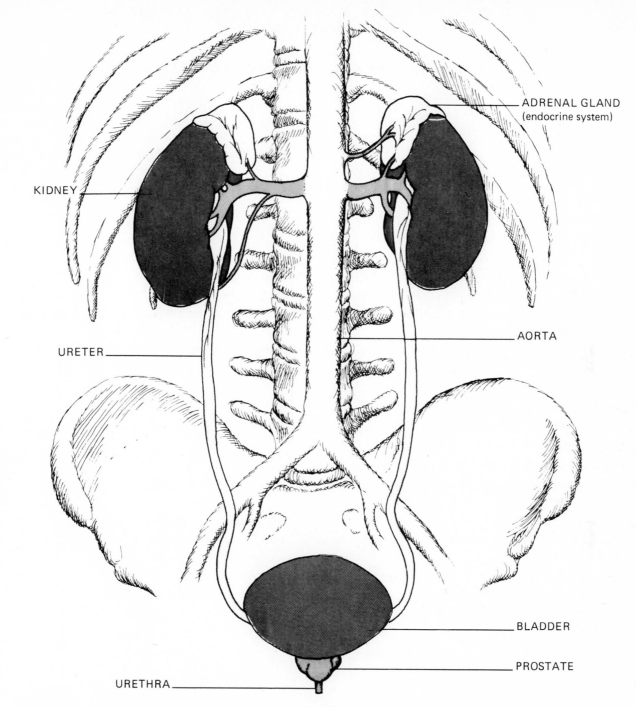

KIDNEY

URETER

ADRENAL GLAND
(endocrine system)

AORTA

BLADDER

PROSTATE

URETHRA

Figure 22–1. Normal urinary tract, showing kidneys, adrenals, ureters, bladder, prostate gland, and urethra, and their positions in relation to bony structures. (Adrenals are part of the endocrine system.) Aorta and renal arteries are shown.

pye*li*tis   inflammation of renal pelvis.

renal failure   due to trauma or any condition that impairs flow of blood to the kidneys; also caused by some toxic substances.

renal transplant   transplanting donor kidney to recipient.

u*re*mia (azo*te*mia)   toxic condition (urine in the blood); nitrogenous wastes not being excreted.

ureter*os*tomy   new opening for drainage of a ureter.

urethritis inflammation of urethra (nonspecific or gonococcal).

UTI urinary tract infection.

Wilms' tumor nephroblastoma; malignant tumor in children (ages 1–5); treated by surgery, radiation, and chemotherapy.

URINARY TERMS: DIAGNOSTIC AND MISCELLANEOUS

albuminuria albumin (protein) in urine; abnormal.

anuria no urinary output.

bladder distention full bladder; patient unable to void.

blood chemistries especially BUN (blood urea nitrogen).

BUN a blood chemistry test that is helpful in diagnosis of kidney disorder.

catheterization emptying bladder with a catheter (tube); may be done to obtain a specimen, to relieve bladder distention, or to measure "residual" urine after patient has voided. Foley (retention) and French catheters are commonly used.

Clinitest (also Testape) convenient, inexpensive method of testing urine for glucose, acetone, albumin, and so on (tablet or specially treated paper are dipped into urine, and color changes occur; ranges are 1+ to 4+).

continent capable of controlling voiding and defecation.

cystoscopy using a **cyst**oscope to examine the bladder.

diuresis increased urinary output, due to medication with a diuretic drug.

dysuria difficult or painful urination.

enuresis bedwetting; not waking up to void.

frequency and urgency frequent, urgent trips to bathroom, but voiding small amounts (painfully); symptoms occur with cystitis.

hematuria blood in the urine (gross or microscopic); should always be investigated.

incontinent inability to control urination (and bowels); stress incontinence with coughing, sneezing, laughing.

I & O intake and output; recording all fluid taken in by mouth or IV, and output.

IVP intravenous pyelogram; introduction of a dye, intravenously, for X-ray examination of renal pelvis.

KUB kidneys, ureters, bladder.

micturate urinate, void.

nocturia, nycturia getting up during the night to void.

oliguria scanty output of urine.

pyuria pus in the urine.

retrograde pyelogram introduction of dye from below, through urethra, for X-ray examination of renal pelvis.

scan (renal) "picture" of kidney after radioactive substance has been given IV; determines function and shape of kidney (renal=kidney).

ultrasonography using high-frequency sound waves, directed into the body and reflected back on to a screen or diagrammed on paper to show organs.

Ua urinalysis (analysis of the urine); routine Ua includes reaction or pH, albumin, glucose, specific gravity (weight as compared to water), and microscopic examination.

urinary retention inability to void; many causes, including loss of muscle tone of bladder from anemia, old age, prolonged operation, psychogenic factors, medication with narcotics, and anesthetics.

vesico combining form meaning bladder; for example, vesicovaginal=pertaining to the bladder and vagina.

void to empty (bladder).

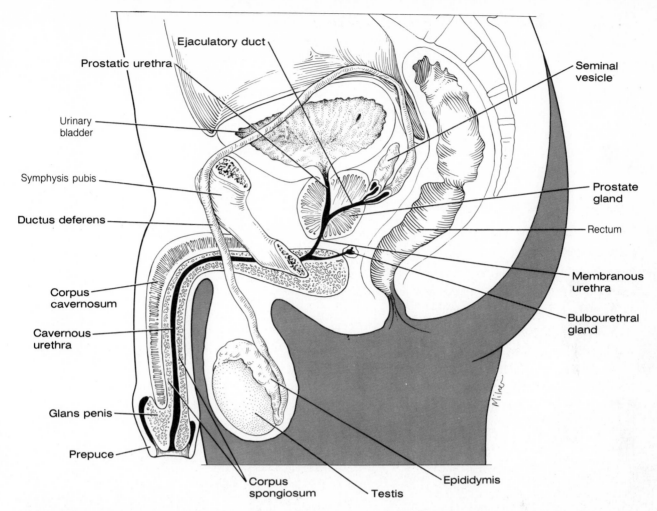

Figure 22–2. Median sagittal section of the male pelvis with a portion of the left pubic bone attached to illustrate the path of the ductus deferens. (From Spence, A.P. and Mason, E.B. 1979. *Human Anatomy and Physiology*, ed. 1. Menlo Park, Calif.: Benjamin/Cummings Publishing Co., p. 762.)

REPRODUCTIVE (GENITAL) ORGANS

men   (see Fig. 22–2).

testes (testis)   also called *testicles*; sex glands located in *scrotum*. They form spermatozoa (sex cells) and secrete the hormone *testos*terone.

ducts

epi**did**ymis   at top of each testis; spermatozoa are stored in these ducts.

vas **def**erens   ductus deferens; excretory duct of the testis.

seminal duct   excretory duct of the seminal vesicle.

e**jac**ulatory duct   canal formed by union of ductus deferens and the excretory duct of the seminal vesicle.

u**re**thra   opening for sperm and urine passage.

accessory glands   secrete alkaline secretions that together with sperm make up *seminal fluid*.

prostate gland   surrounds urethra; secretes alkaline fluid that forms part of semen. Tends to enlarge in older men and may block flow of urine.

external genital**ia**   *scrotum* and *penis*.

women   (see Fig. 22–3).

ovaries   sex glands, located in pelvis. They form *ova* (ovum) – sex cells. *Ovu**la**tion* – ovum leaves ovary. Follicles secrete hormones: **es**trogens and *pro**ges**terones*.

ducts   fallopian tubes, where fertilization occurs.

uterus   top part called the fundus; the neck (cervix) opens into the vagina.

vagina   birth canal; vaginal in**tro**itus, entrance to vagina.

Bartholin's glands   accessory mucous glands.

external *gen*itals   organs of generation; *vulva* or *pu**den**dum* (labia maj**or**a and min**or**a).

breasts   lactation controlled by hormones.

MALE REPRODUCTIVE DISORDERS AND SURGICAL PROCEDURES

BPH   benign pros**tat**ic hy**per**trophy.

*cir*cumcision   cutting around head of penis, removing foreskin.

crypt**orch**idism   "hidden testes"; undescended.

epididy**mi**tis   inflammation of epi**did**ymis (ducts where sperm are stored).

*hy*drocele   hernia (of fluid) in testes.

orchi**ec**tomy   castration.

*or*chiopexy   operative transfer of undescended testis into scrotum and suturing it there; also called or**chi**dopexy, **or**chidoplasty, orchi**or**rhaphy.

or**chi**tis   inflammation of testes; may be due to trauma, mumps, or infection elsewhere in body.

prosta**tec**tomy   excision of prostate; may be done in several ways: transu**reth**ral, supra**pub**ic, peri**ne**al.

*var*icocele   varicose veins near testes.

va**sec**tomy   male sterilization procedure.

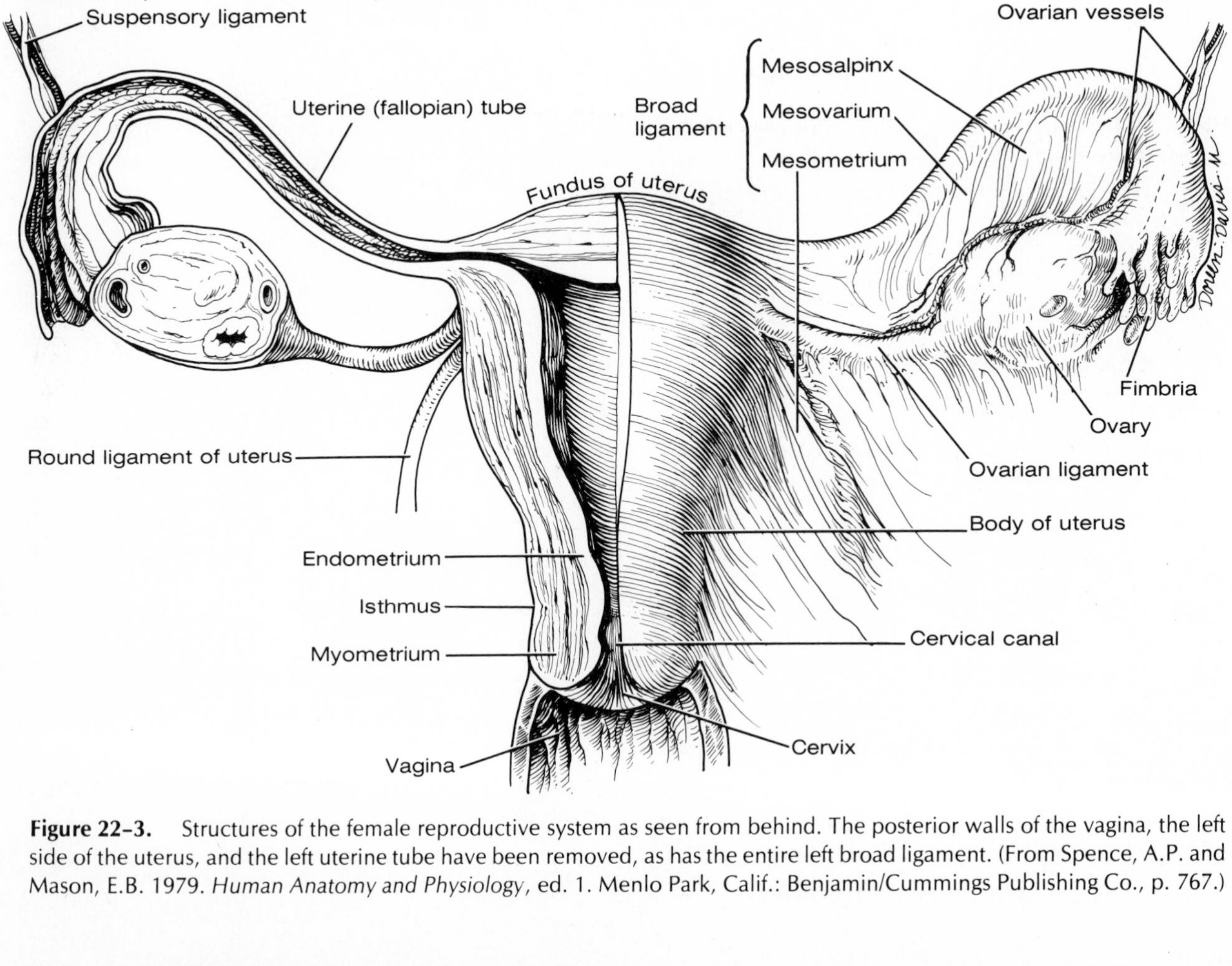

Figure 22–3.   Structures of the female reproductive system as seen from behind. The posterior walls of the vagina, the left side of the uterus, and the left uterine tube have been removed, as has the entire left broad ligament. (From Spence, A.P. and Mason, E.B. 1979. *Human Anatomy and Physiology*, ed. 1. Menlo Park, Calif.: Benjamin/Cummings Publishing Co., p. 767.)

FEMALE REPRODUCTIVE DISORDERS: DIAGNOSTIC AND SURGICAL PROCEDURES

AB (abortion or miscarriage)   interruption of pregnancy before fetus is viable (able to live); spontaneous (as in miscarriage), therapeutic, criminal, threatened; see medical dictionary for other terms.

Bartholin cyst or abscess   inflammation of Bartholin's gland (chronic or acute).

col*por*rhaphy   surgical repair of vagina; also called A & P repair (anteroposterior); to correct cystocele, rectocele.

col*pos*copy   procedure of using **col**poscope for magnified view of the cervix.

cys*tocele   hernia of the bladder.

D & C   dila*ta*tion and curet**tage**; dilating cervix and using a curette to scrape inner surface of uterus; to produce abortion, to diagnose uterine disease, and for incomplete abortion.

endometri*o*sis   cells of the inner lining of uterus spreading into pelvis (peritoneal cavity).

***fi*broids**   benign tumors of uterus.

***fis*tula**   an abnormal passageway, such as a vesicovaginal (between bladder and vagina) or vesicouterine (between bladder and uterus) fistula.

hydro*sal*pinx   fluid collection in tubes, causing distention.

hyste*rec*tomy   excision of uterus; HSO is hysterosalpingo-oophorectomy, excision of all reproductive organs (also called a panhysterectomy).

hysterosal*ping*ogram   "picture" of uterus and tubes to determine whether tubes are **pa**tent (open; pronounced **pay**tent); dye or air may be used.

lapa*ros*copic   sterilization; "band-aid surgery"; patency of tube is destroyed, as in tubal ligation.

leukor*rhe*a   white vaginal discharge.

Marshall Marchetti   surgical repair of cystocele (for stress incontinence).

miscarriage   see abortion.

Mo*nil*ia, moni*li*asis   yeastlike fungous infection (vaginal and other parts of body).

oopho*rec*tomy   excision of ovaries, female castration.

pelvic exam   using **spec**ulum to dilate vagina for inspection of cervix and to take sloughed off cells for Pap (Papanicolaou) smear to detect early carcinoma.

PID   pelvic inflammatory disease, which may cause obstruction of tubes and sterility.

prolapse of uterus   or proci**den**tia; uterus dropping down into vagina.

salpin*gec*tomy   excision of fallopian tube; performed for ectopic pregnancy in tube.

salpin*gi*tis   inflammation of fallopian tube; may cause sterility owing to adhesion formation.

Tricho*mon*as   or trichomon*i*asis; parasite-caused vaginitis, with severe itching and foul discharge.

tubal ligation   "tying" fallopian tubes; sterilization.

vaginal *spec*ulum   see pelvic exam; a dilating instrument.

MALE/FEMALE (ADDITIONAL TERMS PERTINENT TO BOTH SEXES)

***bi*opsy**   tissue obtained for examination, especially the cervix, bladder, prostate, breast.

carci*no*ma   malignant tumor of any of the GU organs, especially cervix, bladder, prostate, breast.

GC smear   test for gonorrhea, a sexually transmitted bacterial disease that may cause sterility; treated with penicillin.

herpes   see STD.

pal*pa*tion   or digital exam; using the hands to feel for ovarian or prostatic hy**per**trophy and breast "lumps."

STD (VD)   sexually transmitted disease; gonorrhea, which may cause sterility; syphilis, which leads to damage of the nervous system if not treated adequately; **her**pes geni**tal**is, which has become prevalent and is not easily treated; some of the vaginal infections and crab lice (pediculosis) are also considered to be STDs.

STS   serological test for syphilis; for example, VDRL (Venereal Disease Research Laboratory), RPR (rapid plasma reagin), Kahn, and so on.

OBSTETRICAL AND NEWBORN TERMS

amniocentesis   taking a sample of amniotic fluid from sac during pregnancy to examine cells for genetic defects.

anesthesia (OB)   regional types (spinal, saddle, caudal); general anesthesia; local, pudendal block.

Apgar (10 points maximum)   numerical expression of the condition of newborn infant; taken at 1 and 5 minutes following birth, maximum 2 points for each: appearance (color); pulse (rate), grimace (response to slap), activity (movement), respirations (breathing, crying, not breathing); for example, Apgar 4–9 (1 and 5 minutes).

BOW   bag of waters (amniotic sac).

bloody show   bloody mucous plug usually passed during late labor.

CPD   cephalopelvic disproportion.

Cesarean (C section)   delivery by an incision into abdomen and uterus.

complications   see placenta and toxemia.

Coombs' test   blood test used to diagnose hemolytic anemias in newborn.

dystocia   difficult labor.

ectopic (extrauterine)   pregnancy outside of the uterus, usually the tube.

episiotomy   incision of perineum to facilitate delivery and avoid laceration (episi/o = vulva).

EDC   estimated date of confinement ("due date").

FHT   fetal heart tones (heard with stethoscope called a fetoscope) or fetal monitoring.

forceps delivery   low-forceps delivery is fairly routine and provides more control; mid- and high-forceps are complicated deliveries.

gestation   period of pregnancy (conception to birth).

gravida   pregnant woman (gravid = pregnant).

ICN   intensive care nursery.

induction   starting labor by artificial means; use of medication to start contractions or by rupturing of membranes.

insemination   impregnating with sperm from mate or donor; "test-tube" baby is a misnomer for procedure in which ovum is taken from ovary and subjected to sperm in a Petri dish; when conception takes place, ovum is implanted in uterus.

LMP   last menstrual period, to determine "due date."

lochia   vaginal discharge following delivery.

meconium   first bowel movement passed by newborn; a black, tarry substance.

multipara   woman who has borne more than one term infant.

neonatal period   first 4 weeks of life.

OB index   Grav, Para, AB, SB (number of pregnancies, term deliveries, abortions, stillborn).

pelvimeter, pelvimetry   instrument to estimate pelvic diameter for delivery (CPD = cephalopelvic disproportion); X-ray pelvimetry and ultrasound are also done.

placenta   the afterbirth; placenta **pre**via and ab**rup**tio placentae are complications of pregnancy (placenta low lying and "coming first" and premature separation of placenta).

postpartum   six-week period following childbirth.

prenatal   before birth; important time for care of pregnant woman, for her and the infant.

primipara   woman who is bearing her first child.

presentation   position infant is in for delivery: vertex is head first (LOA, ROA, left or right occiput anterior; LOP, ROP, left or right occiput posterior); breech is usually buttocks first but may be footling also.

stillborn (sb)   fetus dead at birth.

test-tube baby   see insemination.

toxemia   of pregnancy (also called eclampsia); characterized by hypertension, edema, sudden weight gain; a serious complication that may be fatal to mother and child if not treated.

***tri*mester** three-month periods in pregnancy; first trimester is the period when virus infections such as rubella can produce fetal anomalies.

***ver*nix case*o*sa** "cheesy" white substance on skin of newborn.

SPECIALISTS Male GU patients usually are treated by a urologist; female patients are treated by gynecologists. Nephrologist is another term for urologist and often is combined with internal medicine (internist). Oncologists treat patients with malignancies. Obstetricians care for women during and following pregnancy and deliver the infants. As soon as the infant is born, a pediatrician or neonatologist examines it. Other specialists may be involved as needed, especially neurologists when premature infants are delivered. Many congenital defects are corrected by various surgeons. Midwives may also deliver babies and handle uncomplicated cases.

REPORTS The following reports should be read, preferably aloud. All new or unfamiliar terms should be written and defined.

CASE HISTORY ONE

intravenous pyelogram Examination of the KUB region shows the kidney and psoas muscle shadows to be normal. Serial study after IV administration of contrast medium shows a good nephrogram bilaterally. Prompt excretion of the dye is seen. A normal pelvis and ureters are seen bilaterally. The contour of the bladder is normal. Postvoiding film shows poor emptying of the bladder.

CASE HISTORY TWO

DISCHARGE SUMMARY

This 70-year-old, married, white male entered the hospital with marked lower urinary tract irritative symptoms. Nonfunction of the right kidney was found. A large bladder tumor involving the right side of the bladder was noted, and this was treated with open electroresection. The lesion was definitely stuck on the right side and on histologic examination proved to be grade IV transitional cell carcinoma. Shortly thereafter cobalt therapy was begun on an outpatient basis in this hospital.

Two days prior to admission the patient felt weak and fell down several times the day prior to admission. On the day of admission he had another episode of transient loss of consciousness. After the episodes he felt perfectly well. He was not incontinent and had no convulsive movements or tongue biting (according to the history). The patient had lost 15 pounds with the present illness.

Physical examination on admission revealed a chronically ill appearing man in no acute distress. Heart and lungs were normal. No abdominal masses were palpable. Rectal examination revealed a slightly enlarged prostate. An ill-defined mass was palpable above the prostate on the right. This mass appeared fixed.

Laboratory work: Hgb 9.1, and subsequently 8.2. Hct 30% and subsequently 27%. WBC 10,500 and 13,000. The red cells were described as normochromic and normocytic by the pathologist. Urine contained 15–20 red cells and was loaded with white cells. FBS was 98, 2 hr pp glucose was 138. BUN was 40 and creatinine 2.1. Blood type O positive.

Course in hospital: The patient continued to be unsteady and had difficulty walking and even fell down once. He experienced some diarrhea and nausea, which were controlled with Lomotil and Torecan. Irritative urinary symptoms were present but not troublesome. The patient was continued on AZO Gantanol, which he had taken prior to admission.

Radiotherapy was continued, and two units of whole blood were given. After this the patient did feel stronger and was much steadier on his feet. His Hgb was raised to 10.2 and Hct to 33% with this maneuver. On the twelfth day the radiologist decided to interrupt radiotherapy for a period of a few weeks because of radiation burns to the skin.

The patient was accordingly discharged on that day, to be followed by his urologist and to continue radiotherapy at a later date. Discharge medication included Azo Gantanol and pain medication the patient had at home.

Final diagnosis: Transitional cell carcinoma of the bladder, grade IV, with nonfunctioning right kidney.

CASE HISTORY THREE

DISCHARGE SUMMARY

chief complaint This is the first Duke Hospital admission for a newly born, first of twins, infant admitted for prematurity.

present illness Called to delivery room for first of twins, 1770 g white male product of a 34-week gestation of a 23-year-old, para O-O-O, A positive, STS negative, GC negative, married white female. Pregnancy was complicated by questionable leakage of membranes three days prior to delivery. It was also complicated by premature labor and premature rupture of membranes 16 hours prior to delivery. There was no meconium staining, foul smell, or maternal fever. Labor was spontaneous with an elective low-forceps delivery. Breathing and crying time were stat, with an Apgar of 8–9. Resuscitation given with bulb syringe and oxygen, and the patient was transferred to the ICN.

physical exam Patient is a small, but well-formed, preterm white male infant in no acute distress, active and pink. Pulse 140, resp 56, B/P 42/22, temp 36.1, length 44 cm, weight 1770 g, head circ 30.6 cm. Head: moderate molding. Ears: decreased cartilage. Breast tissue 2–3 mm in diameter. Abdomen: liver down 1.5 cm. Genitals: normal uncircumcised male with testes descended bilaterally; however, right testicle was in the lower part of the canal and not quite in scrotum. The rest of the exam was completely WNL.

accessory laboratory data Venous hct 44%; capillary hct 56%; Dextrostix 90–130; blood gas: pH 7.16, bicarb 21 mEq/L, PCO_2 of 60; gastric aspirate gram stain showed rare polys and no bacteria. CBC: Hgb 15.3; Hct 50%; white cell count 7900; 53 polys; 21 lymphs; 16 monos; 5 eos; 4 stabs; 1 metamyelocyte; 5.8% reticulocytes. Micro chem 12: glucose 130; BUN 9; sodium 140 mEq/L; potassium 5.1 mEq/L; chloride 100 mEq/L; CO_2 of 27 mm/L; total protein 4.4; albumin 2.9; calcium 7.6; phosphorus 5.6; total bilirubin 3.4; direct bilirubin 0.1. Urinalysis was unremarkable; blood type, A negative; direct Coombs, negative.

HOSPITAL COURSE

impression

1. Preterm infant, 34 weeks GA first of twins.
2. Status/post intrapartum hemorrhage, with secondary hypotension, resolved.
3. Hypocalcemia.
4. Metabolic acidosis.
5. Right corneal opacity.

disposition

1. Continue 20 cal Enfamil gavage feedings 45 mL q3h.
2. Neo-Calglucon 250 mg tid po.
3. Sodium bicarbonate 1 mL tid po.
4. Return to special care clinic in one month and be seen by ophthalmology for corneal opacity.

worksheet

Fill in the blank:

1. Name four organs of the urinary system: _____ _____

   _____ _____

2. Incontinent means _____

3. A catheter is used to _____ or to _____

4. Inflammation of the renal pelvis is called _____

5. Cystoscopy means _____

6. D and C stands for _____ _____ _____

   It means _____

   Give two reasons why it may be done: _____

   _____

7. LOA, ROA, LOP, and ROP are abbreviations used to describe vertex _____

8. Four "urine terms" are _____ _____

   _____ — _____

9. Ua means _____ Three tests done in routine Ua are _____

   _____ _____

10. The top part (body) of the uterus is the _____, and the lower (neck) part the

    _____

11. Blood is normally slightly _____ (reaction).

12. Kidney cells are called _____

13. The female sex gland is the _____ The female sex cell is the _____

Define:

14. EDC _____

15. trimester _____

16. ectopic pregnancy _____

17. void _____

18. pudendum _____

19. sperm _____

20. Pap smear or test _____

Give a word for:

21. time when female sex cell leaves ovary _____

22. incision to facilitate vaginal childbirth _____

23. the "afterbirth" _____

24. male sterilization procedure _____

25. abdominal incision and incision into uterus for delivery _____

Use the root word for these and give a complete word:

26. ovaries _____

27. fallopian tubes _____

28. bladder _____

29. prostate _____

30. uterus _____

Give the meaning of:

31. Foley catheter _____

32. LMP (obstetrical term) _____

33. UTI _____

34. cystoscopy _____

35. IVP _____

36. pyuria _____

37. gestation _____

38. Name three urinary tract diseases _____   _____

   _____

39. Diagram KUB:

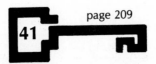

page 209

<h1>chapter 23</h1>
<h1>nervous system</h1>

<h2>outline</h2>

CENTRAL NERVOUS SYSTEM (CNS)   The CNS coordinates and controls all of the body's activities and, together with the endocrine system, helps to maintain homeostasis.

brain   (see Fig. 23–1).

> **cerebrum**   (largest part); *lobes*: frontal, parietal, **tem**poral, and occipital; *function*: consciousness, mental processes, sensations, emotions and voluntary movement.

> **cerebellum**   occupies posterior cranial fossa (shallow depression) behind brain stem; *function*: maintains equilibrium, normal postures, coordination.

> **brain stem**   pons and medulla oblongata. An enlarged extension of the spinal cord. Contains the vital centers: cardiac, vasomotor, and respiratory centers. *Function*: controls rate and strength of heart beat, constriction and dilatation of blood vessels, and rate and depth of respirations.

spinal cord   lies inside the spinal column (vertebral column) from the occipital bone through the foramen **mag**num down to the first lumbar vertebra. *Function*: conducts impulses between the brain and other parts of the body and serves as a center for reflexes.

meninges (singular is **meninx**)   are membranes that cover the spinal cord and brain (see Fig. 23–2).

> **dura mater**   tough outer covering.

> **arachnoid**   middle layer.

> **pia mater**   internal layer, directly covering brain and cord.

cerebrospinal fluid   fluid that circulates around the cord and the brain, in the subarachnoid space (see Fig. 23–1).

AUTONOMIC NERVOUS SYSTEM (PERIPHERAL NERVOUS SYSTEM)

cranial nerves   12 pairs.

1. Olfactory (sense of smell).
2. Optic (vision).
3. Oculomotor (movement of eyes).
4. Trochlear (muscle of eyes).
5. Trigeminal (facial movements).
6. Abducens (eye muscles that turn eye outward).
7. Facial (muscles of face, ears, scalp).
8. Auditory (hearing and equilibrium).
9. Glossopharyngeal (secretion of parotid gland, taste).
10. Pneumogastric, vagus (voice and swallowing).

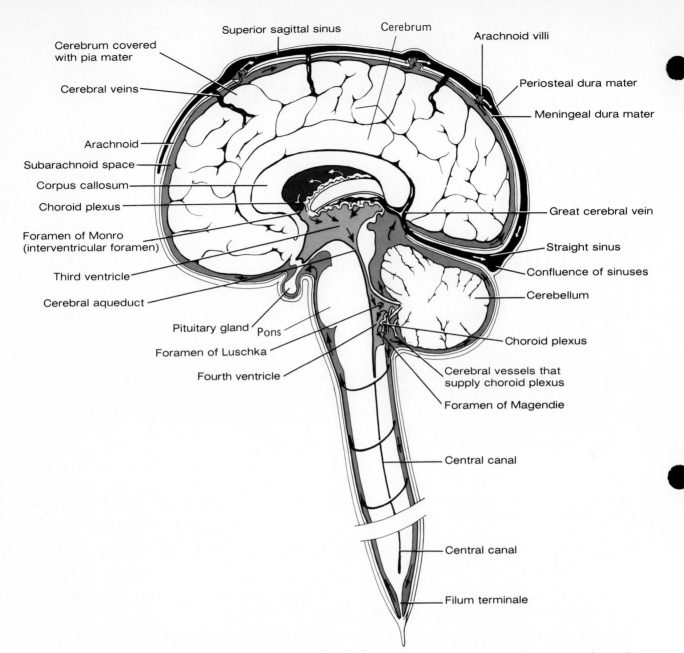

Figure 23-1. The location of the cerebrospinal fluid that surrounds the brain and spinal cord. The arrows indicate the direction of the flow of the fluid. (From Spence, A.P. and Mason, E.B. 1979. *Human Anatomy and Physiology*, ed. 1. Menlo Park, Calif.: Benjamin/Cummings Publishing Co., p. 317.)

11. Spinal (neck muscles).

12. Hypo**glos**sal (tongue).

A crutch to help memorize these: "On old Olympus torrid top, a Finn and German picked some hops." (That is, if you wish to learn them.)

spinal nerves   31 pairs attached to spinal cord. Numbered according to the section of the spinal column; for example, C-1 is first cervical, T-8 is eighth thoracic, and so on. Co is the coccyx.

The autonomic nervous system is called "involuntary" because we do not control it (circulation, for example). It conducts impulses out from the brain stem or spinal cord to smooth muscle, cardiac muscle, and so on. (Autonomic means self-governing.)

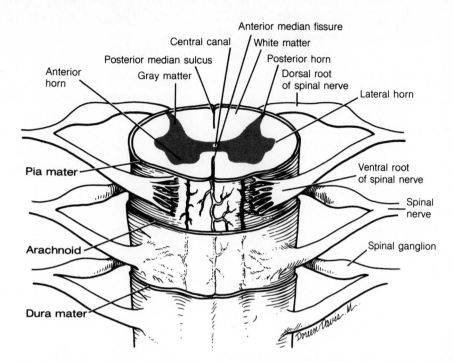

Figure 23-2. The meninges that surround the spinal cord. (From Spence, A.P. and Mason, E.B. 1979. *Human Anatomy and Physiology*, ed. 1. Menlo Park, Calif.: Benjamin/Cummings Publishing Co., p. 323.)

The autonomic nervous system is further divided into two divisions:

sympa*thet*ic   (cell bodies originate in thoraco**lum**bar sections T-1 to L-2) assists the body in emergencies, defense, and survival.

parasympa*thet*ic   (cell bodies originate in cranio**sac**ral sections) brings the body functions back to normal, after the stressful situation has ended.

In general, these two divisions have opposing functions; they are important in maintenance of the body's homeo**stat**ic condition. Following are *some* examples of their action:

Sympathetic (adrenergic nerves)		Parasympathetic (cholinergic nerves)
Constrict	Cerebral arteries	Dilate
Dilate	Pupils	Constrict
Increased	Metabolic rate	No action
Dilate	Bronchi	Constrict
Constrict	Pulmonary arterioles	Dilate
Rate increased	Heart	Rate decreased
Decreased	Stomach/GI motility	Increased

■ **Note:**   Although it has been thought that we have no control over the autonomic functions, experience with bio**feed**back in recent years is changing our attitudes somewhat. It has been shown that blood pressure, body temperature, and some other "involuntary" functions can be altered.

NERVE CELLS (NEURONS)   respond to stimuli (stimulus-response) and specialize in transmitting impulses. Nervous tissue is extremely delicate and is well protected by bones of the cranium and spinal column. Further protection is provided by the membranes (meninges) and the cerebrospinal fluid.

SPECIALISTS   Patients with neurological disorders or injury to the brain or cord are usually treated by neurologists and neurosurgeons. Other involved specialists are internists, radiologists, psychiatrists, and physiatrists.

THE NEUROLOGICAL EXAMINATION

mental status   intellect; **af**fect (mood or emotional state); disordered thought, such as delusions, hallucinations, illusions; insight; consciousness; language function.

cranial nerves   tested separately for taste, touch, temperature, visual acuity, position sense, and so on.

spinal cord and peripheral nerves

1. Motor function: muscles, adequate strength, quick contraction, prompt relaxation; flaccid and spastic paralysis.

2. Sensory function: touch, pain, position, vibration.

3. Complex functions: involved movement, coordination, reflexes (including Babinski), balance (Romberg).

DISEASES, ANOMALIES, TRAUMA

Alzheimer's disease (presenile dementia)   early senility, cause unknown, leading to severe deterioration.

ALS (amyo*troph*ic lateral scle*ro*sis)   progressive disease, cause unknown, starting with loss of coordination and leading to extensive disability.

***ab*scess (brain)**   secondary to infection in body (ear, sinuses, for example).

anen*ceph*aly   congenital absence of brain ("monster"); always die in 1–2 days.

Bell's palsy   paralysis of one side of face, inflammation of seventh cranial nerve.

***cer*ebral palsy**   paralysis resulting from developmental defects or trauma; variety of symptoms; may be spastic, flaccid, athetoid (writhing movements).

CVA (cerebrovascular accident)   any interruption of blood supply to the brain causes brain damage, with resulting neurologic symptoms. (CVA, TIA, and so on are covered in Chapter 19.)

con*cus*sion   usually involves loss of consciousness due to blow to head; there may be damage without loss of consciousness.

con*vul*sion (seizure)   sudden disturbances in mental functions and body movements, some with loss of consciousness.

encepha*li*tis   inflammation of the brain; many types; can be caused by bacterial or viral infection; some types borne by mosquito; can occur following some vaccinations.

***ep*ilepsy**   seizure disorder; may be caused by injury; often the cause is unknown; treated but not cured with medication; grand mal and petit mal are terms to describe type of seizure.

fracture (skull)   usually comminuted with bony fragments in brain, making surgery imperative; trauma to the skull may be due to birth injury, falls or blows to the head, gun shot wounds, and so on.

hema*to*ma   "blood tumor" (clot), may be sub**du**ral, suba**rach**noid, epi**du**ral or intra**cer**ebral; if large enough to cause pressure on brain, it must be removed.

herpes zoster   "shingles": an acute inflammatory reaction in spinal or cranial nerve due to dormant viral infection in body; common in older people and with some carcinoma patients.

hydro*ceph*alus   "water in the head": increased accumulation of CSF in ventricles of the brain; may be due to trauma, tumor, anomaly, or infection; causes mental retardation.

***Hun*tington's chorea**   hereditary disorder; progressive; purposeless movements, constant and uncontrolled, leading to dementia.

***Kor*sakoff's syndrome**   vitamin D deficiency usually secondary to alcoholism; characterized by memory deficits progressing to complete amnesia.

menin*gi*tis   inflammation of meninges due to bacterial, viral, or fungal infection; may be secondary to disease of sinuses, ear, mastoid; aseptic meningitis is a nonpurulent form.

me*nin*gocele (myelome*nin*gocele)   hernia of meninges (and cord) to surface of the back; a congenital anomaly; may be repaired surgically, but some disability will remain.

multiple scle*ro*sis (MS)   brain and cord contain areas of degenerated myelin; symptoms and course of the disease are variable, but visual problems are common; manifested by tremors, slurred speech, eventual disability; no really effective treatment.

neu*rop*athy (neu*ri*tis)   disease of peripheral and cranial nerves; motor, sensory, and reflex impairment.

organic brain syndrome (chronic brain syndrome)   group of symptoms of the senile variety; these diagnoses are used when nothing else "fits," and the patient has brain damage (possibly due to alcoholism or syphilis).

***Par*kinson's disease**   usually occurs after age of 50 years; manifested by expressionless face, slow movement, muscular tremors, stooped posture, shuffling-type gait, rigidity; L-dopa medication is helpful; usually cause is unknown, but occasionally it is a sequel to encephalitis.

poliomye*li*tis   viral infection, affecting all areas of the brain, brain stem, and cord; paralytic type is most severe; prevention is the key with vaccination of the oral type (Sabin).

sci*at*ica   severe pain in the leg along the course of sciatic nerve, felt at back of thigh running down inside of the leg; may be associated with herniated disk.

shunts   types of bypass, via catheter, for drainage of CSF from the ventricles in the brain to the spinal canal or the thoracic cavity; for example, ventriculo**pleur**al, ventriculocistern**os**tomy, ventriculo**at**rial; used in treating hydrocephalus.

spinal cord injuries   compression or transection; inevitably leave permanent dysfunction depending on the level of cord damage; contusion (rapid edematous swelling of cord) *may* leave some residual disability (paraplegia, quadriplegia).

tumors (cord, brain)   benign or malignant, primary or metastatic; may be classified by location, tissue type, or degree of malignancy (grades I to IV); may be intracerebral, extracerebral, intradural, extradural; detailed discussion is beyond the scope of this text. Some common tumors are gli**o**mas (astrocy**to**ma, glioblas**to**ma, oligodendrogli**o**ma, ependy**mo**ma), hemangioblas**to**ma, medulloblas**to**ma, spongioblas**to**ma, meningi**o**ma, neu**ro**mas (schwann**o**ma, neurilem**mo**ma, neurofi**bro**ma, neuri**no**ma). Metastatic lesions often come from lung, breast, prostate. All tumors, benign or malignant, may be lifethreatening because they may be inaccessible surgically.

"whiplash"   imprecise term for injury to cervical vertebrae and adjacent soft tissues (sudden jerking producing hyperextension of neck).

DIAGNOSTIC AND SURGICAL TERMS

***an*giogram (ar*ter*iogram), cerebral**   radiopaque substance injected into arteries in neck, then X-ray films are taken.

Ba*bin*ski's sign   reflex response; when sole of the foot is stroked, big toe turns up instead of down (normal in newborn, but pathologic later on).

brain scan   radioactive element given and later observed in brain tissue.

burr holes   small openings made with a trephine in the bone of the skull to permit access, obtain biopsy, evacuate hematoma, and for insertion of drains or monitoring devices.

cor*dot*omy   cutting of nerve fibers to relieve intractable pain.

crani*ot*omy   incision to gain access to the brain when burr holes are not adequate for the procedure.

EEG (electroen*ceph*alogram)   record of electrical activity of the brain.

EEG (echoen*ceph*alogram)   use of ultrasound to show displacement of brain structures; both EEGs are useful in diagnosis of seizure disorders and in locating area of damage.

laboratory procedures   examination of cerebrospinal fluid (cell counts, cultures, blood, and so on).

lami*nec*tomy   excision of the arches of vertebrae to view spinal cord (discussed in Chapter 18).

lumbar puncture (LP), spinal tap   insertion of needle into subarachnoid space to measure pressure, get lab sample, inject dye for myelography, and administer regional anesthesia.

lumbar sympa*thec*tomy   cutting fibers of sympathetic nerves that contract walls of blood vessels of the lower leg to relieve poor peripheral circulation.

myelogram (myelography) a "picture" produced after the injection of a dye into subarachnoid space to detect tumors or herniated disks.

nerve block injection of anesthetic into nerve to produce loss of sensation.

pneumoencephalogram (PEG) "picture" of brain after air has been injected into subarachnoid space by lumbar puncture; useful in diagnosis of hydrocephalus, tumors, and so on.

rhizotomy cutting roots of spinal nerves to relieve incurable pain.

Romberg test checking balance by having person touch tip of nose with index finger with eyes closed; arms are outstretched with eyes closed; observer watches for "drift."

trephination drilling hole in skull to evacuate clots or inject air for diagnostic procedure.

vagotomy cutting vagus nerve as treatment for peptic ulcer (lessens secretion of hydrochloric acid in stomach).

ventriculography injection of air directly into ventricles when PEG cannot be done because of massive lesion or increased intracranial pressure.

RELATED TERMS

aphasia loss of ability to speak; "without speech."

ataxia lack of muscle coordination.

biofeedback training to develop ability to control autonomic nervous system (B/P, heart rate, and so on).

cauda equina "horse's tail": the end of the spinal cord, the group of nerves that supply the rectal area (below L-2); **cau**dal refers to this area (caudal anesthesia, for example).

comatose in a deep stupor; cannot be aroused.

contrecoup occurring on the opposite side; injury in which brain literally bounces back and forth, causing injury to side opposite the blow to the head.

DTR (deep tendon reflex) body movement at unconscious level.

encephalon the brain.

fissure deep furrow in the brain (fissure has some other meanings).

flaccid flabby; poor muscle tone.

foramen magnum opening in occipital bone through which cord passes.

ganglion a "knot" of many cell bodies outside the cord and brain.

gyrus, gyri (plural) convolutions of the cerebrum.

hemisphere either half of the brain.

ipsilateral on the same side; affecting the same side.

limbic system "edge or border of a part," refers to that part of the brain having to do with emotional behavior and attitudes.

manometer apparatus to measure pressure (of spinal fluid).

myelin white fatty substance that surrounds certain nerve fibers (white matter).

neurilemma (sheath of Schwann) membrane enveloping peripheral nerves.

paralysis inability to use muscles due to nerve damage.

paresis incomplete or partial paralysis.

paresthesia abnormal sensation, such as numbness and tingling without apparent cause; heightened sensitivity; occurs in central and peripheral nerve lesions/disorders.

plexus a network of nerves (or blood vessels).

reflex involuntary response to stimulus.

spastic having forceful uncontrollable contractions.

stimulus anything that brings about a response; an irritant such as a pinprick.

sulcus, sulci (plural) deep furrows in the brain (grooves).

syncope fainting; loss of consciousness.

ventricle (brain)   cavity in the brain; there are four.

SOME PSYCHIATRIC TERMS

af fect   emotional reaction, either inappropriate or completely absent.

aggression   hostile attitude; may be due to insecurity or feeling of inferiority.

am*biv*alence   opposing feelings, such as love and hate.

am*nes*ia   loss of memory.

au tism   complete withdrawal; not able to communicate.

cata*ton*ic   does not talk, move, or react; observed in schizophrenia.

delusion   false belief, such as megalo**man**ia.

de*lir*ium   mental confusion or excitement.

depression   all bodily functions slowed down; lack of hope; ECT may be helpful.

echo*la*lia   repetition of anything that is said instead of answering.

ECT, EST   electroconvulsive (shock) therapy.

hallucination   auditory or visual; hearing or seeing things not really present.

hypo*chon*dria   preoccupation with body; imaginary illnesses.

hys*ter*ia   extremely emotional state; also hysterical blindness, and so on.

involutional melan*cho*lia   mental illness in menopause; depression.

ma*ling*ering   making believe; pretending (to be ill, for example).

manic depressive   major psychosis; periods of elation and profound depression.

megalo*man*ia   delusions of being someone important.

neu*ro*sis   having a feeling of extreme anxiety and sometimes hypochon**dri**asis; person with a neurosis is still in touch with reality.

neuras*then*ia   ill-defined weakness; weak, tired feeling that rest does not alleviate.

***par*anoid**   having feelings of persecution.

pho*bia   exaggerated fear (for example, inability to leave the house); some medical dictionaries list all phobias.

psy*cho*sis   mental illness in which person is out of touch with reality.

REM   rapid eye movements; occur during periods of dreaming.

schizo*phre*nia   major mental illness (several types) affecting usually young people.

(tests)   Bender Visual Motor Gestalt Test, MMPI (Minnesota Multiphasic Personality Inventory), Rorschach Inkblot Test, Stanford-Binet Intelligence Scales, TAT (Thematic Apperception Test), WAIS (Wechsler Adult Intelligence Scale), WISC (Wechsler Intelligence Scale for Children).

■ **Note:**   The term "functional" when referring to mental illness usually means there is no organic cause for it or there is not apparent brain damage present. The term "organic" usually means there *is* brain damage that is causing the symptoms.

Read the following reports and look up any words you do not know. You may also want to look back to the musculoskeletal system in which some neuromuscular disorders are presented.

CASE HISTORY ONE

procedure: skull radiograph   Four views of the skull are obtained. Two burr holes are demonstrated in the left and right frontal parietal regions. Otherwise the bony calvarium is intact. There is no evidence of fracture. No abnormal intracranial calcifications are identified. The sella appears normal.

CASE HISTORY TWO

procedure: cervical spine radiograph   AP, lateral, and oblique views of the cervical spine were obtained. The vertebral bodies and disk spaces appear well maintained. There is no evidence of fracture or dislocation. Minimal degenerative changes are noted.

CASE HISTORY THREE

procedure: myelogram   Contrast was injected into the lumbar subarachnoid space, and appropriate films were obtained. There was excellent demonstration of the lumbar subarachnoid space. Again evident is the left L4–5 extradural defect, as demonstrated on April 18, 1979, showing no appreciable change. There continues to be slight compression of the L5 nerve rootlet on that side. Impingement into the anterior subarachnoid space is observed on the upright cross-table lateral view. Interpretation: L4–5 extradural defect compatible with a disk bulge is observed, as demonstrated previously, with no significant change.

CASE HISTORY FOUR

procedure: brain scan   Neuroanatomic structures reviewed include cerebellar hemispheres; temporal, frontal, parietal, and occipital lobes; brain stem; ventricles; subarachnoid spaces and cisterns. Bilateral parietal bony defects are noted, and subjacent to the left parietal defect the brain is slightly more dense, although there is no contrast enhancement or mass effect. There is a slight widening of the left sylvian fissure and slight reduction in the left temporal density above that region, again subjacent to bone. Ventricles are normal. Midline is undisplaced with minimal widening of cerebral sulci over the convexities. Impression: Minimal left temporal atrophy. Bilateral bony defects consistent with patient's prior surgical history.

CASE HISTORY FIVE

electroencephalogram report   Most of this tracing was obtained while the patient was awake, but there are several periods of drowsiness or light sleep. Dominant rhythms include well-formed symmetrical 9–10 cycle per second alpha rhythm and beta activity, which is usually in the 20–30 cycle per second frequency range. Occasional theta waves are present. There are prominent eye blink artifacts. Hyperventilation produced no significant change. There are no spikes, paroxysms, or persistent asymmetries. Conclusion: normal EEG.

worksheet

Fill in the blank:

1. The cerebrum is the _____ part of the _____

2. The dura mater, arachnoid, and pia mater are _____

3. The cranial nerves for vision are _____; sense of smell _____;

   and hearing _____

4. Write the abbreviation for the fourth thoracic spinal nerve: _____; third cervical

   _____; and first coccygeal _____

5. The bony protection for the brain is the _____ and for the spinal cord _____

   The fluid protection for the brain and cord is _____

6. Neurons are _____ The encephalon is the _____

7. Name two tumors of the nervous system: _____

8. A weakness on one side of the body is called _____

9. Paralysis on one side of the body is called _____

10. Define:

    gyri _____

    sulci _____

    Write the singular form of both: _____   _____

11. Ventricles in the brain are _____; if they are distended, the condition resulting is

    _____

12. A stimulus is followed by a _____ when the nervous system is intact.

13. CSF is obtained by performing a spinal tap, also called a _____

    This fluid may be required for examination for _____ purposes.

14. Caudal anesthesia is injected into _____

15. Meningitis is _____

16. The sympathetic and parasympathetic are divisions of the _____ nervous system.

17. Match the words in the left column with those in the right column.

    a. no speech   _____   shock treatment

    b. flaccid   _____   response

    c. Babinski   _____   hyperextension

    d. craniotomy   _____   convulsion

    e. Romberg   _____   paralysis

    f. myelogram   _____   skull incision

    g. palsy   _____   to view cord

    h. seizure   _____   balance

    i. whiplash   _____   flabby

    j. ipsilateral   _____   aphasic

    k. stimulus   _____   same side

    l. ECT   _____   without cause

    m. functional   _____   foot reflex

18. Name and describe briefly two nervous system conditions not mentioned in this worksheet

    _____

    _____

19. What are the three types of "rhythms" or "waves" mentioned in the EEG report? _____

    _____   _____

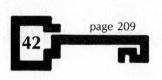

page 209

42

chapter 24
eyes, ears, and teeth

---

outline

EYES   rest in eye sockets; orbital ridge of cranium (eyebrow area).

PARTS OF THE EYE   (see Fig. 24–1).

*scle*ra   outer covering (rear part is the white of the eye; clear front part is the *cor*nea).

conjunc*ti*va   mucous membrane covering of eye; also lines eyelids.

choroid   dark-brown layer between sclera and retina (five layers); it is part of the ***u*vea** (iris, ciliary body, and choroid).

iris   colored band of choroid surrounding the pupil.

pupil   a "hole" in the **iris**; the iris regulates the size of the pupil.

lens   transparent, colorless structure encapsulated and held in place behind the pupil by a ligament attached to the ciliary muscle.

***cil*iary muscle**   changes the shape of the lens when it contracts and relaxes.

a queous humor   watery liquid in anterior chamber in front of the lens; it circulates through the anterior and posterior chambers of the eye.

***vit*reous humor**   jellylike transparent substance inside eyeball.

retina   innermost (third layer of the eye) that receives images formed by the lens; contains sensitive nerve fibers; connected with optic nerve.

Muscles attached to the outside of the eyeball provide eye movements. The optic nerve transmits images to the brain. Lacrimal glands and ducts (tear glands) are located at the outer upper aspect of the eyes (called the lacrimal apparatus).

EYE AND VISION DISORDERS

ambly*o*pia   "lazy eye"; one eye not being used; treatment is by patching the used eye to force use of the lazy eye; if not treated early (preschool), unused eye will lose visual acuity.

a*stig*matism   irregularity of the curvature of the eye (cornea and lens); corrected with lenses.

blepha*ri*tis   inflammation of the eyelids (blephar = eyelids).

blepharop*to*sis   drooping of the upper eyelids.

cat aract   opaque lens (instead of clear); most are of the senile type, especially in diabetics; can also be congenital or a result of trauma. Treatment is surgery to extract lens; this may include intraocular lens implant, or person may wear glasses following surgery.

chal*az*ion ("kalazion")   mei **bo**mian cyst on eyelid (enlarged sebaceous gland); may need surgical removal.

color blindness   most cases are congenital (in males) but can be caused by injury, disease, or drugs; may be limited to red/green only.

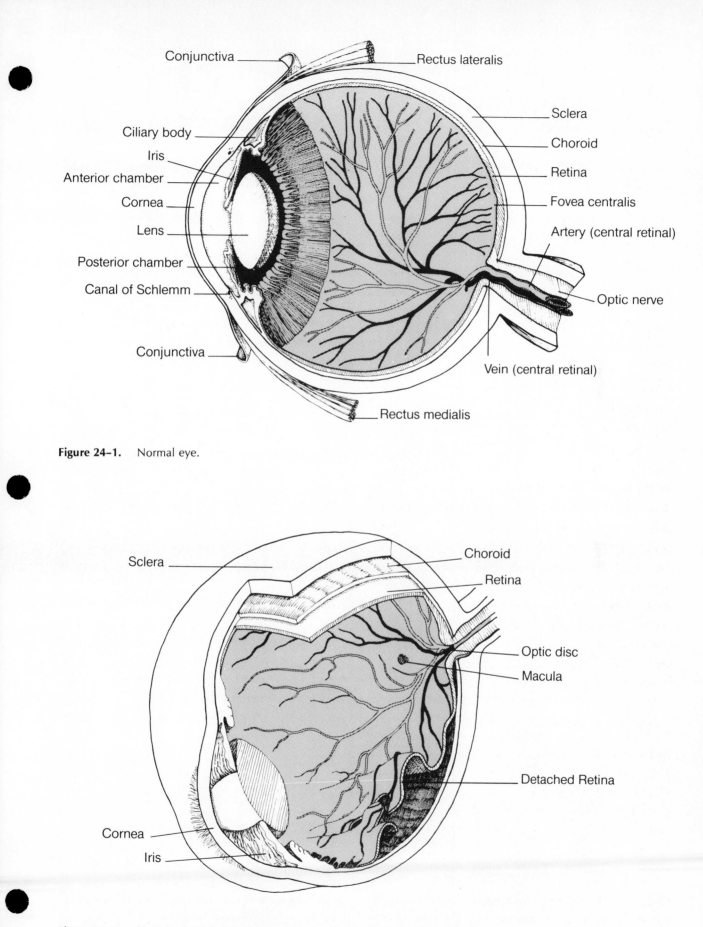

Figure 24–1. Normal eye.

Figure 24–2. Detached retina. (Courtesy of Stanley R. Shorb, M.D., Phoenix, AZ.)

conjuncti*vi*tis   inflamed conjunctiva (membrane covering the front of the eyeball and lining eyelids); acute type called "pink eye"; other types result from irritation from swimming pools and allergies.

corneal ulcer   usually the result of injury or inflammation; contact lenses may also be partial cause.

dacryoade*ni*tis   inflammation of the lacrimal (tear) gland.

dacryocys*ti*tis   inflammation and obstruction of lacrimal sac following nasal trauma, deviated septum, nasal polyps (any prolonged obstruction).

***dac*ryolith**   a "stone" in the lacrimal duct.

detached retina   may be a small detachment or involve almost the entire retina; occurs in myopics frequently; may be the result of injury; treatment is to use a laser to "reattach" (see Fig. 24–2).

"floaters" (in vitreous)   common complaint among older people; bits of protein or cells floating in vitreous fluid that cause visual disturbances; there is no treatment; not considered significant in itself.

foreign bodies in eye   if imbedded they may require surgery; chemicals in the eye should be washed out immediately; safety goggles could prevent many of these types of injuries.

glau*co*ma   increase in intraocular pressure due to closing of canal of Schlemm; fluid cannot circulate, and pressure builds up; usually occurs after age of 40 years and may be asymptomatic; diagnosis is made with ton*om*etry; treated with miotic drugs (pilo**car**pine); several types of surgery are also possible if needed.

herpes zoster (ophthalmic)   involvement of the fifth cranial nerve (face, eye, and nose) with the herpes virus; a serious form of herpes.

hemorrhages (subconjunc*ti*val)   blood under the membrane as a result of injury; can also occur spontaneously; usually resolves itself.

hyper*o*pia   farsightedness; cannot see at close range (to read, for example); see presbyopia.

injuries   foreign body, lacerations, contusions (black eye), and burns.

i*ri*tis   inflammation of the iris; acute or chronic; cause may be unknown but is often associated with rheumatic diseases, diabetes, and trauma; treatment consists of medications and warm compresses.

kerato*co*nus   cone-shaped cornea causing severe myopia; contact lenses may improve vision for a time; corneal transplant is performed when vision deteriorates.

mei*bo*mian cyst   see chalazion.

nys*tag*mus   rapid, side-to-side movement of eyeball (usually due to nervous system or inner ear disturbance).

papille*de*ma   swelling of the optic nerve (choked disk); usual cause is intracranial pressure; can be observed with ophthalmoscope.

presby*o*pia   affliction of older-age people; lens loses elasticity (loss of accommodation); treatment is reading glasses or bifocals (presby = old).

reti*ni*tis   many types, including ac*tin*ic; reti*ni*tis pigmen**to**sa is hereditary; chronic progressive degeneration of retina.

retinoblas*to*ma   malignant gli*o*ma of retina.

retin*op*athies   any disorder of retina; arteriosclerotic, hypertensive, diabetic, solar, syphilitic.

stra*bis*mus   "crossed" eyes; any deviation from normal (convergent or divergent); also called squint; muscle defect that is correctable by surgery with good results.

stye (hor*de*olum)   inflammation of sebaceous gland of eyelid.

tra*cho*ma   chronic infection of conjunctiva and cornea; not common in the United States except in some American Indian populations.

uve*i*tis   inflammation of iris and blood vessels.

SURGICAL AND DIAGNOSTIC EYE TERMS

cataract extraction   with or without intraocular lens implant, the lens is removed surgically; see cryoextraction and phakoemulsification.

cryoextraction   standard procedure requiring a rather large incision where cornea meets sclera (cryo = cold); use of liquid nitrogen, which forms an ice ball attaching the lens to the probe.

cryo*ret*inopexy   fixation of detached retina cold. (Retinopexy also can be done with laser.)

eye muscle surgery   shortening and/or lengthening muscles that regulate eye movement for correction of deviation; such as crossed eyes.

dacryocyst*ot*omy   incision of the lacrimal sac.

enuclea tion   surgical removal of eye.

fund*os*copy, fund*us*copy   examination of the inner eye with ophthalmoscope or funduscope; this examination enables the viewer to see the blood vessels clearly and can aid in early diagnosis of hypertension; if vessels in the eye show damage, it can be assumed other vessels are also suffering damage.

goni*os*copy   using a special optical instrument to inspect the angle of the anterior chamber, useful in diagnosing closed-angle glaucoma.

iri*dec*tomy   excision of part of the iris; one type of surgery used in glaucoma to allow fluid to circulate.

iriden*clei*sis   similar to above (iridectomy); used for glaucoma.

ker atoplasty   corneal transplant (using donor cornea).

laser photocoagu*la*tion   laser produces intense heat; used in treatment of retinal detachment.

pte*ryg*ium surgery   the "p" is silent in this word; growth of conjunctiva over inner portion of eye (an abnormal growth that can be removed surgically).

slit lamp examination   slit lamp produces a narrow beam of high intensity, and a microscope makes it possible to view various parts of the eye.

ton*om*etry (ton*om*eter)   instrument for measuring pressure within eyeball for diagnosing glaucoma before it destroys vision; several types of tonometers are used (Schiötz tonometer is a popular one).

trabecu*lec*tomy   excision of fibrous bands (connective tissue).

vit*rec*tomy   aspiration of vitreous fluid and replacement with saline solution or vitreous to clear opaque vitreous.

RELATED TERMS

accommodation   ability of the eye to adjust to seeing at different distances with ease (near/far).

aniso*cor*ia   unequal pupils

Braille   raised alphabet in books for the blind.

canal of Schlemm   opening through which aqueous humor must flow out, or pressure in eye increases.

cc   with correction (lenses).

can thus, canthi (plural)   corner of the eye; inner and outer canthi.

cry oprobe   surgical instrument used with liquid nitrogen.

cys totome   instrument for cutting anterior lens capsule. Also spelled cystitome.

di*op*ters   unit of measure for lenses.

emme*tro*pia   normal vision.

eye bank   for donor corneas.

fundus   of the eye is the backpart.

***fun*duscope**   spelled with a "u" or an "o" (fundoscope); ophthalmoscope.

guide dogs   formerly called seeing-eye dogs; for the blind.

lacri*ma*tion   production of tears by lacrimal apparatus.

laser   acronym for light amplification by stimulated emission of radiation (if you care to know).

len*som*eter   device for obtaining prescription of eyeglasses.

mi*ot*ic (my*ot*ic)   drug used to contract pupil (either spelling is correct); for example, pilocarpine.

mydri*at*ic   drug that dilates pupil; for example, atropine or cocaine.

OD   right eye (oculus dexter).

OS   left eye (oculus sinister).

OU   both eyes (oculi unitas).

oph*thal*moscope   same as funduscope; instrument for looking into the eye.

peripheral vision vision out to the side (at the outer edges).

PERLA pupils equal, react to light and accommodation; PERRLA (extra "r" means "round").

refractive errors vision disorders that are correctable with lenses.

sc without correction (glasses).

Snellen eye chart with letters, or "illiterate E" chart (for vision screening).

visual acuity (VA) clearness, sharpness of vision.

20/20 vision *not* perfect vision; only means person can see at 20 feet what most people see at 20 feet; a screening term meaning the person is not nearsighted.

SPECIALISTS The ophthalmologist (sometimes called oculist) is the primary person treating eye disorders. In eye surgery they tend to specialize; one does cornea transplants, one does mostly cataracts or detached retina cases, and so on. The optometrist (not a medical doctor) is qualified to fit glasses or contact lenses. The internist may treat some eye infections, and in some cases a neurologist may be involved.

■ **Note:** The three leading causes of blindness are glaucoma, cataract, and trachoma. It is important to have eye examinations regularly (especially after the age of 40 years), as there may be no symptoms with certain eye conditions and only regular testing will help in early diagnosis, thereby saving visual acuity.

EARS (see Fig. 24–3).

external ear **aur**icle, or pinna, and ear canal.

middle ear lined with mucous membrane; three bones: **mal**leus, **in**cus, **sta**pes.

inner ear **ves**tibule, semi**cir**cular canals, and **coch**lea.

tympanic membrane ear drum or my**rin**ga; separates middle ear from external ear.

cerumen wax in ear canal.

eustachian tubes from middle ear to pharynx (throat); equalize pressure.

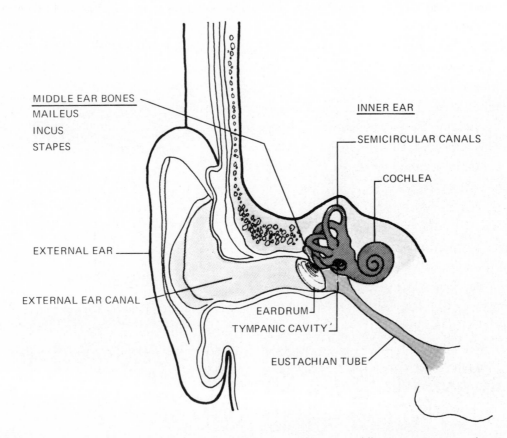

Figure 24–3. Ear, showing outer ear canal, eardrum (tympanic membrane), middle ear, inner ear, and eustachian tube. (Adapted from Sloane, S.B.: The medical word book, Philadelphia, 1973, W.B. Saunders Company.)

EAR DISORDERS

deafness   hearing impairment is the preferred term; hearing loss may be conductive (sound waves cannot be transmitted) or perceptive (nerve damage); causes may include injury, disease, toxic drugs, congenital defects.

eustachian salpin*gi*tis   inflammation of Eustachian tube.

foreign body in ear   such as insects, beans, and so on; insect in ear may be flushed out with oil; in case of beans, peas, and so on never instill water or fluid that would cause the bean to swell.

furuncu*lo*sis   and other skin-type infections can affect ear canal as well.

impacted cerumen   hard, dry wax in outer ear canal.

labyrin*thi*tis   otitis interna; inner ear disturbance.

mastoi*di*tis   inflammation of the mastoid process, which is a process of the temporal bone.

Meniere's disease   or syndrome; cause usually unknown; characterized by tinn**i**tus, dizziness, feeling of pressure in ear; recurrent and progressive.

myrin*gi*tis   inflammation of the ear drum due to infection or trauma.

otitis *me*dia   middle ear inflammation; common infection in children, usually treated with antibiotics.

otitis externa   bacterial, fungal ear canal infection.

otoscle*ro*sis   anky*lo*sis of the stapes (one of the middle ear bones) causing deafness, especially in low tones.

presby*cu*sis   form of nerve deafness in older people.

trauma   cauliflower ear is a neglected hematoma; trauma can occur to any part of the ear as a result of a blow to the head or from inserting objects into the ear.

SURGICAL PROCEDURES

fenes*tra*tion   artificial opening is made to bypass the damaged middle ear, allowing sound waves to pass and reach inner ear (in otosclerosis).

mastoi*dec*tomy   excision of mastoid cells; since the use of antibiotics, this procedure is seldom necessary (ear infections are treated before mastoid is involved).

myrin*got*omy   incision into eardrum; when eardrum is in danger of rupturing spontaneously, this may be done and may include insertion of tube for drainage.

o*toplasty   plastic surgery on the ear (pinna).

stape*dec*tomy   excision of stapes (middle ear bone) to restore hearing; an artificial stapes is inserted.

tympano*plas*ty   plastic surgery on eardrum.

tympa*not*omy   see myringotomy.

RELATED TERMS

acoustic mea*tus   opening or passage in the ear.

AD, AS, AU   right ear, left ear, both ears.

auditory, acoustic   pertaining to the ear or hearing.

audi*om*eter   device for testing hearing.

audi*om*etrist   person who performs hearing tests.

dec*ibel   unit of measure for sound.

electronystag*mog*raphy   method of testing vestibular function by assessing eye motion.

hearing aids   types include bone conduction receiver and air conduction receiver.

hearing-ear dogs   dogs trained to respond to sounds and alert the hearing-impaired person.

o*toscope, o*tos*copy   instrument and procedure for looking into ear.

sign language   use of hands to communicate.

tin*ni*tus   "ringing" and other sounds in the ear.

tuning fork   a forklike steel instrument used in testing hearing.

ver*tigo   sensation of whirling motion, dizziness.

SPECIALISTS   Ear disorders may be treated by an otolaryngologist, an otologist, and an internist. Surgery is done by an otologist, with the use of microscopes (microsurgery) for better visualization of tiny structures.

TEETH

de*cid*uous teeth   deciduous means "falling away"–baby teeth; total of 20, start at 6 months with two lower central incisors.

permanent teeth   total 32, including third molars (wisdom teeth); start at age 6 years.

DENTAL TERMS

***ab*scess**   localized pus collection.

***car*ies**   cavities.

extractions   odontectomy; oral surgery.

gingi*vi*tis   inflammation of the gums (gingivae).

impaction   tooth embedded in the al**ve**olus so that its eruption is prevented; requires extraction.

maloc*clu*sion   poor alignment of teeth, such as overbite.

plaque   buildup of hard material between teeth and around gum line, causing gums to retract and teeth to become loose (also called tartar or calculus).

pyor*rhe*a   pus-pocket formation around tooth; gum disease.

prophy*lac*tic dental care   brushing, flossing, cleaning by dentist or hygienist at regular intervals; fluoride treatments.

restorative dentistry   fillings, inlays, crowns, bridge work, and dentures.

tooth surfaces   buccal (pronounced "buckle"), labial, lingual, mesial, occlusal, proximal, and distal (buccal refers to the cheek; you should be able to figure out the others).

DENTAL PRACTITIONERS

DDS   Doctor of Dental Surgery.

DMD   Doctor of Dental Medicine.

specialists   oral surgeon, ortho**don**tist, pedo**don**tist, perio**don**tist, prostho**don**tist (prosthesis is a "false part," such as dentures).

Dental hygienist

Chairside assistant

Dental laboratory technician   (makes dental appliances).

worksheet

Fill in the blank:

1. Nearsightedness is also called _____

2. The instrument for measuring pressure within the eyeball is the _____

3. The abbreviation for the right eye is _____ for both or each eye _____

   for the left eye _____; for right ear _____

4. The medical term for clouded lens is _____

5. Tear glands and ducts are part of the _____ apparatus.

6. Side vision is called _____

7. The specialist who treats refractive errors with glasses (not an MD) is (a, an) _____

8. Ear wax is also called _____

9. Give two words meaning eardrum _____ _____

10. Inflammation of the middle ear is called _____

11. Tubes from middle ear to pharynx are the _____

12. The machine used to measure hearing ability is the _____

13. _____ is the unit of measure for sound.

14. The nerve to the ear is the _____ nerve.

15. Tartar around teeth is called _____

16. Inflammation of gums may be called _____ or _____

17. Baby teeth are _____ teeth.

18. False teeth are called _____

19. "Any disease" of the retina is called _____

20. Inflammation of the mucous membrane of the eye is called _____

Identify:

21. ophthalmologist _____

22. otologist _____

23. ENT _____

24. DDS _____

25. orthodontist _____

26. periodontist _____

Define:

27. glaucoma _____

28. accommodation _____

29. PERLA _____

30. prophylactic dental care _____

31. papilledema _____

32. restorative dentistry _____

33. caries _____

34. ophthalmoscope _____

35. prosthetic dentistry _____

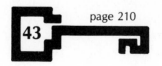

page 210

43

Read the following reports and look up any words you do not know. Write the words and the definitions.

CASE HISTORY ONE

preoperative dx   cataract, right eye.

postoperative dx   same.

operation   cataract extraction, right eye.

description   The right eye was prepared and draped in the usual sterile fashion for ocular surgery and 10 minutes of ocular massage done to soften the eye. Next, lid drapes and speculum were placed, and the intraocular pressure checked and found to be less than 10 mmHg. A superior rectus fixation suture was placed of 4-0* black silk and a fornix-based conjunctival flap prepared. Next, limbal groove was made with a 64 Beaver blade at the surgical limbus and the anterior chamber entered at 12 o'clock with a Sparta blade. A 180-degree corneal scleral section was then done with scissors and two postplaced 10-0 nylon sutures inserted superiorly and looped out of the way. Peripheral iridectomy was done at 2 o'clock with peripheral iridotomy at 10 o'clock. Zolyse was placed into the posterior chamber and irrigated after one minute.

   The cataractous lens was extracted with the Amoils cryophake without difficulty or vitreous loss. The two nylon sutures were drawn up and tied and Miochol and an air bubble placed in the anterior chamber. Next a total of seven more interrupted 10-0 nylon sutures were used to close the wound. An air bubble and balanced salt solution was placed in the anterior chamber and the wound tested for tightness. Finding it to be so, the rectus suture was removed and the conjunctiva repaired with two wing sutures of 8-0 chromic. Atropine 1% drops were placed on the cornea along with some Maxitrol ointment, the eye doubly patched, and the patient returned to the recovery room in good condition. There were no complications.

CASE HISTORY TWO

preoperative dx   chronic erythema and edema with pain of the ear canal skin and drum.

postoperative dx   same as above.

operation   tympanoplasty with resection of canal skin and drum and grafts.

procedure   With appropriate premedication, the patient was taken to the operating room and placed in the supine position and given general endotracheal anesthesia. The left ear was placed uppermost and prepped with Betadine and draped in routine fashion. Inspection disclosed erythema of the handle of the malleus and of the posterior two thirds of the drum, with marked thickening, perhaps three to four times its normal size. The skin also had raised ridges on the posterior quadrant and bleeding of the posterior canal wall.

   A retroauricular incision was made, with deepening to the temporalis fascia, a large segment of which was taken and allowed to dry. The canal skin was elevated from the retroauricular position and then incised at the level of the fibrous annulus and elevated anteriorly. The drum was elevated from the fibrous annulus. The fibrous annulus was allowed to remain intact, and the drum posteriorly was resected to the anterior margin of the handle of the malleus. Care was taken to dissect it cleanly off the malleus by sharp dissection; the lateral process of the malleus was also dissected off. In entry into the mastoid cortex, I found a small black piece of material, which was of undetermined origin, that measured approximately 0.5 cm. It seemed very hard. This may be the foreign body of which he was complaining. It was sent to pathology, and the immediate report was that it was nonspecific material.

   The temporalis fascia segment was rehydrated and placed on a bed of Gelfoam and Hydeltrasol and clipped with Wegner's microclips to the anterior tympanic membrane remnant and led out the posterior canal wall. The posterior skin was then draped over this, and a parachute dressing of Owen's silk was applied through the canal. The retroauricular incision was closed with 4-0 chromic and 6-0 nylon, continuously locked, with a rubber band drain led off the inferior segment of the wound. A mastoid dressing was applied. He was then awakened and returned to the recovery room in good condition.

---

*The zero is referred to as "aught" so in dictation—four aught.

chapter 25
endocrine system

---

outline

FUNCTION   to regulate body activity and, together with the nervous system, help maintain homeostasis.
All of the organs in the endocrine system are glands (see Fig. 25–1). They are called ductless glands because they have no ducts. (A duct is a narrow tube that carries secretions.) *Ductless glands* secrete hormones internally, *directly into the blood stream*, instead of into ducts. Hormones affect many body functions.

Endocrine glands	*location, function*
pi*tu***itary** (**hy***po***physis**; anterior and posterior)	deep in cranial cavity; called master gland, as it affects all others.
***thy*roid** (shaped "like a shield")	aside and in front of larynx (neck); alters metabolic rate and secretes thyroxine (high in iodine).
***par*athyroids** (four)	behind thyroid; regulate calcium and phosphorus content of blood and bones.
a*dre***nals** (cortex, outer; medulla, inner)	one atop each kidney; secrete steroids (corticoids) and help body cope with stress.
***pan*creas**	behind stomach; controls use of sugar and starch. Islands of Langerhans secrete insulin (beta cells).
sex glands (gonads)	ovaries secrete estrogens and progesterone; testes secrete testosterone.
***pin*eal gland**	base of brain (little is known about it).
***thy*mus**	pleural cavity (mediastinum); decreases in size in adult (may have some function in immune responses).

ENDOCRINE DISEASES   occur when a gland secretes too much or too little hormone.

Hypersecretion	*Hyposecretion*
Pituitary	
Acro**meg**aly	Dwarfism (congenital)
Gi**gant**ism	Simmonds' (adults)
Thyroid	
Exoph**thal**mic or toxic goiter (Graves' disease)	Goiter (simple) due to lack of iodine
	Cretinism (children)
	Myxe**de**ma (adults)

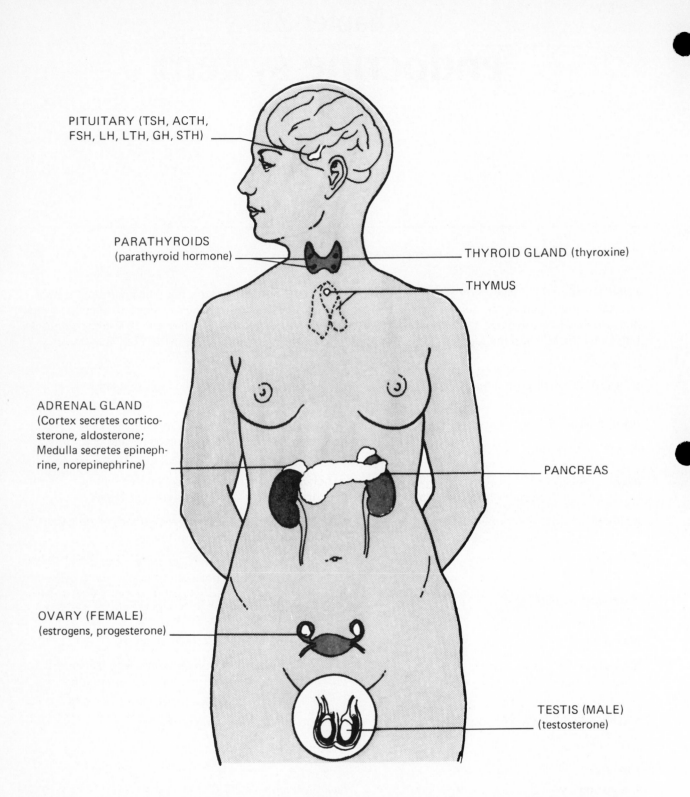

PITUITARY (TSH, ACTH, FSH, LH, LTH, GH, STH)

PARATHYROIDS (parathyroid hormone)

THYROID GLAND (thyroxine)

THYMUS

ADRENAL GLAND (Cortex secretes cortico-sterone, aldosterone; Medulla secretes epineph-rine, norepinephrine)

PANCREAS

OVARY (FEMALE) (estrogens, progesterone)

TESTIS (MALE) (testosterone)

Figure 25–1.   Endocrine glands, small but very important ductless glands that secrete hormones directly into the blood stream. Hormones produced are shown in parentheses. (See abbreviations in Appendix h for Pituitary hormones.)

Parathyroids

    Loss of calcium from bones (increased fragility)   Tetany (low Ca level); neuromuscular hyperexcitability

Adrenals

    Cushing's (cortex hormone)   Addison's disease

    Pheochromocy**to**ma (medulla)

Pancreas

    Hypogly**ce**mia   Dia**be**tes mel**li**tus / **mel**litus (you will hear both pronunciations)

Ovaries and testes

    Overdevelopment of sex characteristics   Inability to carry through a pregnancy

TESTS FOR ENDOCRINE FUNCTION

Blood chemistry tests are done to determine the amount of a particular hormone in a blood sample. Urinalysis (especially 24-hour urine tests) are used in many cases. X-ray examination may be helpful in diagnosing tumors of glands. The most frequently used tests are:

thyroid function studies T_3 and T_4; PBI (protein-bound iodine) and BMR (basal metabolism rate) are older tests (new tests for thyroid function rapidly replace older ones); RAIU (radioactive iodine uptake); thyroid scan; ultrasound (ech**og**raphy); needle biopsy.

pancreatic function studies   GTT (glucose tolerance test), FBS (fasting blood sugar), PP blood (post-prandial, after meal), urinalysis.

MAJOR DISEASES

acro*meg***aly**   enlarged and distorted extremities and face, especially the jaw; monsterlike appearance; partial hypophy**sec**tomy, which may be done "transphenoidally," or radiotherapy are treatments of choice.

Addison's disease   weakness, weight loss, jaundice, hypoglycemia; treatment is with cortisone drugs.

cre*tinism   (in children)   slow, physically and mentally; treatment is with thy**rox**ine.

Cushing's disease   weak, obese, hypertensive, hyperglycemic, moon facies (moon face, edematous); if caused by tumor, treatment is adrenalectomy.

dia*be***tes mel***li***tus**   poly**dip**sia (thirst), poly**u**ria, weakness, and fatigue are early symptoms; see discussion at end of this listing; treatment is with diet, oral hypoglycemic drugs, insulin.

exoph*thal***mic goiter**   (Graves' disease or toxic goiter); swelling of the thyroid gland in neck; tachycardia, weight loss, protruding eyes, diapho**re**sis, shaking, mental symptoms; treatment is with surgery or antithyroid drugs.

goiter   (simple)   caused by lack of iodine in diet; treatment is with iodine, surgery.

myxe*de***ma**   obesity, sluggishness, dry puffy skin due to mucous accumulations under skin; myx/o means mucous; treatment is with thyroxine.

pheochromocy*to***ma**   "pheochromo" means dusky color; a tumor of the adrenal medulla, producing hypertension, weight loss, personality changes, diaphor**e**sis, tachy**car**dia; treatment is with surgery and antihypertensive medications.

Simmonds' disease   exhaustion, emaciation, cachexia; treatment is with various hormones whose release is dependent upon pituitary function because the pituitary is no longer functioning in this disorder.

tetany   severe muscle and nerve weakness causing spasm, twitching, convulsions; opis**thot**onos (severe arching of back type of spasm); treatment is with calcium.

RELATED TERMS

aci*do***sis**   disturbance of acid-base balance; accumulation of acids or excessive loss of bicarbonate (diabetic coma).

ano*rex***ia**   loss of appetite.

cachexia ("kakexia")   a state of malnutrition and wasting, emaciation.

cataract   clouding of the lens of the eye; surgical extraction is the treatment.

convulsions   involuntary muscular contractions.

diaphoresis   excessive perspiring.

emaciation   wasting; extremely thin condition.

gangrene   death of tissue due to inadequate circulation; amputation is the treatment.

gland   any organ that secretes something; glands that are not "endocrine" are "exocrine" (sweat and salivary glands, for example).

oral medications (hypoglycemic)   medications used by some non-insulin-dependent diabetics; these drugs are not insulin; many physicians feel they are not useful (that people who take them would do just as well with diet and exercise alone).

hypophysectomy   excision of pituitary gland, partial usually; may be done through sphenoid (transphenoidal hypophysectomy).

insulin   first produced for commercial use in 1923; an antidiabetic hormone made from a combination of beef and pork sources. Regular insulin is shortacting; Protamine, Zinc and Iletin; NPH Iletin; Lente are names for longer-acting types. Insulin syringes are special types of syringes, U-40, U-80, U-100, for the different concentrations (units) of insulin. A portable insulin pump has become available and can be worn by the diabetic; it delivers a constant supply of insulin to the patient.

ketosis   accumulation of ketone bodies due to incomplete metabolism of fatty acids (consumption of more fat than can be burned completely by the body; the unburned fats produce an acid chemical substance called ketone); excessive ketone produces a form of acidosis in diabetics (vinegary odor to the breath).

neuropathy   "any disease of nerves," observed often in diabetes. Examples are loss of Achilles tendon reflex; sensory disorders, such as increased sensation (hyperesthesia), peculiar sensations (paresthesia), or loss of feeling, especially in lower extremities; footdrop, and so on; impotency; postural hypotension.

MORE ABOUT DIABETES MELLITUS   *the major disease* of this system. There are two major types (and the terminology keeps changing): juvenile-onset (insulin-dependent), in which insulin is not produced, and maturity-onset (non-insulin-dependent) diabetes, in which insulin may be produced, but the body cannot use it. One theory is that interaction between sugar and insulin takes place in cells called insulin receptors. These receptors also attract fat and can only accommodate *fat* or *insulin*. Fat gets to receptors first, and insulin has nowhere to go.

statistics   The life span of diabetics is 30% lower than that of nondiabetics. Diabetes is the leading cause of new cases of blindness (retinopathy and cataract). It is the major cause of kidney disease and neurologic disorders, cardiovascular mortality, peripheral vascular disorders, impotence, nonaccidental amputation, and psychologic damage.

diet, exercise, and normal weight maintenance   These are the important issues in diabetes. This is a chronic, incurable disease; it *can be* controlled in most cases. A "brittle" diabetic is one whose condition is difficult to control.

COMPLICATIONS

	Diabetic coma (not enough insulin)	Insulin shock (too much insulin)
Symptoms	Slow onset, polyuria, thirst, anorexia, nausea, flushed dry skin, abdominal pain, low blood pressure and eyeball tension, air hunger, "sweet" breath	Sudden onset, hunger, nervousness, dizziness, moist pale skin, shallow breathing, mental confusion
Treatment	Insulin	Food, juice, candy
Recovery	Slow	Rapid

Either of the above can proceed to death if not treated in time. Patients who take insulin must learn to recognize early signs and seek necessary treatment.

OTHER COMPLICATIONS (long term)

susceptibility to infection   Even minor lesions can lead to gangrene. Elevated blood glucose makes it difficult for diabetics to heal properly. During pregnancy diabetics are more likely to have problems. (Reread "statistics" for other complications.)

drugs   Insulin (many types) must be injected, *at least* daily, in insulin-dependent patients (more often in some cases). Oral drugs do not replace insulin and can only be used in maturity-onset diabetes. Their use is controversial presently. Some physicians feel that patients who do not require insulin can do just as well with diet and exercise as with the "pills."

insulin pump   This is a new device worn by the patient (attached to belt). It dispenses insulin automatically as the body's need arises. It holds about a 2-week supply.

This report should be read and new words underlined and defined. It is a good example of diabetic complications as well as of eye terminology.

CASE HISTORY

history and physical

present illness   Patient is a 79-year-old diabetic gentleman who underwent cataract surgery to his left eye in 1968 and had excellent vision results recorded recently. Approximately 1 month ago, he lost the vision in his left eye while straining to dig a ditch from his wheelchair. He saw a large red blob with streaks of black in his visual field followed by flashes of light. Since that time he has no clearing evident in his visual acuity, which is obscured by a diagnosed vitreous hemorrhage. He has poor vision in his right eye due to a dense cataract.

past history   Amputations of both legs due to diabetic small vessel disease. Hernia surgery, fractured hip. Medications: 26 U of NPH insulin dialy. Allergies: penicillin. General health: He is an alert, active gentleman considering his advanced years and his disability coincident with the below-the-knee amputations bilaterally.

ocular exam   Vision in the right eye is light perception only due to a dense cataract and what was found on B-scan ultrasonography to be a scatter of intermittent echoes, suggesting vitreous hemorrhaging in the right eye. The left eye had vision of hand motion with light projection into all four quadrants. There is a full superior iridectomy, and the left eye shows no evidence of rubeosis. Intraocular pressures are 18 and 14 in the right and left eyes respectively. Fundus examination of the left eye reveals white stalklike emanating tissue from the region of the optic nerve obscuring all fundus view. The ultrasonography of the left eye reveals multiple linear echoes suggestive of vitreous bands and hemorrhage, but there is no evidence of retinal detachment on the B scan dynamically or in the photographs.

impression   Cataract, right eye, with probably vitreous hemorrhage. Vitreous hemorrhage, left eye. Surgical aphakia, left eye.

The patient is to undergo vitrectomy via the pars plana under general anesthesia February 29. (The pars plana is the thin part of the ciliary body, called the ciliary disk; it connects the choroid and the iris.)

worksheet

Fill in the blank:

1. Hormones are secreted only by _____ glands.

2. Another name for glands of internal secretion or endocrine glands is _____

3. The male hormone is called _____; and female hormones are _____

   and _____

4. Describe the location of the following:

pituitary gland _____

_____

thyroid gland _____

_____

Islands of Langerhans _____

_____

5. Name two tests for thyroid function: _____ _____

6. Name two tests for glucose (blood tests): _____ _____

7. _____ is essential for thyroid function.

8. The hormone secreted by pancreas special cells is _____

9. In diabetic coma, the onset is _____

and the treatment is _____

10. The treatment for insulin shock is _____

11. A goiter is an enlarged _____

12. Sometimes a blood test is done after a meal instead of during fasting. The term for a test done two hours

after eating is _____

13. In endocrine disorders, the gland is usually producing too much or not enough. The words for this are

_____ and _____

14. The pancreas is located _____

15. Excision of the pancreas is called _____

16. Another name for the pituitary is _____

17. In acromegaly (pituitary dysfunction), the _____ are enlarged.

18. Some other diseases of the endocrine system not mentioned in this worksheet are _____

and _____

19. Name the frequent complications in diabetes: _____

_____

20. Define: a. hypophysectomy _____

b. neuropathy _____

c. diaphoresis _____

d. goiter _____

e. tachycardia _____

f. cataract _____

g. anorexia _____

h. cachexia _____

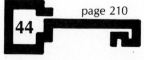

page 210

44

appendix a
answer keys

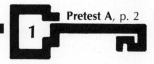

Pretest A, p. 2

1. an instrument for looking at microscopic objects (to magnify size). **2.** excision of the tonsils. **3.** excision of the appendix. **4.** a "break" in a bone (kinds of fractures include simple, compound, greenstick, and comminuted). **5.** inflammation of the skin. **6.** a cut made with a scalpel or knife (for surgical purposes). **7.** womb, female reproductive organ in which embryo develops. **8.** care before birth, during pregnancy. **9.** lung infection; inflammation of the lungs. **10.** free of all contaminants (bacteria, and so on). (We do not usually speak of a person as being sterilized; we say "he is sterile.") **11.** microorganisms; the term "germs" is not a good one because it implies all bacteria are "bad," when in fact many are used in the food industry, and so on. *Pathogenic* bacteria cause disease. **12.** This word literally means "against life." The action of an antibiotic is against the life of the bacteria causing a disease. **13.** Miscarriage and abortion are used interchangeably. When something is aborted, it is not carried to completion; in this case, the fetus. **14.** picture or record produced by an electrocardiograph machine showing electrical impulses of the heart action. **15.** "contagious" disease, or one that is readily passed from one person to another. **16.** infection caused by staphylococcus, a specific type of bacterium. (This organism is capable of causing many different diseases, for example, skin infections and food poisoning.) **17.** throat infection caused by streptococcus, a specific type of bacterium. (Not all sore throats are caused by this organism.) **18.** aspirin. **19.** menstruation.

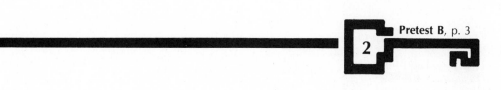

Pretest B, p. 3

1a. study or science of life. **1b.** study or science of microorganisms (bacteria). **1c.** study or science of microorganisms. **1d.** study or science of terms. **2a.** study of body structure. **2b.** study of body function. **2c.** study of the nature and causes of disease; also, condition produced by disease; etiology means study of cause of disease. **3.** heart, arteries, veins, lungs, bronchial tubes, esophagus, stomach, small intestines, large intestines, bladder, liver, and so on. **4.** circulatory, respiratory, digestive, urinary, and so on. (You will learn some other names for some of these systems.) **5.** pediatrician, obstetrician, gynecologist, and so on. **6.** arthritis, pneumonia, bronchitis, diabetes, and so on. **7.** appendectomy, tonsillectomy, hysterectomy, tracheotomy, and so on.

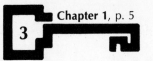

Chapter 1, p. 5

1. a word part, at the beginning of a word (can change the word to opposite meaning). **2.** a word part, at the end of a word. **3.** main part of a word, to which may be added a prefix, a suffix, or another root word. (In medicine, many root words are derived from Latin, Greek, etc.) **4.** two or more root words plus suffix. **5.** root word plus /o used when two or more root words are combined. **6.** before maturity or ahead of time. **7.** excessively active. **8.** study or science of the "mind." **9.** excision of tonsils. **10.** inflammation of the bronchial tubes. **11.** instrument for looking at microscopic objects. **12.** treatment with water. **13.** infection in lungs and bronchial tubes. **14.** pertaining to heart and vessels. **15.** pertaining to stomach and intestines. **16.** "without blood" (low red blood count). **17.** to cut out. **18.** excessive amount of urine. **19.** heart inflammation in sac around heart (peri = around).

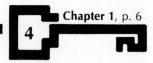

Chapter 1, p. 6

1. excision of the tonsils. **2.** excision of the appendix. **3.** excision of the adenoids. **4.** excision of the thyroid gland. **5.** excision of the spleen. **6.** excision of the uterus (womb). **7.** excision of the gallbladder. **8.** excision of hemorrhoids (commonly called piles), actually are varicose veins at anal opening. **9.** excision of the gums (dental surgery for diseased gums). **10.** removal of breast. **11.** excision of the adrenal gland. **12.** excision of the pancreas. **13.** excision of the colon (large intestine). **14.** excision of a nerve. **15.** excision of the duodenum (first part of small intestine, follows stomach). **16.** excision of the larynx (watch pronunciation: **lar**inks). **17.** excision of the ureter (tubes from kidney to the bladder). **18.** excision of the stomach. **19.** excision of the cervix (of the uterus; extends down into vagina). **20.** excision of the eardrum (tympanum). **21.** excision of the ovary. **22.** excision of the urinary bladder or cystic duct of the gallbladder; can also mean excision of a cyst.

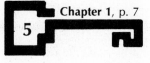

Chapter 1, p. 7

1. tonsillectomy. **2.** adenoidectomy. **3.** thyroidectomy. **4.** adrenalectomy. **5.** appendectomy. **6.** hysterectomy. **7.** hemorrhoidectomy. **8.** colectomy. **9.** laryngectomy. **10.** gastrectomy. **11.** cervicectomy.* **12.** tympanectomy. **13.** cholecystectomy. **14.** cystectomy. **15.** mastectomy. **16.** splenectomy. **17.** neurectomy. **18.** duodenectomy. **19.** odontectomy. **20.** pancreatectomy. **21.** cutting out. **22.** cutting into. **23.** cavity is a hollow space; a body cavity, any space that holds organs (chest cavity, abdominal cavity, cranial cavity). It can also mean a natural body opening, such as the oral cavity (mouth) or the nasal cavity (nose).

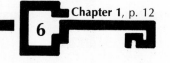

Chapter 1, p. 12

1. adenoidectomy: excision of adenoids. **2.** gingivectomy: excision of gum tissue. **3.** splenectomy: excision of spleen. **4.** gastrectomy: excision of stomach. **5.** cholecystectomy: excision of gallbladder. **6.** laryngectomy: excision of larynx. **7.** lobectomy: excision of lobe of lung. **8.** pancreatectomy: excision of pancreas. **9.** duodenectomy: excision of duodenum. **10.** nephrectomy: excision of kidney. **11.** neurectomy: excision of a nerve. **12.** oophorectomy: excision of an ovary. **13.** thyroidectomy. **14.** adrenalectomy. **15.** hysterectomy. **16.** tonsillectomy. **17.** hemorrhoidectomy. **18.** appendectomy. **Extra:** tonsillectomy and adenoidectomy.

---

* The word *cervix* means neck. The neck of the uterus, or the part that extends down into the vagina, is the cervix. The vertebrae in the neck are also called *cervical* vertebrae.

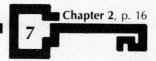

1. new permanent opening into the colon. **2.** new permanent opening into the stomach. **3.** new permanent opening into the ileum. **4.** new permanent opening into the trachea. **5.** new permanent opening into the bladder. **6.** new permanent opening into the intestine. **7.** new permanent opening into the jejunum. **8.** incision into the abdomen. **9.** incision into the trachea.

10. incision into the vein. **11.** incision into the stomach. **12.** incision into the bladder. **13.** incision into a lobe. **14.** herniorrhaphy, nephrorrhaphy, and so on. **15.** nephropexy, salpingopexy, and so on. **16.** rhinoplasty, arthroplasty, and so on. **17.** lithotripsy, neurotripsy, and so on. **18.** abdominocentesis, thoracocentesis, and so on.

1. gastrectomy. **2.** tracheostomy. **3.** cystotomy. **4.** arthroplasty. **5.** nephropexy. **6.** oophorectomy. **7.** neurotripsy. **8.** ileostomy. **9.** colostomy. **10.** cholecystectomy. **11.** thoracocentesis (or thoracentesis). **12.** herniorrhaphy. **13.** arthrocentesis. **14.** appendectomy: excision of appendix. **15.** gastrotomy: incision into stomach. **16.** abdominocentesis: "tapping" of abdomen to remove fluid. **17.** salpingectomy: excision of fallopian tube. **18.** tracheotomy: incision into trachea. **19.** nephropexy: fixation of kidney. **20.** splenectomy: excision of spleen. **21.** gastroduodenostomy: new permanent opening between stomach and duodenum. **22.** herniorrhaphy: repair of a hernia. **23.** hysterectomy: excision of uterus. *Go back and rework drill (p. 13) with root words.*

1. psychosis. **2.** appendicitis. **3.** neuralgia. **4.** cystocele. **5.** adenopathy. **6.** neurosis. **7.** menorrhagia. **8.** dermatitis. **9.** dentalgia. **10.** acidosis. **11.** hysteropathy: any disease of the uterus. **12.** rectocele: hernia of rectum. **13.** myalgia: pain in muscles. **14.** nephrosis: condition of kidneys. **15.** hepatitis: inflammation of the liver. **16.** sclerosis: condition of "hardening." **17.** hemorrhage: heavy, uncontrollable bleeding. **18.** myodynia. **19.** otitis: inflammation of the ear. **20.** nephropathy: any disease of the kidney. **21.** peritonitis: inflammation of peritoneum. **22.** spondylopathy: any disease of vertebrae. **23.** dentodynia: pain in a tooth. **24.** atelectasis: incomplete dilatation of lung (collapse). **25.** redness, heat, swelling, pain.

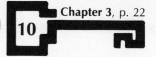

1. aseptic: "without sepsis," or in other words, sterile. (Aseptic technique is used in surgery.) 2. afebrile: "without fever," or normal temperature. 3. anemic: "without blood," condition in which there are not enough red blood cells. 4. arrhythmic: "without rhythm," such as the normal rhythm of the heart beat. 5. adduction: toward the midline of the body; the opposite of abduction. 6. adhesion: a growing together of tissues that should not be connected. 7. abduction: away from the midline of the body. 8. abnormal: away from the "normal"; deviant in some way. 9. anteflexion: bending forward or tipped forward (uterus anteflexed, for example). 10. antibiotic: "against life" of the bacteria; a drug that inhibits or destroys bacterial life. 11. antiseptic: "against sepsis" or contamination; combats contamination or infection. 12. anticonvulsive: "against convulsions," a drug used to inhibit convulsions. 13. antineoplastic: "against" new growths; drug used to treat cancerous growth. 14. contraindicated: "not indicated," not advisable or recommended. (Certain drugs are contraindicated for diabetics, for example.) 15. cytometer: device that counts cells (blood cells). 16. cystocele: hernia or rupture of the bladder;

bladder "dropping down" into vagina in the female. 17. disease: "from ease," or the lack of ease; any abnormal entity. 18. dysuria: painful urination. 19. dysmenorrhea: painful menstruation. 20. dysentery: "painful intestines," severe type of diarrhea. 21. dyspnea: difficult, labored breathing. 22. hemostasis: stopping bleeding or controlling of bleeding, especially in surgery (for example, good hemostasis maintained). 23. hemiplegia: "half paralyzed," one side of body paralyzed. 24. hypertension: high blood pressure. 25. hypertrophy: excessive growth. 26. hypoactive: low activity; sluggishness. 27. hypodermic: under dermis (skin) (as in hypodermic needle, for example). 28. intercostal: between the ribs (for example, intercostal muscles). 29. intramuscular: within a muscle (for example, many medications are injected intramuscularly). 30. intravenous: within the vein. 31. intrathecal: within spinal canal. 32. sepsis: a state of putrefaction (putrid); infected, contaminated, dirty. 33. bladder: any hollow sac, usually holds fluid. 34. hernia: a rupture or swelling; projection of an organ or a part from normal place.

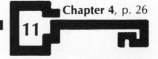

1. otoscope, otoscopy.* 2. gastroscope, gastroscopy. 3. sigmoidoscope, sigmoidoscopy. 4. bronchoscope, bronchoscopy. 5. ophthalmoscope, ophthalmosopy. 6. rectoscope, proctoscope, proctoscopy. 7. anoscope, anoscopy. 8. laparoscope, laparoscopy. 9. adenectomy. 10. appendicitis. 11. cardialgia. 12. cystocele. 13. hysteropathy. 14. otoscope. 15. dermatome. 16. neurosis. 17. cholecystitis. 18. electrocardiograph. 19. myelogram. 20. thyroidectomy. 21. gastroscope. 22. nephritis. 23. cephalalgia. 24. electroencephalogram. 25. bronchoscope. 26. colostomy. 27. pyelogram. 28. gastrectomy (partial or subtotal). 29. hemorrhage: uncontrolled bleeding. 30. angiogram: X-ray film of vessels (after dye is

injected). 31. speculum: dilating instrument. 32. electrocardiography: procedure of taking electrocardiogram. 33. echocardiography: cardiogram produced using ultrasound. 34. ileostomy: new permanent opening into the ileum. 35. ophthalmoscope: instrument for looking into eye. 36. bronchoscopy: procedure of using a bronchoscope. 37. stethoscope: instrument for listening. 38. hemiplegia: one side paralyzed. 39. instrument for dilating the opening of a cavity so that it can be seen. (Since there is no light attached to it, a flashlight or overhead lamp is used.) Examples are the *vaginal speculum*, used for pelvic exam, and the *nasal speculum*, used for examining interior of nostrils.

1. thermometer. 2. adenitis. 3. neuralgia. 4. tonsillectomy. 5. ileostomy. 6. bronchoscopy. 7. electroencephalograph. 8. gastrectomy. 9. arthritis. 10. electrocardiogram. 11. speculum. 12. hysterectomy. 13. cholecystitis. 14. laparotomy. 15. nephrosis. 16. T. 17. F (for looking into the ear). 18. F (of the brain). 19. T. 20. T. 21. T. 22. F (may be external or internal bleeding). 23. T. 24. T. 25. T. 26. instrument

used to make an opening larger. 27. instrument used to dilate a natural body orifice (vagina, anus, ear, nose). 28. instrument used to dilate a stricture (a part that has been closed off). 29. instrument to be introduced into a cavity or to dilate a stricture (to detect a foreign body). **Extra:** -ograph suffix usually refers to a machine; in this word it means the X-ray picture.

---

* Accent is always on os- in oscopy. Pronounce the words in 1–8.

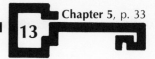

1. internist, pediatrician. 2. gynecologist, internist. 3. urologist, internist, gynecologist (for women). 4. orthopedist. 5. surgeon. 6. allergist, internist, pediatrician. 7. dermatologist, internist, pediatrician. 8. otologist, otorhinolaryngologist, internist, pediatrician. 9. gastroenterologist, internist, pediatrician. 10. endocrinologist, internist, psychiatrist; also new specialty for obesity: bariatrics. 11. ophthalmologist. 12. obstetrician. 13. psychiatrist, internist. 14. cardiologist, internist. 15. internist, orthopedist, gerontologist. 16. internist, endocrinologist. 17. internist, surgeon, oncologist. 18. pediatrician, internist. 19. neurologist, internist. 20. ophthalmologist, neurologist. 21. physician still in training, doing practical work. 22. physician who has completed internship, usually getting more experience and may be working toward a specialty. 23. "one who practices." 24. physician (DO) who attends different kind of medical school than MD student, with more emphasis on the importance of the "skeleton," does some manipulative procedures. 25. A radiologist specializes in X-ray treatment and diagnosis. 26. An internist often treats children. 27. A referral to a medical specialist usually comes from a GP, pediatrician, or other specialist. 28. A variety of practitioners ranging from MDs to naturopaths. 29. hematologist.

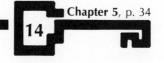

Examples (name any ten): 1. internist, internal medicine: all nonsurgical cases; no obstetrics. 2. orthopedist, orthopedics: skeletal, muscular problems; fractures. 3. obstetrician, obstetrics: prenatal, delivery, postpartum. 4. gynecologist, gynecology: diseases of female reproductive system. 5. urologist, urology: urinary tract; diseases of male reproductive system. 6. cardiologist, cardiology: heart and vessels. 7. endocrinologist, endocrinology: disease of endocrine system; glands. 8. oncologist, oncology: cancerous tumors. 9. pediatrician, pediatrics: children; prevention and treatment of childhood diseases. 10. psychiatrist, psychiatry: mental disorders.* 11. optometrist. 12. chiropractor. 13. podiatrist. 14. psychologist. 15. T. 16. T. 17. F (Although an osteopath does some manipulation, this individual has more education and is qualified to do everything an MD does.) 18. T. 19. T. 20. T. 21. F (There are "doctors" in every field, such as education and business.) 22. T.

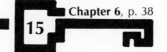

1. without fever (normal temperature). 2. without breathing (periods of no breathing). 3. slow heart beat. 4. rapid heart beat. 5. remove water or fluid. 6. replace fluid (in dehydrated subject). 7. flowing through (of feces). 8. increased output of urine. 9. one side paralyzed (although the prefix hemi- means one half, in this word it always means one side). 10. destruction of blood cells. 11. red color in blood (iron-containing pigment). 12. attraction to members of same sex. 13. condition of staying the same. (That is, the body strives to maintain homeostasis or constancy.) 14. high blood pressure. 15. excessively active. 16. low blood pressure. 17. under the skin (hypodermic injection). 18. treatment with water. 19. "water in the head" (increased amount of cerebrospinal fluid in ventricles of brain). 20. fear of water. (Dog with hydrophobia, or rabies, will not drink.) 21. tumor of fat. 22. excessive amount of urination. 23. many cysts. 24. before surgery. 25. before birth. 26. foreknowledge; prediction of outcome of disease. 27. running before; symptom indicative of approaching disease (pertains to initial stage). 28. following surgery. 29. following childbirth.

---

* There are other possibilities; they should follow this format.

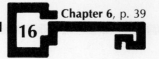

1. without fever (normal temperature). **2.** without fever. **3.** not typical. (Atypical cells are abnormal cells or cells undergoing some changes.) **4.** without a voice; unable to speak. **5.** without breathing; periods of no breathing. **6.** without development (or a wasting away, as with muscles not used). **7.** without feeling (a state produced by anesthetics, used for surgical procedures). **8.** without pain (analgesic drugs relieve pain).

9. without air. (Some bacteria can thrive in anaerobic conditions, without oxygen, such as tetanus.) **10.** without rhythm (cardiac arrhythmia). **11.** without contamination (sterile). **12.** without symptoms. **13.** no menstruation (first sign of pregnancy). **14.** without oxygen or not enough oxygen. **15.** without trauma (injury). **16.** "without eating"; unable to swallow. **17.** without vessels. **18.** without appetite.

1. T. **2.** F (Hemoplegia would be paralyzed blood; hemiplegia means one side paralyzed.) **3.** T. **4.** F (Dyspnea is difficult breathing; apnea is periods of no breathing.) **5.** T. **6.** T. **7.** antihistamine. **8.** hypodermic. **9.** tachycardia. **10.** prenatal. **11.** hemiplegia. **12.** anemia. **13.** without air (oxygen). **14.** without growth (wasting away). **15.** without pain (pain relieving). **16.** remove water. **17.** high blood pressure.

18. treatment with water. **19.** "knowledge before," predicted outcome. **20.** after surgery. **21.** "much urine," excessive urination. **22.** fast heart beat. **23.** "without blood," low red blood count. **24.** running before (early symptoms). **25.** destruction of blood (cells). **26.** excessive heat; raising bodily temperature: to destroy cancer cells before radiation; to kill certain types of bacteria.

1. vertebrae. **2.** ova. **3.** diagnoses. **4.** thrombi. **5.** apices. **6.** enemata. **7.** cocci. **8.** media. **9.** nuclei. **10.** bursae. **11.** bacterium. **12.** datum. **13.** crisis. **14.** prognosis. **15.** uterus. **16.** speculum. **17.** carcinoma. **18.** gingiva. **19.** focus. **20.** appendix.

21. patent, lumen. **22.** perforated. **23.** os, introitus, orifice. **24.** vasoconstriction. **25.** stoma. **26.** vasodilators. **27.** media. **28.** appendices. **29.** cervix. **30.** petechiae.

1. F (The doctor uses a speculum). **2.** F (It is an inflammation of the mouth.) **3.** T. **4.** T. **5.** T. **6.** T. **7.** F (They are bones in palm of the hand.) **8.** T. **9.** F (Excision of the pancreas is pancreatectomy or pancreectomy.) **10.** T. **11.** T. **12.** T. **13.** T. **14.** T. **15.** process of "straightening teeth," treating malocclusion. **16.** plastic surgery on the nose. **17.** incision of the ear drum (tympanic membrane). **18.** surgical puncture of

the chest (tapping) to remove fluid. **19.** inflammation of the ureter. **20.** excision of the ovary. **21.** incision into the abdomen. **22.** inflammation of the pleural membrane (chest). **23.** instrument for measuring pelvis. **24.** above pubes. **25.** inflammation of cartilage. **26.** cervical. **27.** thoracic or dorsal. **28.** lumbar. **29.** sacral. **30.** coccygeal.

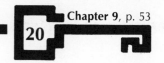

The -oma words are difficult, as are their definitions; do not concern yourself too much with the exact meanings. Just remember that -oma is a new growth or tumor that serves no useful purpose.

1. tumor of a gland (epithelial tissue). **2.** cancerous tumor. **3.** tumor of fibrous (connective) tissue. **4.** tumor of glia cell (nerve cell). **5.** tumor of liver. **6.** lymph tissue tumor. **7.** granulation tissue tumor (at site of injury or ulcer) **8.** tumor originating in bone marrow (malignant). **9.** tumor in muscle tissue. **10.** malignant tumor in connective tissue (cancer). **11.** blood tumor (clot). **12.** increased pressure in eyeball. (Literal meaning is "gray swelling"; this is not really a tumor.) **13.** difficult or labored breathing. **14.** no breathing; patients sometimes have short periods of apnea. **15.** able to breathe only when sitting upright (usually with trunk of body resting on overbed table, and so on). **16.** rapid breathing. **17.** slow breathing.

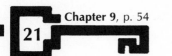

1. lipoma. **2.** hematoma. **3.** mucoid. **4.** hypertrophied. **5.** dyspnea. **6.** tachypnea. **7.** hemiplegia. **8.** paraplegia. **9.** pyorrhea. **10.** diarrhea. **11.** osteomalacia. **12.** hemolysis. **13.** carcinoma, sarcoma. **14.** apneic. **15.** orthopneic. **16.** the same throughout; particles dispersed evenly. **17.** all four limbs paralyzed. **18.** resembling fat. **19.** unit of heredity. **20.** one-sided weakness. **21.** organs of reproduction. **22.** tumor of gland. **23.** inflammation of the lungs. **24.** overgrowth of cells. **25.** disease producing. **26.** yes. **27.** in position; not spread to surrounding tissue. **28.** metastatic cancer spread from another site. **29.** new growth; tumor.

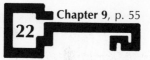

1. inflammation of skin of extremities. **2.** pointed head. **3.** living in presence of oxygen. **4.** living without oxygen. **5.** condition of cells of unequal size. **6.** difficult labor. **7.** exaggerated feeling of depression. **8.** easy labor. **9.** exaggerated feeling of well being. **10.** easy death. **11.** attraction to those of opposite sex. **12.** of unlike natures; composed of unlike substances. **13.** attraction to those of same sex. **14.** uniform in structure, composition or nature. **15.** condition of cells being equal in size. **16.** same tension or tone; isotonic solution: one that contains same salt concentration as body fluids. **17.** equal temperature. **18.** ill at ease. **19.** poorly aligned; not coming together evenly. **20.** enlarged extremities. **21.** enlarged heart. **22.** cessation of menstruation. **23.** painful menstruation. **24.** voiding during the night (*not bedwetting*). **25.** epidemic of great proportions; world-wide. **26.** pus exuding from; pyogenic lesion produces pus. **27.** flow of pus; in common usage, pus from the gums. **28.** group of symptoms characteristic of a certain disease; for example, carpal tunnel (wrist), shoulder hand (shoulder).

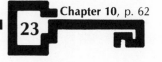

1. e**ryth**rocyte. **2.** cya**no**sis. **3.** mela**no**ma. **4.** leu**ke**mia. **5.** carci**no**ma. **6.** hydro**ther**apy. **7.** li**po**ma. **8.** throm**bo**sis. **9.** pa**thol**ogy. **10.** staphylo**coc**ci. **11.** strepto**coc**ci. **12.** ba**cil**li. **13.** woman having her first child. **14.** injury, physical or emotional. **15.** hardening of the arteries. **16.** control of bleeding. **17.** gallstones (condition of); -iasis similar to -osis. **18.** condition of "dead tissue." **19.** heating through. **20.** without feeling or sensation. **21.** study or science dealing with the blood. **22.** urine in the blood (components of urine in the blood stream, due to kidney malfunction). **23.** woman who has been pregnant three times, has had two full-term births. **24.** T. **25.** T. **26.** T.

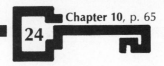

1. white blood cell. **2.** condition of "eating cells" (cells that engulf bacteria, and so on). **3.** mental illness, "split personality." **4.** treatment with water. **5.** control of bleeding. **6.** paralysis of *one side* of the body. **7.** "without blood," condition in which red blood count is low. **8.** urine components in the blood. **9.** mania in which person has highly inflated opinion of self. **10.** study or science dealing with the blood. **11.** cancerous or malignant tumor. **12.** nearsightedness. **13.** spasm of a nerve. **14.** enlarged colon. **15.** blood in the urine. **16.** prog**no**sis: predicted outcome of a disease. **17.** he**mol**ysis: destruction of blood (cells). **18.** di**plo**pia: "double vision," seeing double.

19. diag**no**sis: "knowing through," studying symptoms and arriving at decision. **20.** hysteror**rhex**is: rupture of the uterus (breaking open). **21.** patho**gen**ic: from which disease arises, disease causing. **22.** syn**drome**: "running together," symptoms that occur together and characterize a certain disease condition. **23.** **coc**ci: round bacteria. **24.** **he**moglobin: a protein in red blood cells; it carries oxygen. **25.** noct**u**ria: urinating during the night; *not* bedwetting. **26.** mul**tip**ara: woman who has borne more than one child. **27.** throm**bo**sis: condition of clotting (in blood vessels). **28.** e**ryth**rocyte: red (blood) cell. **29.** gravid: pregnant. **30.** staphylo**coc**cus: round bacteria growing in cluster formation.

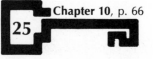

1. diagnosis, symptoms. **2.** streptococcus. **3.** antibiotic. **4.** prognosis. **5.** myopia, cannot. **6.** hydrotherapy, diathermy, cryotherapy. **7.** leukocytes, erythrocytes. **8.** WBC, RBC. **9.** pathogens, cocci, bacilli.

10. primipara. **11.** five pregnancies, two term births. **12.** preoperative (preop), anesthetic, postoperative (postop).

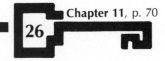

1. movement away from midline (of body); think of kidnapping. **2.** movement toward midline. **3.** "cutting around" penis (foreskin). **4.** not indicated (certain drugs not indicated in pregnancy, for example). **5.** arising from outside (body). **6.** same as 5. **7.** out of place, as a pregnancy outside uterus. **8.** secreting externally through a duct. **9.** secreting internally directly into bloodstream. **10.** arising from within. **11.** scope for looking inside body. **12.** area over the stomach. **13.** outside the uterus (same as ectopic). **14.** below the sternum. **15.** below normal. **16.** on the same side. **17.** in the middle of the sternum. **18.** suturing of

mesentery. **19.** spread of cancer cells (change or transformation). **20.** tissue change; conversion of food to heat and energy. **21.** "beyond ankle" (bones of the foot). **22.** "near or beside" medical. **23.** similar to typhoid. **24.** two like parts paralyzed (lower extremities). **25.** around the teeth (gums). **26.** around tonsils. **27.** around the heart. **28.** around the "wastes" (between genitals and rectum). **29.** behind the peritoneum. **30.** turned backward. **31.** through, or by way of, the urethra. **32.** through, or by way of, the vagina (normal delivery).

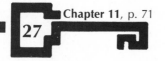

1. standing. **2.** bending. **3.** lying. **4.** straightening. **5.** distal; lateral; bilateral. **6.** lying. **7.** cephalic; caudal. **8.** lithotomy. **9.** inside; outside. **10.** anteroposterior; posteroanterior, and left lateral of chest (X-ray pictures taken from front to back; from back to front, and from left side). **11.** T. **12.** T. **13.** F (Caudal

anesthesia is injected into the tail end of the spinal cavity.) **14.** T. **15.** T. **16.** F (In the peritoneal cavity, not perineum; perineum is area between anus and vulva.) **17.** T. **18.** T. **19.** F (Hemiplegia is paralysis on one side; paraplegia involves lower half of the body.) **20.** T. **21.** T. **22.** T. **23.** T. **24.** T.

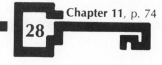
1. addicted. **2.** abduction. **3.** ectogenous. **4.** ectopic. **5.** retroperitoneal. **6.** transurethral. **7.** quadrants. **8.** ambivalence. **9.** tricuspid. **10.** lithotomy. **11.** bilateral. **12.** bilateral. **13.** partially in a coma. **14.** woman who has borne more than one child. **15.** double vision. **16.** over the stomach. **17.** arising from within the organism (body). **18.** toward the midline. **19.** below the sternum. **20.** "around the wastes," area between anus and vulva. **21.** on left side, left knee flexed. **22.** one side. **23.** "around the teeth," gums. **24.** bending. **25.** coccus, round bacteria found in pairs. **26.** OD; grain; g.* **27.** cc; +; mg.* **28.** AP.

Chapter 12, p.78

29

1. termination of pregnancy before fetus is viable. **2.** area of body from below ribs to pubis. **3.** from below ribs (adjective). **4.** localized collection of pus. **5.** sudden, severe, usually not long-lasting (disease). **6.** growing together (tissues adhering where they should not). **7.** accessory parts of a structure, for example, adnexa uteri. **8.** process of listening for sounds (see no. 43). **9.** instrument for sterilizing (steam under pressure). **10.** armpit. **11.** abnormality. **12.** examination of live tissue. **13.** suture material. **14.** a tube, usually for withdrawing fluid, such as that for withdrawing urine from the bladder. **15.** pertaining to the neck, for example, cervical vertebrae (neck area); also, cervix of the uterus. **16.** long-lasting, usually not curable, disease. **17.** type of suture material; chromic catgut. **18.** tail bone. **19.** present at birth (born with). **20.** process of stretching or opening up. **21.** edema: fluid in body tissues (leaves a "pit" with pressure); ascites: fluid in peritoneal cavity; anasarca: generalized, severe edema; dropsy: an obsolete term for edema. **22.** blood clot, floating freely in blood stream. **23.** vomiting. **24.** introduction of fluid into rectum (for cleansing purposes, for example). **25.** waste matter, elimination. **26.** recurrence or flare-up of symptoms after period of remission. **27.** connective tissue (supports and separates muscles). **28.** feverish; elevated temperature. **29.** quivering type of heart beat; ineffective in pumping blood; restore rhythm (defibrillation). **30.** profuse bleeding, internal or external. **31.** jaundice: pigment coloring skin and membranes. **32.** preventive measure to prevent disease. **33.** inability to control urination (and bowels). **34.** tissue reaction to injury: signs are redness, heat, swelling, pain (loss of function possible). **35.** insufficient supply of blood; for example, ischemic area. **36.** yellowing of skin, whites of eyes, membranes, body fluids due to bile pigment resulting from excessive bilirubin (pigment in bile) in the blood. It is a symptom, not a disease. Coomb's: test to diagnose hemolytic anemias. **37.** spread to other parts of the body, especially cancer cells. **38.** thick, slippery substance secreted by mucous membranes. mucous (adjective); mucosa=mucous membrane. **39.** fat, excessive overweight. **40.** able to be felt. **41.** inability to move a part (usually caused by nerve damage). **42.** forming the wall of a cavity; for example, parietal pleura. **43.** tapping to produce sounds (percussion and auscultation or P and A). **44.** area between anus and genitals. **45.** membranous lining of abdominopelvic cavity (peritoneal cavity). **46.** membranous lining of chest cavity (pleural cavity). **47.** dropping down, out of place; for example, prolapsed uterus (dropping into vagina). **48.** preventive measure; for example, prophylactic dental care—brushing and cleaning, fluoride treatment. **49.** full of pus, producing pus. **50.** period when symptoms disappear temporarily. **51.** acute and chronic condition, sore stiff muscles. **52.** having the nature of serum; membrane that produces serumlike substance. **53.** secretion from deep down in bronchial tubes (not saliva). **54.** material used to stitch up incisions or injuries; also suture lines in cranium. **55.** infectious agent, smaller than bacteria. **56.** abdominal organs. **57.** to empty bladder; urinate.

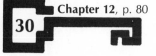

Chapter 12, p. 80

30

1. F (It is an acute disease.) **2.** T. **3.** F (It is one a person is born with.) **4.** T. **5.** F (An incontinent person is one who canot control voiding.) **6.** T. **7.** T. **8.** T. **9.** F (A **bi**opsy is the examination of *live* tissue.) **10.** T. **11.** emesis. **12.** edema, ascites, anasarca. **13.** enema. **14.** axilla. **15.** inflammation. **16.** abdominal. **17.** sputum. **18.** embolism. **19.** viscera. **20.** immunization. **21.** emptied (bladder). **22.** pus producing, draining. **23.** sagging, dropped down. **24.** able to be felt. **25.** prevention. **26.** excessive fluid in peritoneal cavity. **27.** severe, generalized edema. (28–32 may be listed in any order) **28.** diphtheria, pertussis, tetanus: DPT (Pertussis is whooping cough.) **29.** rubeola (hard measles). **30.** rubella (German or three-day measles). **31.** poliomyelitis. **32.** parotitis (mumps). **33.** influenza, pneumonia; typhoid.

---

*Still used, but obsolete, are the following abbreviations: grain=gr; gram=gm or Gm; milligram=mgm.

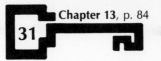

1. 600,000 units intramuscularly every eight hours. **2.** 30 milligrams by mouth every four hours, as needed-for headache. **3.** grains 1½ at bedtime as needed. **4.** 100 milligrams by mouth, at bedtime. **5.** nothing by mouth after midnight. **6.** 1000 cubic centimeters of 5% glucose in distilled water, intravenously, immediately. **7.** twice a day, out of bed. **8.** give patient plenty to drink; keep record of intake and output. **9.** tid. **10.** gr. **11.** g. **12.** c̄. **13.** ƺ. **14.** dc. **15.** H₂O. **16.** O₂. **17.** ac.

18. BRP (bathroom privileges). **19.** GI. **20.** ss̄. **21.** intravenous pyelogram. **22.** 4 times a day. **23.** units. **24.** quantity not sufficient. **25.** suppository. **26.** normal saline. **27.** tender loving care. **28.** intravenously. **29.** electrocardiogram. **30.** temperature, pulse, respirations. **31.** temperature, pulse, respirations, B/P. **32.** computerized axial tomography: series of "pictures"; more detailed information than from X-ray films. **Extra:** See note No. 3, p. 83.

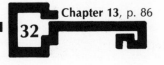
Chapter 13, p. 86
32

1. ER or A & D. **2.** OR, RR, surg. **3.** X-ray. **4.** ER or OPD. **5.** CCU or ICU. **6.** OB, labor, nursery, postpartum ward. **7.** peds. **8.** CS. **9.** lab. **10.** PT. **11.** MR.

12. morgue. **13.** SS. **14.** NP. **15.** ENT or MOR. **16.** OT or PM & R. **17.** CS.

What other departments can you think of? _____

_____

_____

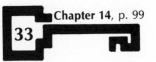
Chapter 14, p. 99
33

1. complete blood count (per cubic millimeter). **2.** white blood count (per cubic millimeter). **3.** red blood count (per cubic millimeter). **4.** hemoglobin (the red coloring in the blood). **5.** hematocrit (volume of red cells in a sample of blood). **6.** fasting blood sugar. **7.** Diff stands for differential, and it means counting each of the different kinds of leukocytes or white blood cells in a blood sample. **8.** *neutrophils, eosinophils, basophils,* lymphocytes, monocytes. (These *leukocytes* are named by the kind of dye they "take." Phil means "to love." Eosin is a kind of acid dye. Eosinophils "love" it. Basophils "love" basic dyes. Neutrophils take "neutral" dye.) **9.** numbers of cells, size, and shape (in other words, how many, how big, and how they look); hematology. **10.** reaction, specific gravity, test for glucose, albumin, and microscopic findings. **11.** Voided specimen is passed by patient, normally. A catheterized specimen is obtained with a sterile catheter after patient has been washed; so a catheterized specimen is cleaner, less likely to be contaminated, and thus more useful for a test. (This is especially true in the female. Any vaginal discharge will contaminate the specimen, and if the patient is menstruating, it is difficult to get a clean urine specimen.) **12.** serology (VDRL, Venereal Disease Research Laboratories test for syphilis). **13.** bacteriology; C & S (culture and sensitivity). **14.** test to detect abnormal (cancer) cells; taken from the cervix of the uterus with a swab or stick; cytology division. **15.** Examination of *live* tissue; a frozen section. **16.** See pp. 89–90. **17.** Fasting means not eating; a fasting blood sugar is taken before breakfast, and the patient has been on NPO since midnight. **18.** PMNs, segs. **19.** monos, eos, basos. **20.** enzyme. **21.** 11–16 g/dL.

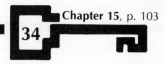

1. *Physician's Desk Reference*: a comprehensive book published yearly, listing all prescription drugs by brand or trade name, generic name (and chemical name) and showing which drug company produces each. Also explains the use of each drug, giving side effects, contraindications, and dosage recommended, among other things. **2.** over the counter: refers to any drug that may be purchased without a prescription. **3.** prescription, recipe; "take." **4a.** increases urinary output. **4b.** relieves pain. **4c.** reduces or relieves nasal congestion. **5.** Generic refers to the chemistry of the drug; the brand name is one chosen by a drug company for its product that falls in a certain generic class. There are many brand name drugs for every generic drug, and prices vary considerably. The pharmacist may substitute the most reasonable buy for the patient if the physician orders specifically by the generic name. He may *not* substitute a generic for a brand name drug. **6.** A drug salesman, representing a certain drug company. **7.** T. **8.** F (All drugs have an expiration date and should be discarded after that date.) **9.** F (Most medical dictionary listings do not contain drugs. The **PDR** is the best reference to use.) **10.** T. **11.** T. **12.** You have probably heard of Darvon, Seconal sodium, Premarin, and others. Examples of classifications are antipruritics, antineoplastics, cardiovascular preparations, antinauseants, anti-inflammatory drugs, hemorrhoid preparations, and so on. *You* write the examples. **13.** A prescription usually reads as follows: Rx: Darvon Compound, 32 mg, Cap T tid prn, for pain **14.** Some words that appear frequently are anorexia, nausea, vomiting, diarrhea, alopecia, thrombocytopenia, pruritus, myelosuppression, idiosyncrasies.

1. peritoneal cavity; thoracic, pleural cavity. **2.** cranial cavity. **3.** cell. **4.** nucleus, cytoplasm or protoplasm, and cell membrane; genes are in the chromosomes (in the nucleus). **5.** cardiovascular. **6.** musculoskeletal. **7.** respiratory. **8.** gastrointestinal. **9.** musculoskeletal. **10.** endocrine. **11.** nervous. **12.** genitourinary. **13.** genitourinary and endocrine. **14.** integumentary. **15.** genitourinary and endocrine. **16.** epithelial, connective, muscle, and nervous. **17.** group, organs. **18.** absorption, storage, and use of foods for growth and repair of tissue, production of energy, elimination of wastes. **19.** tissues. **20.** muscle (dome shaped). **21a.** divides body into equal right and left sides. **21b.** divides body into anterior and posterior. **21c.** divides body into superior and inferior. **22.** cell division (means of multiplying). **23.** legs. **24.** striped (this is voluntary muscle or skeletal muscle). **25.** release of a substance. **26.** taking in. **27.** process of excreting or expelling. **28.** study of diseases; diseased state. **29.** state of constancy.

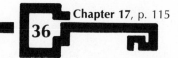

1. dermatologist. **2.** protection, receptor, temperature regulator, excretion (any two answers would be sufficient). **3.** epidermis. **4.** sudoriferous. **5.** sebaceous. **6.** impetigo, scabies, psoriasis, and so on. **7.** corium; blood vessels, nerves, sweat and oil glands. **8.** herpes simplex. **9.** contact dermatitis, eczema, neurodermatitis. **10.** paronychia. **11.** Mantoux: tuberculosis; Dick: susceptibility to scarlet fever; and so on. **12.** T. **13.** T. **14.** T. **15.** T. **16.** F (A vesicle is a blister.) **17.** T. **18.** F (It is a loss of pigment and is not infectious.) **19.** dermatome. **20.** urticaria. **21.** nevi; mole. **22.** erythema. **23.** syphilis, measles (rubeola), varicella (chickenpox). **24.** louse. **25.** acne vulgaris. **26.** papule, macule, bulla, and so on.

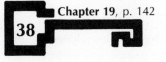

1. cranium. 2. sinuses. 3. sutures. 4. fontanels. 5. cervical, thoracic, lumbar, sacral, coccygeal. 6. movement toward the midline. 7. connective fibrous tissue holding one bone to another. 8. connective fibrous tissue holding muscle to bone. 9. small sac filled with fluid, at joints to cushion them. 10. greenstick: bone broken, but not separated; simple: bone broken, not protruding through skin; compound: bone broken and piercing through skin. 11. orthopedist, osteopath, chiropractor. 12. straight; literally, means "straight child," but actually means treatment of bone disorders. 13. another kind of physician who uses all MD methods, but also may use manipulation (more importance placed on "spinal column" alignment). 14. bending; straightening. 15. sternum; vertebral column. 16. inability to move part. 17. wasting away (from disuse). 18. excessive development. 19. knee cartilage: superior aspect of tibia. 20. frontal, occipital, parietal, temporal, and so on (any three). 21. ribs. 22. bones (skeleton). 23. diaphragm. 24. striated, smooth, cardiac. 25. osteoarthritis, osteomalacia, rickets. 26. by form, function, attachments, and so on. 27. bones. 28. axial, appendicular. 29. larger head proportionately; fontanels in skull; softer bones (cartilage). 30. see Fig. 18–1.

Chapter 19, p. 142

1. disease of the heart and/or blood vessels. 2. cerebrovascular accident; rupture or blockage of artery in brain. 3. pulmonary; systemic. 4. pulmonary artery and lungs; left atrium, pulmonary vein. 5. aortic valve; aorta. 6. tricuspid; mitral. 7. superior vena cava; inferior vena cava. 8. keep blood from backflowing (blood can move in forward direction only). 9. blood vessels. 10. collateral (circulation). 11. oxygen; nutrients; carbon dioxide; wastes. 12. dividing wall between right and left sides of heart. 13. heart ventricles contract; top number in B/P. 14. heart ventricles relax; bottom number in B/P. 15. heart muscle. 16. procedure done before transfusion to be sure of compatibility. 17. study or science of the blood. 18. without oxygen. 19. twisted, tortuous, dilated. 20. arteries that supply heart muscle (myocardium) with blood. 21. A, B, AB, O. 22a. erythrocytes. 22b. leukocytes. 22c. thrombocytes or platelets. 22d. neutrophils, eosinophils, basophils, lymphocytes, monocytes. 23. Rh negative or Rh−. 24. pacemaker. 25. cardiologist; hematologist. 26. coronary occlusion, coronary thrombosis, myocardial infarct or infarction. 27. pericardium; endocardium. 28. electrocardiogram; coronary care unit. 29. exercise or lack of it; eating or fasting; emotions; amount of blood, thickness of blood, condition of arteries. 30. cardio; phlebo; arterio; (hem) angio; thrombo; embolus. 31. type O. 32. prevents antibody production. 33. aneurysm, leukemia, atrial septal defect, transient ischemic attack, and so on. 34a. myocardial infarct. 34b. congestive heart failure. 34c. cerebrovascular accident. 34d. atrial septal defect. 34e. transient ischemic attack. 35. attain normal weight, exercise, cut down on use of salt.

Chapter 20, p. 150

1. thoracic, pleural. 2. nares, pharynx, larynx, trachea, bronchi, bronchioles, lungs (alveoli). 3. diaphragm; it moves down; makes more room; during inspiration. 4. epiglottis. 5. pharynx; from pharynx to middle ear; equalize pressure. 6. tiny air sacs in lungs where gaseous exchange takes place. 7. pleurisy. 8. O_2 and CO_2 (oxygen and carbon dioxide). 9. nares; septum. 10. apex; apices; base. 11. sinuses. 12. in front of (It would not be possible to do a tracheotomy if it were in back of esophagus.) 13. radiologist or roentgenologist. 14. oto(rhino)laryngologist or ENT specialist. 15. tracheostomy. 16. diaphragm. 17. atelectasis; tuberculosis. 18. amount of air that can be forcibly expelled after deep inspiration. 19. emphysema. 20. dyspnea. 21. orthopnea. 22. apnea. 23. pharyngitis, sinusitis, tonsillitis, and so on. 24. upper respiratory infection. 25. short of breath. 26. intermittent positive pressure breathing. 27. anterior-posterior and side, X-ray. 28. expectorants; aerosols. 29. rales. 30. carcinoma of lung (bronchogenic carcinoma). 31. fast breathing. 32. secretions from bronchial tubes. 33. allergic disorder with severe wheezing. 34. cough that produces sputum. 35. machine used to check vital capacity. 36. scope for looking into bronchi. 37. breathing in. 38. tapping chest to remove fluid. 39. both lungs involved. 40. bronchi.

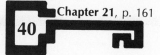
1. digestive; peritoneal, abdominopelvic. 2. liver; appendix. 3. teeth, tongue, salivary glands, pancreas, liver, gallbladder. 4. duodenum, jejunum, ileum. 5. esophagus; peristalsis. 6. cecum, ascending colon, transverse colon, descending colon, sigmoid colon, rectum (anus). 7. anus. 8. feces, stool. 9. upper GI series, lower GI (barium enema), GB series; stool to lab, proctoscopy, biopsy, gastric analysis, gastroscopy, and so on. 10. liver; gallbladder; aids in digestion of fats; cystic, hepatic, common. 11. choledoch; cholecyst; cholangiography or choledochography. 12. introduction of solution into rectum, for cleansing or for X-ray, for example. 13. tiny projections that line small intestine, increase surface area. 14. circular (purse string type) muscle (anal sphincter, for example). 15. instrument for looking into the rectum. 16. fats, carbohydrates, proteins; 9, 4, 4. 17. proteins. 18. right and left hypochondria, right and left lumbar, right and left inguinal; epigastric, umbilical, and suprapubic should be shown in a drawing (see p. 154). 19. peritoneal; greater, lesser. 20. feeding by tube inserted into stomach. 21. washing out stomach. 22. inflammation of the mouth. 23. inflammation of the tongue. 24. excision of the gallbladder. 25. new permanent opening into colon. 26. inflammation of the liver. 27. condition of gallstones. 28. loss of appetite. 29. within normal limits. 30. small intestine, villi. 31. appendectomy, ileostomy, anastomosis, and so on. 32. peptic or duodenal ulcers, colitis, appendicitis, esophagitis, and so on.

1. kidneys, ureters, bladder, urethra. 2. unable to control voiding and/or bowels. 3. obtain a urine specimen (sterile); to relieve distended bladder when person is unable to void. 4. pyelitis. 5. looking into the bladder with a cystoscope. 6. dilatation and curettage; dilating cervix and scraping uterus; diagnostic purposes or to produce miscarriage. 7. presentations of infant at delivery (head). 8. hematuria, dysuria, anuria, polyuria, and so on. 9. urinalysis; reaction, specific gravity, glucose, and so on. 10. fundus; cervix. 11. alkaline. 12. nephrons. 13. ovary; ovum. 14. estimated date of confinement (delivery). 15. three-month period (especially in a pregnancy). 16. pregnancy outside of uterus; usually in fallopian tube. 17. empty (bladder). 18. vulva. 19. male sex cell. 20. test to detect malignant cells, especially cervix. 21. ovulation. 22. episiotomy. 23. placenta. 24. vasectomy. 25. cesarean section. In 26–30, any appropriate word is acceptable; for example: 26. oophoritis. 27. salpingopexy. 28. cystocele. 29. prostatectomy. 30. hysterorrhexis. 31. a tube used to retain continuous drainage of urine; a retention catheter. 32. last menstrual period before pregnancy. 33. urinary tract infection. 34. procedure of looking into bladder with "scope." 35. intravenous pyelogram (X-ray procedure). 36. pus in the urine. 37. period of pregnancy; time required for development of offspring. 38. nephrosis, cystitis, pyelonephritis, etc. 39. diagram of kidneys, ureters, bladder (see Fig. 22–1).

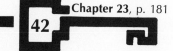
1. largest, brain. 2. exterior, middle, and interior layers of the meninges (membranes that cover brain and spinal cord). 3. optic, olfactory, auditory. 4. T4, C3, Co-1. 5. cranium, vertebral column; cerebrospinal fluid. 6. nerve cells; brain. 7. gliomas, meningiomas. 8. hemiparesis. 9. hemiplegia. 10. convolutions of the brain; deep furrows in brain; gyrus, sulcus (singular form). 11. cavities through which CSF circulates; hydrocephalus. 12. response. 13. lumbar puncture; diagnostic. 14. the sacrococcygeal area. 15. inflammation of the meninges (membranes). 16. autonomic. 17. l, k, i, h, g, d, f, e, b, a, j, m, c. 18. For example, parkinsonism affects older people with severe tremor and masklike facies; herpes zoster is a viral infection that causes lesions along course of a nerve. 19. alpha, beta, theta.

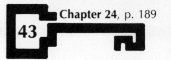

1. myopia. **2.** tonometer. **3.** OD, OU, OS, AD. **4.** cataract. **5.** lacrimal. **6.** peripheral vision. **7.** optometrist. **8.** cerumen. **9.** tympanum, myringa. **10.** otitis media. **11.** eustachian. **12.** audiometer. **13.** decibel. **14.** auditory. **15.** plaque. **16.** gingivitis, pyorrhea. **17.** deciduous. **18.** dentures. **19.** retinopathy. **20.** conjunctivitis. **21.** MD or DO eye specialist. **22.** MD or DO ear specialist. **23.** ear, nose, and throat. **24.** general dentist; Doctor of Dental Surgery. **25.** dental specialist, treats malocclusion, and so on. **26.** dental specialist, treats gum disease. **27.** increased intraocular pressure, leads to blindness (not a tumor). **28.** ability to adjust quickly to near and far vision. **29.** pupils equal, react to light and accommodation. **30.** brushing, flossing, fluoride, dental checkups. **31.** edema of optic nerve where it enters eye. **32.** all types of dental repair (fillings, for example). **33.** dental cavities. **34.** instrument for looking into eye. **35.** use of appliances: false teeth (dentures) and bridge work, for example.

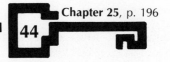**Chapter 25**, p. 196

1. endocrine (ductless). **2.** ductless glands. **3.** testosterone; estrogens, progesterone. **4.** in the cranial cavity at base of brain; in the neck, anterior, below thyroid cartilage; in the pancreas (behind stomach). **5.** PBI, protein-bound iodine; RAI, radioactive iodine. **6.** FBS, fasting blood sugar; GTT, glucose tolerance test. **7.** iodine. **8.** insulin. **9.** slow; insulin. **10.** food (sugar or juice, for example). **11.** thyroid. **12.** two-hour postprandial. **13.** hyperfunction, hypofunction. **14.** behind the stomach (LUQ). **15.** pancreatectomy or pancreectomy. **16.** hypophysis. **17.** extremities. **18.** myxedema, giantism, dwarfism, thyrotoxicosis. **19.** early arteriosclerosis, vision and dental problems, gangrene, infection. **20a.** excision of pituitary. **20b.** any disease of nerves. **20c.** excessive perspiring. **20d.** enlarged thyroid gland. **20e.** rapid heart beat. **20f.** clouded lens of eye. **20g.** without appetite. **20h.** severe wasting, emaciation.

appendix b
disease report outline

Your instructor may assign topics or may allow you to choose one that interests you. Reports may be written or given orally, if time permits. Use the outline below; be concise.

etiology   the cause of the disease (such as bacterial, viral, and degenerative factors). Cause may be unknown, but some theories certainly are prevalent and these can be mentioned.

population affected   factors of age, sex, and race, for example. (Who gets the disease?)

signs and symptoms   what does the patient complain of? What does the physician see (subjective and objective)? Special diagnostic tests necessary for diagnosis can be included here, GB series, GI series, and IVP, for example.

treatment   general kinds of treatment available, for example, surgery, medication, diet, bedrest, radio-therapy, and physical therapy (not too detailed).

prognosis   predicted outcome. Is the prognosis good, fair, guarded, or poor? Are there any sequelae (after effects), is complete cure likely, is this a terminal condition, or is it a chronic condition in which the patient may need help to cope with disability?

community resources available   for example, lung associations for emphysema or TB, heart associations for cardiovascular diseases, and special groups such as "ostomy" clubs. (These associations usually have free literature available; see Appendix d.)

bibliography   include at least two articles or readings.

appendix c
using your medical dictionary

Your medical dictionary can be very helpful if you learn how to use it. Look through it to see what it contains. Some dictionaries have a table of contents or index at the front of the book. Some have instructions for use at the front and a table of contents just before the appendix at the back of the book.

All medical dictionaries contain lists of arteries, veins, muscles, and nerves in the appendix. Some also include listings of joints and ligaments and a great variety of other tables, such as weights and measures, signs and symbols, first aid, poisons and antidotes, medical emergencies, phobias, fractures, calorie lists, root words, prefixes, suffixes, plural endings, communicable diseases, immunization schedules, laboratory tests, and normal values.

It is important to learn what your dictionary contains and to become familiar with other medical dictionaries that you may need to use from time to time. Most dictionaries contain some excellent diagrams and illustrations. A picture often tells you more than a definition. In addition to pictures in the text of the book, you may find a section of "plates" showing each of the body systems.

When looking up a word, such as a certain disease, test, or syndrome, you may find it listed under the name of the disease or under "disease"; for instance, it may be listed under "Addison's disease" or "disease—Addison's." It will probably be listed in both places.

Dictionaries contain information on body systems. Look under the name of the system. You will learn that some systems have more than one name; for instance, the cardiovascular system is also the circulatory system, and the reproductive system is included in the genitourinary system.

Some abbreviations will be listed alphabetically, and usually there will also be a list of abbreviations in the appendix. There are so many medical abbreviations that you will find separate books of abbreviations used in the medical world.

Before purchasing a particular medical dictionary, look it over carefully. You may find that a large comprehensive dictionary is more confusing than helpful for your purposes. Be sure that the definitions are given in a manner that is understandable to you. There are many medical dictionaries available; it is merely a matter of picking the one that is best suited for you.

Your dictionary, in most cases, will be helpful to you in learning correct pronunciation. However, pronunciation is best learned by actually practicing saying the words in class and as you work with them in written work.

Your instructor may suggest a dictionary for this class. There is also a list of dictionaries in the reference material suggested in Appendix e.

appendix d
organizations offering free literature

Alcoholism Information Center
American Cancer Society
American Diabetes Association
American Heart Association
American Red Cross
Arthritis Foundation
Association for deaf (state)
CARES (Epilepsy)
Council of blind (state)
Cystic Fibrosis National Research Foundation
Department of health (state)
Easter Seal Society for Crippled Children and Adults
-Ectomy Clubs (Mastectomy, Laryngectomy)
Epi-Hab
Family planning council (state)
Foundation for Blind

Hemophilia Association
Huntington's Chorea
Kidney foundation (state)
Leukemia Society of America
Lions Vision Center
Lung association (state)
Medical societies (county and state)
Mental health associations (local and state)
Mental retardation associations
March of Dimes
Multiple Sclerosis Society
Muscular Dystrophy Association of America
Myasthenia Gravis
-Ostomy Clubs (Colostomy)
Retired physicians' associations
United Cerebral Palsy Association

See the Yellow Pages of phone directory under "Associations," or the white pages.

appendix e
reference materials

1. Ask your instructor about books that may be available in the department library. Your instructor may also have medical journals and other publications you can use.

2. Remember that there is no point in reading some highly technical book or article that you do not understand. It is more important to read, at least at the beginning of your medical career, books and articles that you do understand. As you learn more, you can gradually start to read more comprehensive material.

3. Watch for special television shows; these are usually shown on educational channels but occasionally may appear on regular channels. Programs such as "General Hospital" will not help you, but occasionally you may learn something even from such programs as "Quincy" and "Medical Center," although these programs usually present rather unrealistic situations and rare diseases.

4. Spend some time in the library to see what is available. Investigate books available in paperback, new or used.

5. Read newspaper "doctor" columns and save interesting articles. These are good because they usually discuss common conditions rather than rare ones.

6. Look for articles about health and medicine in popular magazines. Look for books in the library or in paperback on such topics as hypertension, heart disease, hypoglycemia, diabetes, arthritis, and cancer. (These books are generally written for the layman.)

7. See the Yellow Pages of your phone book; under "Associations" you will find state and national health agencies. Visit some of these to see what free literature they offer. Especially helpful are the cancer, heart, and lung associations.

The following reference material has been divided into nine categories, although some books will fall into more than one category.

BODY SYSTEMS

American Medical Association. *The Wonderful Human Machine*. 525 N. Dearborn Street, Chicago, IL 60610. (Worth sending for; good illustrations; price $1.25.)

Anthony, C. P. 1980. *Structure and Function of the Body*. St. Louis: C. V. Mosby Co.

Asimov, I. 1963. *The Human Body: Its Structure and Operation*. Boston: Houghton Mifflin Co. (There are many other books by Asimov, plus one paperback.)

Best, C. H., and Taylor, N. B. 1958. *The Living Body: A Text in Human Physiology*. New York: Holt, Rinehart and Winston.

Carlson, A., Johnson, V., and Cavert, H. M. 1961. *The Machinery of the Body*. Chicago: University of Chicago Press.

Cooley, D. G. (editor). 1973. *Family Medical Guide*. Des Moines: Better Homes and Gardens Books.

Ferris, E., and Skelley, E. 1979. *Body Structure and Function*. Albany, N.Y.: Delmar Publishers.

Fishbein, M. (editor). 1981. *The New Illustrated Medical and Health Encyclopedia*. New York: H. S. Stuttman Co., Inc. (Eighteen volumes; good; simply written information on systems and diseases.)

Guyton, A. C. 1976. *Textbook of Medical Physiology*. Philadelphia: W. B. Saunders Co. (Very technical.)

Memmler, R. L. 1977. *The Human Body in Health and Disease*. New York: Harper & Row, Inc.

Memmler, R. L., and Wood, D. L. 1977. *Structure and Function of the Human Body*. New York: Harper & Row, Inc.

Nilsson, L. 1974. *Behold Man*. Boston: Little, Brown & Co., Inc. (Excellent illustrations and photographs.)

Taylor, J. W., and Ballenger, S. 1980. *Neurological Dysfunctions and Nursing Interventions*. New York: McGraw-Hill, Inc.

Other body system references: anatomy and physiology books, biology books, health books, encyclopedias, medical dictionaries, and family health books.

DISEASES

Berkow, R. (editor). 1977. *Merck Manual of Diagnosis and Therapy*. Rahway, N.J.: Merck, Sharp and Dohme Research Laboratories, Merck & Co., Inc. (Excellent resource for diseases and treatment; very technical.)

Boyd, W., and Sheldon, H. 1980. *An Introduction to the Study of Disease*. Philadelphia: Lea & Febiger.

Miller, B. F. 1978. *The Complete Medical Guide*. New York: Simon & Schuster, Inc. (Excellent family health book.)

Myers, J. S. 1966. *Orientation to Chronic Disease and Disability*. New York: Macmillan, Inc. (Especially helpful for the degenerative diseases.)

Rothenberg, R. E. 1976. *The Complete Surgical Guide*. New York: Weathervane Books.

Walter, J. B. 1977. *An Introduction to the Principles of Disease*. Philadelphia: W. B. Saunders Co.

Young, C. G., and Barger, J. D. 1973. *Introduction to Medical Science*. St. Louis: C. V. Mosby Co.

Other disease references: pathology books and books written for the layperson on certain diseases, such as heart attack, hypertension, cancer, diabetes, and arthritis; popular magazines including *Family Health* and *Today's Health* (now incorporated in *Health*); medical and nursing journals—*American Journal of Nursing*, *R. N. Journal*, *Nursing 83* (and 84, 85, and so on; current year); and newspaper "doctor" columns.

ABBREVIATIONS

Cole, F. 1970. *The Doctor's Shorthand*. Philadelphia: W. B. Saunders Co.

Medical Abbreviations: A Cross Reference Dictionary. 1967. Ann Arbor, Mich.: Special Studies Committee of the Michigan Occupational Therapy Association.

Steen, E. B. 1971. *Medical Abbreviations*. Philadelphia: F. A. Davis Co.

Steen, E. B. 1978. *Abbreviations in Medicine*. New York: Macmillan, Inc.

MEDICATIONS

Graedon, J. 1980. *People's Pharmacy*. New York: Avon Books.

Physician's Desk Reference. 1982. Oradell, N.J.: Medical Economics Co. (Published yearly with supplements during the year. This book lists all prescription drugs and drug companies and gives information about each drug. Your instructor should have this, or ask your doctor to save an old copy for you.)

SURGICAL AND MEDICAL TERMINOLOGY

Coleman, F. 1978. *Guide to Surgical Terms*. Oradell, N.J.: Medical Economics Co. (Terms pertaining to surgical procedures and operations are listed by systems [specialties—for example, orthopedic surgery, ear surgery], and it names surgical and other instruments.)

Chabner, D-E. 1981. *The Language of Medicine*. Philadelphia: W. B. Saunders Co. (A worktext explaining medical terms.)

Ehrlich, A. 1977. *The Medical and Health Sciences Word Book*. Boston: Houghton Mifflin Co.

Franks, R. 1972. *Reverse Medical Secretary*. Oradell, N.J.: Medical Economics Co. (Suffixes, all words with -ectomy, for example; glossaries listed under eye, heart, diseases, drugs, signs, specialties, surgery, abbreviations, and laboratory.)

Frenay, A. C. 1977. *Understanding Medical Terminology*. St. Louis: Catholic Hospital Association.

Lorenzini, J. A. 1978. *Medical Phrase Index—A One-Step Reference to the Terminology of Medicine*. Oradell, N.J.: Medical Economics Co.

Rothenberg, R. E. *Understanding Surgery*. New York: Trident Press.

Sloane, S. B. 1978. *Medical Word Book*. Philadelphia: W. B. Saunders Co. (Symbols, abbreviations, terms by systems, laboratory terms, surgical terms, and illustrations.)

Szulec, J. A. 1980. *A Syllabus for the Surgeon's Secretary*. Detroit: Medical Arts Publishing Co.

Young, C. G., and Austrin, M. G. 1979. *Learning Medical Terminology Step by Step*. St. Louis: C. V. Mosby Co.

MEDICAL OFFICE PROCEDURES   (medical secretaries, medical assistants, medical receptionists, transcribers and unit clerks)

Bredow, M., and Cooper, M. G. 1978. *The Medical Assistant: A Guide to Clinical, Secretarial and Technical Duties*. New York: McGraw-Hill, Inc. (Contains information for assisting the specialist in ECG, physical therapy, minor surgery, and laboratory; deals with medical law.)

Bredow, M. 1973. *Medical Secretarial Procedures*. New York: McGraw-Hill, Inc.

Doyle, J. M. and Dennis, R. L. 1978. *The Complete Handbook for Medical Secretaries and Assistants*. Boston: Little, Brown & Co.

Frederick, P. M., and Kinn, M. E. 1981. *The Office Assistant in Medical Practice*. Philadelphia: W. B. Saunders Co.

LaFleur, M., and Starr, W. 1979. *Unit Clerking in Health Care Facilities, A Textbook of Theory and Practice*. Philadelphia: W. B. Saunders Co.

MEDICAL TESTS

Fox, M., and Schnabel, T. 1979. *It's Your Body—Know What the Doctor Ordered—Your Complete Guide to Medical Testing*. Bowie, Md.: Charles Press Publishers.

Klein, A. 1977. *Medical Tests and You*. New York: Grosset & Dunlap.

MEDICAL DICTIONARIES

Blakiston's Gould Medical Dictionary. 1979. New York: McGraw-Hill, Inc.

Dorland's Pocket Medical Dictionary. 1977. Philadelphia: W. B. Saunders Co. (Also *Dorland's Illustrated Medical Dictionary*.)

Melloni's Illustrated Medical Dictionary. 1979. Baltimore: Williams & Wilkins Co.

Miller, B. F., and Keane, C. B. 1978. *Encyclopedia and Dictionary of Medicine, Nursing, and Allied Health*. Philadelphia: W. B. Saunders Co.

Rothenberg, R. E. 1975. *Medical Dictionary and Health Manual*. New York: Signet Classics (Paperback $3.50; excellent diagrams and understandable definitions, but no pronunciation; many tables and other information, useful for the entire family.)

Stedman's Medical Dictionary. 1972. Baltimore: Williams & Wilkins Co.

Taber's Cyclopedic Medical Dictionary. 1981. Philadelphia: F. A. Davis Co.

SPARE TIME READING

Barnard, C. 1978. *In the Night Season*. New York: Popular Library. (Other books by Christian Barnard.)

DeKriuf, P. 1945. *Microbe Hunters*. New York: Pocket Books.

Eiseman, B. 1980. *What Are My Chances?* (of getting well). Philadelphia: W. B. Saunders Co.

Harris, C. 1975. *One Man's Medicine*. New York: Harper & Row, Inc.

Morgan, E. 1982. *Solo Practice—A Woman Surgeon's Story*. Boston: Little, Brown & Co.

Nolan, W. A. 1972. *The Making of a Surgeon*. New York: Pocket Books. (Also by the same author: *A Surgeon's World*, *Healing*, and *Surgeon Under the Knife*. All excellent reading and very informative.)

appendix f
chapter tests, review tests, and final exam

Your instructor will decide on which tests will be given; some instructors may choose to use their own tests.

chapter 1
medical words: -ectomy

points: 100

_____

name

_____

course or section no.

---

test

Spell: (4 points each)

1. _____

2. _____

3. _____

4. _____

5. _____

6. _____

7. _____

8. _____

9. _____

10. _____

11. _____

12. _____

Define any eight: (2 points each)

_____

_____

_____

_____

_____

_____

_____

_____

_____

_____

_____

_____

_____

_____

_____

_____

_____

_____

_____

_____

_____

_____

Build a word: (6 points each; if correct word but misspelled, only 3 points)

13. Excision of the adenoids _____

14. Excision of the spleen _____

15. Excision of the stomach _____

chapter tests, review tests, and final exam **219**

16. Excision of the pancreas _____

17. Excision of the larynx _____

18. Excision of a nerve _____

Test Key 1, Instructor's Guide

chapter 2
other surgical procedures: suffixes

points: 100

_____
name

_____
course or section no.

test

Spell: (2 points each)   **Define all:** (2 points each)

1. _____

2. _____

3. _____

4. _____

5. _____

6. _____

7. _____

8. _____

9. _____

10. _____

11. _____

12. _____

13. _____

14. _____

15. _____   _____

   _____

Build a word: (4 points each; if correct word but misspelled, only 2 points)

16. Excision of the appendix _____

17. New permanent opening into the stomach _____

18. Crushing of a "stone" (litho) _____

19. Fixation or suturing a fallopian tube _____

20. Incision into the abdomen _____

21. Excision of an ovary _____

22. Surgical repair of a kidney _____

23. Surgical puncture (tapping to remove fluid) of abdomen _____

24. New (emergency) opening into (incision into) trachea _____

25. Excision of the pancreas _____

Test Key 2, Instructor's Guide

**chapter 3
diseases or conditions:
prefixes and suffixes**

points: 104

name _____

course or section no. _____

_____

test

_____

Give a word for: (4 points each)

1. Excision of the uterus _____

2. Inflammation of the ear _____

3. A new permanent opening into the colon _____

4. Tapping (puncture) of the chest to remove fluid _____

5. Repair of a hernia _____

6. Rupture (hernia) of the bladder _____

7. Condition of the skin _____

8. "Any disease" of the glands _____

9. Incision into the trachea _____

10. Fixation of a kidney _____

11. Excision of the spleen _____

12. Pain along a nerve _____

13. A hollow sac or organ _____

14. An infected state or condition _____

15. High blood pressure _____

Spell: (2 points each)

16. _____

17. _____

18. _____

19. _____

20. _____

21. _____

Define: (2 points each)

_____

_____

_____

_____

_____

_____

_____

_____

_____

_____

_____

_____

22. _____   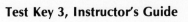 _____
                                 _____

23. _____   _____
                                 _____

24. _____   _____
                                 _____

25. _____   _____
                                 _____

26. _____   _____
                                 _____

Test Key 3, Instructor's Guide

chapters 1–3

points: 100

_____
name

_____
course or section no.

review test

True/False: Circle the number of the *true* statements only. Defend your answers. Explain what is "untrue" in the false statements. (3 points each)

1. Hysterectomy means excision of the uterus.

2. Stomatitis is inflammation of the stomach.

3. Spondylopathy involves vertebrae.

4. The -itis ending is sometimes spelled -idis.

5. Cystocele is a hernia or rupture of the bladder.

6. A new permanent opening into the colon is called a colostomy.

7. Plastic surgery of the nose is called rhinoplasty.

8. A mastectomy is surgical excision of a mastoid.

9. A temporary, emergency incision into the trachea is a tracheotomy.

10. Cerebral hemorrhage means bleeding in a part of the brain.

11. Dysuria is painful or difficult breathing.

12. Hypotension is high blood pressure.

Correct spelling: Mark an **X** *after* the *correctly* spelled words (1 point each).

13. antibiotic _____   antebiotic _____

14. hemaplegia _____   hemiplegia _____

15. herniorrhaphy _____   herniorraphy _____

16. splenectomy _____   spleenectomy _____

17. tonsillectomy _____   tonsilectomy _____

18. inflamed _____   inflammed _____

19. intervenous _____   intravenous _____

20. appendicitis _____   appendicitus _____

21. tracheodomy _____   tracheotomy _____

22. colocystitis _____   cholecystitis _____

Spell: Define first five. (spelling, 3 points; definition, 2 points)

23. _____   _____

_____

24. _____ _____

25. _____ _____

26. _____ _____

27. _____ _____

28. _____

29. _____

30. _____

31. _____

32. _____

33. _____

34. _____

Define three: bladder, sepsis, hernia, inflammation, cavity, abdomen (3 points each)

35. _____

_____

36. _____

_____

37. _____

_____

Test Key 4, Instructor's Guide

chapter 4
medical instruments
and machines

points: 100

name _____

course or section no. _____

test

1. Name five "scope" instruments used *for looking into* body parts and name the body part:

   Scopes (3 points each)   *Body part* (2 points each)

   _____   _____

   _____   _____

   _____   _____

   _____   _____

   _____   _____

2. Name two "scopes" used *for listening*:

   Scopes (3 points each)   *Body part* (2 points each)

   _____   _____

   _____   _____

Fill in the blank: (2 points each)

3. Electrocardi**og**raphy is a procedure similar to electroencepha**log**raphy, except that the first concerns the
   _____ and the second, the _____

4. An electrocardiogram is placed in the patient's file. It is a _____ of heart action. A
   thermometer records _____

5. There are many kinds of dilators. One that is used to dilate the vaginal orifice is called a _____
   (during pelvic examination).

6. List at least 15 *suffixes* you have learned and place them under the proper heading: (1 point each)

cutting or surgical procedures	diseases or conditions	medical instruments and machines and their use

chapter tests, review tests, and final exam

Spell: (2 points each)   **Define:** (2 points each)

7. _____   _____

                                    _____

8. _____   _____

                                    _____

9. _____   _____

                                    _____

10. _____   _____

                                    _____

11. _____   _____

                                    _____

12. _____   _____

                                    _____

13. _____   _____

                                    _____

14. _____   _____

                                    _____

15. _____   _____

                                    _____

16. _____   _____

                                    _____

Test Key 5, Instructor's Guide

chapters 1–4

points: 100

name _____

course or section no.

---

alternate review test

Spell: (2 points each)

1. _____

2. _____

3. _____

4. _____

5. _____

6. _____

7. _____

8. _____

9. _____

10. _____

Define: (2 points each)

_____
_____
_____
_____
_____
_____
_____
_____
_____
_____
_____
_____
_____
_____
_____
_____
_____
_____
_____
_____

Define: (2 points each)

11. hyste**rec**tomy _____

12. **cys**tocele _____

13. co**los**tomy _____

14. hyper**ten**sion _____

15. lapa**rot**omy _____

16. ade**nop**athy _____

17. thoracocen**te**sis _____

18. sal**ping**opexy _____

19. cholecys**ti**tis _____

20. derma**to**sis _____

Write a word for: (3 points each)

21. Pain along a nerve _____

22. Condition of the nerves _____

23. Plastic surgery on the nose _____

24. Surgical repair of a hernia _____

25. Incision into the stomach _____

Spell: (2 points each)   **Define five:** (1 point each)

26. _____   _____

27. _____   _____

28. _____   _____

29. _____   _____

30. _____   _____

31. _____   _____

32. _____   _____

33. _____   _____

34. _____   _____

35. _____   _____

Test Key 6, Instructor's Guide

chapter 5
medical specialties and specialists:
-ology, -ologist

name _____

points: 101

course or section no. _____

test

Name the medical or osteopathic specialist: (4 points each) Must be spelled correctly.

1. Prenatal care, delivery, and postpartum _____

2. All kinds of nonsurgical conditions _____

3. Children only _____

4. Interpreting and diagnosing by X-ray procedures _____

5. Skin conditions and diseases _____

6. Mental illness _____

7. Eye diseases and eye surgery _____

8. Diseases and injuries, nervous system _____

9. Heart (and blood vessel) diseases _____

10. Hearing disorders _____

True/False: Circle the number of the *true* statements only. Defend your answers. Explain what is "untrue" in the false statements. (3 points each)

11. Many kinds of different specialists perform surgery; general practitioners also perform surgery.

12. An optometrist treats refractive errors by prescribing glasses.

13. An osteopathic physician has an equal number of years of education as a medical doctor.

14. A psychologist is an MD.

15. Foot disorders can be treated by an MD or a podiatrist.

16. False teeth are called dentures; they are a prosthetic device.

Identify: (3 points each) (spell out)

17. DO _____

18. DDS _____

19. RN _____

20. LPN _____

21. MD _____

Fill in the blank: (4 points each)

22. The dental specialist who straightens teeth is the _____

23. The dental specialist who treats gum diseases is the _____

Spell: (2 points each)   **Define:** (2 points each)

24. _____,_____   _____

          _____

25. _____   _____

          _____

26. _____   _____

          _____

27. _____   _____

          _____

28. _____   _____

          _____

Test Key 7, Instructor's Guide

**chapters 4–5
instruments
specialties**

name
_____

points: 101

course or section no.
_____

test

Name five "scopes" used for looking into body parts, and name the body part: (points: 2, 1)

_____   _____

_____   _____

_____   _____

_____   _____

_____   _____

Name two "scopes" used for listening, and name the body parts: (points: 2, 1)

_____   _____

_____   _____

Fill in the blank: (Each blank 2 points unless otherwise shown.)

An electrocardiogram is placed in the patient's file. It is a _____ of heart action. A

thermometer records _____. (2 points)

Electrocardiography is a procedure similar to electroencephalography, except that the first concerns the

_____ and the second, the _____.

One type of dilator used to dilate the vaginal orifice is called a _____ (in pelvic exam).

Identify: (spell out)

DO _____   RN _____

DDS _____   MD _____

LPN _____

The dental specialist who straightens teeth is an _____; who treats gum disease is a

_____

Name the physician specialist for:

a. Prenatal care, delivery _____

b. Any nonsurgical condition _____

c. Children only _____

d. Skin conditions and diseases _____

e. Mental illness _____

f. Eye surgery and other care   _____

g. Heart and blood vessel diseases   _____

h. Diseases/injuries of nervous system   _____

i. Ear surgery, hearing loss   _____

j. X-ray interpretation and treatment   _____

Write and define 15 suffixes: (1–2 word definition) (1 point each)

_____   _____   _____   _____

_____   _____   _____   _____

_____   _____   _____   _____

_____   _____   _____   _____

_____   _____   _____   _____

_____   _____   _____   _____

_____   _____

Circle incorrectly spelled words: (1 point each)

coloscopy   orthroscope   myogram   radiograph

spirometery   anjiogram   microtome   mylography

Spell and define: (1 point each)

_____   _____

_____   _____

_____   _____

_____   _____

_____   _____

Test Key 8, Instructor's Guide

**chapters 6
more medical prefixes
and review**

points: 100

name

course or section no.

test

True/False: Circle the number of the *true* statements only. Defend your answers. Explain what is "untrue" in the false statements. (3 points each)

1. A medication given before surgery is called a postoperative medication.

2. Prognosis is the predicted outcome of a disease.

3. The six-week period following delivery is called postpartum.

4. A patient who cannot void may be said to have polyuria.

5. Dysmenorrhea means painful menstruation.

6. A general anesthetic produces loss of all sensation.

7. An antiseptic helps to prevent infection.

8. Hyperactive people would not be as likely to be overweight as those who are hypoactive.

9. Fear and excitement often cause bradycardia.

10. Lipoma means a tumor on the lip.

Spell: (3 point each)

11. _____

12. _____

13. _____

14. _____

15. _____

16. _____

17. _____

18. _____

Define: (3 point each)

_____
_____

_____
_____

_____
_____

_____
_____

_____
_____

_____
_____

_____
_____

_____
_____

19. _____   _____

_____

20. _____   _____

_____

Define: (2 points each)

21. ar**rhyth**mia _____

22. dys**u**ria _____

23. hypo**der**mic _____

24. antico**ag**ulant _____

25. he**mol**ysis _____

Test Key 9, Instructor's Guide

chapters 1–7

_____
name

points: 102

_____
course or section no.

review test

Build a word that means: (3 points each)

1. Excision of the uterus _____

2. Incision into the trachea _____

3. A new permanent opening into the colon _____

4. Plastic surgery on the nose _____

5. A condition of "tubercles" _____

6. Inflamed liver _____

7. Any disease of the glands _____

8. Pain in a nerve _____

9. Hernia of the bladder _____

10. Surgical crushing of a "stone" _____

Name the specialist in each field: (1 point each) Must be spelled correctly.

11. obstetrics _____

12. urology _____

13. gynecology _____

14. orthopedics _____

15. internal medicine _____

Write the plural of: (2 points each)

16. diagnosis _____

17. apex _____

18. focus _____

19. vertebra _____

20. diverticulum _____

21. lumen _____

22. phalanx _____

Spell: (1 point each)

Define any 23 words: (1 point each)

23. _____

24. _____

25. _____

26. _____

27. _____

28. _____

29. _____

30. _____

31. _____

32. _____

33. _____

34. _____

35. _____

36. _____

37. _____

38. _____

39. _____

40. _____

41. _____

42. _____

43. _____

44. _____

45. _____

46. _____

47. _____

48. _____

49. _____

50. _____

Test Key 10, Instructor's Guide

chapter tests, review tests, and final exam

chapter 9
more suffixes and prefixes

points: 102

_____
name

_____
course or section no.

test

Spell dictated words: After supplying the correctly spelled word, fill in the blanks to complete sentences. Blanks may contain more than one word. (Spelling, 2 points each; fill in the blank, 2 points each, but only 1 if word is misspelled)

1. _____ is a _____ or _____

2. _____ means _____ _____

3. _____ of muscles results from _____ _____

4. _____ is difficult _____

5. Right _____ is _____ of the right _____ of the body.

6. _____ means _____ breathing.

7. _____ occurs because of dietary deficiency. It means _____ of _____

8. _____ occurs with most illnesses. It means general _____

9. _____ can cause loss of sleep. It means _____ during the _____

10. _____ means a group of _____ that generally occur together.

11. _____ is the opposite of _____ (bad feeling).

12. _____ occurs at about age 50. It means _____

13. _____ lesions are producing _____

14. _____ people are _____ to people of the _____

15. _____ solutions have an amount of salt equal to that of _____

16. _____, when painful, is called _____

17. _____ is disfiguring. A person with this condition has _____ _____

18. _____ means (literally) a condition of _____ _____

19. _____ is best treated by a dentist called an _____

20. _____ means (literally) _____ It refers to frequent watery _____

21. _____ means that a malignant tumor has not _____

Test Key 12, Instructor's Guide

chapters 1–9

points: 100 + 5 bonus points

name _____

course or section no. _____

---

review test

Define: (2 points each)

1. tonsillectomy _____

2. mastectomy _____

3. cholecystectomy _____

4. colostomy _____

5. tracheotomy _____

6. abdominocentesis _____

7. herniorrhaphy _____

8. spondylosis _____

9. appendicitis _____

10. hysteropathy _____

Give a word for the following: (2 points each)

11. "Any disease" of glands _____

12. Incision into the abdomen _____

13. Recording (picture) of heart impulses _____

14. Instrument for looking into ear _____

15. Process of making a record of brain waves _____

16. Inflammation of the liver _____

17. "Crushing" of a nerve _____

18. Inflammation of the nose _____

19. Excision of the stomach _____

20. Pain in a tooth _____

Name five medical specialists (DOs or MDs) and tell what kinds of cases or patients they treat: (2 points each)

21. _____   _____

22. _____   _____

23. _____   _____

24. _____   _____

25. _____   _____

chapter tests, review tests, and final exam

Spell: (1point each)

Define any 20: (1 point each)

26. _____

27. _____

28. _____

29. _____

30. _____

31. _____

32. _____

33. _____

34. _____

35. _____

36. _____

37. _____

38. _____

39. _____

40. _____

41. _____

42. _____

43. _____

44. _____   _____

_____

45. _____   _____

_____

46. _____   _____

_____

47. _____   _____

_____

48. _____   _____

_____

49. _____   _____

_____

50. _____   _____

_____

51. _____   _____

_____

52. _____   _____

_____

53. _____   _____

_____

54. _____   _____

_____

55. _____   _____

_____

Bonus: Name the five sections of the vertebral column, in order (1 point each)

_____

_____

_____

_____

_____

Test Key 13, Instructor's Guide

**chapter 10
bacteria, colors, and
other root words**

points: 100

name _____

course or section no. _____

test

Define: (2 points each)

1. a**ne**mia _____
2. acro**meg**aly _____
3. ther**mom**eter _____
4. noct**u**ria _____
5. hema**tol**ogy _____
6. phagocy**to**sis _____
7. hysteror**rhex**is _____
8. prog**no**sis _____
9. **syn**drome _____
10. he**mol**ysis _____
11. hyper**o**pia _____
12. patho**gen**ic _____
13. mul**tip**ara _____
14. choleli**thi**asis _____

Spell: After supplying the correctly spelled word, fill in the blanks to complete the sentences. (2 points each)

15. _____ is a term for _____

_____ _____

16. _____ is a condition of being _____ in color.
17. _____ is a malignant or _____ _____
18. _____ means (literally) _____ _____
19. _____ means a condition of _____ _____
20. _____ is a mental _____
21. _____ is _____ tissue.
22. _____ means without _____
23. _____ is a _____ of _____
24. _____ is important in surgery. It means _____
25. _____ is a bacterium that causes illness. It is _____ in shape and

grows in _____

26. _____ is a rod-shaped _____

27. _____ is an injury, _____ or _____

28. Draw a picture of staphylococci and a picture of the bacterium referred to in Question 25. (2 points for each drawing)

Test Key 14, Instructor's Guide

chapter 11
directional, positional, and
numerical terms

_____

name

points: 100

_____

course or section no.

_____

test

_____

Fill in the blanks: (4 points each)

1. The opposite of flexion is   _____

2. Distal is the opposite of   _____

3. The front surface of the body is   _____

4. The back surface of the body is   _____

5. The abdomen is divided into four areas called _____ for describing the area involved.

6. Cephalic means toward the head; _____ means toward the tail (base of the spine).

7. Bedsores are called _____ ulcers because they are caused by lying in bed.

8. Bilateral pneumonia means pneumonia in _____   _____

9. A primipara is a woman who is having her _____   _____

10. Seeing double is called   _____

11. Semicomatose means in a partial   _____

12. A tubal pregnancy is one "out of place" and is called   _____

True/False: Circle the number of the _true_ statements only. Defend your answers. Explain what is "untrue" in the false statements. (2 points each)

13. Dorsal recumbent position is lying on back, face up.

14. Epigastric pain is pain over the stomach area.

15. An AP X-ray film of the chest is taken from the back of the patient.

16. Periodontal disease is a gum disease that causes teeth to become loose.

17. Sound is measured in decibels.

18. The abbreviation for grams is gr.

19. A fever is a temperature over 98.6F; a temperature below 98.6F is considered to be a subnormal temperature.

20. Internal hemorrhage is bleeding somewhere inside the body.

21. Rotation means turning.

22. Lenses (eyeglasses) are measured in diopters.

Define: (3 points each)

23. extrauterine   _____

24. lithotomy position   _____

chapter tests, review tests, and final exam   **251**

25. hemiplegia _____

26. abduction _____

Spelling: (2 points each)

27. _____ 32. _____

28. _____ 33. _____

29. _____ 34. _____

30. _____ 35. _____

31. _____ 36. _____

Test Key 15, Instructor's Guide

chapter 12
important words

_____
name

_____
course or section no.

points: 101

---

test

True/False: Circle the number of the *true* statements only. Defend your answers. Explain what is "untrue" in the false statements. (3 points each)

1. The terms "ascites" and "anasarca" refer to excessive fluid accumulation in the body tissues.

2. Routine immunizations include DPT, polio, MMR (measles, mumps, rubella) and flu shots.

3. Many disease conditions are characterized by periods of remission and exacerbation.

4. If a patient is afebrile, he has a fever.

5. A palpable lesion is one that can be seen.

6. Immunizations are prophylactic measures.

7. Serous drainage is "similar to serum."

8. Adnexa uteri are the ovaries, fallopian tubes, and ligaments.

9. Auscultation has to do with listening to sounds from within the body.

10. Percussion is done along with auscultation. It means tapping or striking to produce sounds.

11. Axillary temperature is taken in the groin.

12. Anomaly means some kind of defect or irregularity.

13. A biopsy involves the examination of dead tissue.

Fill in the blank: (4 points each)

14. Abortion means premature expulsion of a nonviable _____

15. Abscess is a localized accumulation of _____

16. An _____ infection usually starts suddenly and is more severe but shorter in duration than a _____ infection.

17. _____ is a word that means "growing together" of tissues that should not be attached.

Define: (2 points each)

18. incontinent _____

19. voided _____

20. edema _____

Spell: (1 point each)   **Define:** (1 point each)

21. _____ _____

22. _____ _____

23. _____ _____

    chapter tests, review tests, and final exam   **253**

24. _____   _____

25. _____   _____

26. _____   _____

27. _____   _____

28. _____   _____

29. _____   _____

30. _____   _____

31. _____   _____

32. _____   _____

33. _____   _____

34. _Underline_ words that are incorrectly spelled. (Correct them for a bonus point.)

dilitation _____

coccygeal _____

sputum _____

cervicle _____

paralyzed _____

pertussis _____

abdomin _____

diphtheria _____

abdomenal _____

fibrilation _____

Test Key 16, Instructor's Guide

chapters 1–12

points: 105

_____

name

_____

course or section no.

_____

review test

_____

Write a word for the following: (2 points each; if correct word but misspelled, only 1 point)

1. Excision of the spleen   _____

2. Inflammation of the bronchial tubes   _____

3. A condition of the nerves   _____

4. Incision into the stomach   _____

5. Difficult or labored breathing   _____

6. Recording or picture of the electrical impulses of the heart   _____

7. Instrument for measuring the pelvic size   _____

8. Any disease of the uterus   _____

9. Instrument for looking into the ear   _____

10. Cancerous tumor (malignant tumor)   _____

True/False: Circle the number of the _true_ statements only. Defend your answers. Explain what is "untrue" in the false statements. (1 point each)

11. The machine that records brain waves is an electroencephalograph.

12. Thoracocentesis is similar to abdominocentesis except it pertains to the chest instead of to the abdomen.

13. Inflammation of the liver is hepatosis.

14. A new permanent opening into the trachea is a tracheotomy.

15. An ophthalmoscope is the instrument used for looking into the eyes.

16. Some diseases are characterized by exacerbations and remissions.

17. A dermatome is an instrument used to cut a thin section of skin.

18. Hematology is the study or science of blood.

19. An intern is a medical specialist whose specialty is called internal medicine.

20. Hydrotherapy is treatment with heat.

21. Pathogenic bacteria are those that cause disease.

Name five medical or osteopathic specialties: (1 point each)

22. _____

23. _____

24. _____

25. _____

26. _____

Write the plural of the following: (1 point each)

27. diagnosis _____ 30. vertebra _____

28. apex _____ 31. coccus _____

29. urinalysis _____

Give the opposite of the following: (1 point each)

32. anterior _____

33. proximal _____

34. caudal _____

35. flexion _____

36. internal _____

Spell out: (1 point each)

37. T & A _____

38. AP, PA (pertaining to X-ray examination) _____

39. RUQ _____

40. P & A (in physical exam) _____

Define: (1 point each)

41. hemolysis _____

42. hypertrophy _____

43. nocturia _____

44. syndrome _____

45. anaerobic _____

46. phebitis _____

47. staphylococcus _____

48. trauma _____

49. prognosis _____

50. erythrocyte _____

51. ectopic _____

52. bilateral _____

53. multipara _____

54. lumen _____

55. heterosexual _____

Spell: (1 point each)

Define 56–70: (1 point each)

56. _____

_____

_____

57. _____

_____

_____

58. _____

_____

_____

59. _____

_____

_____

60. _____

_____

_____

61. _____

_____

_____

62. _____

_____

_____

63. _____

_____

_____

64. _____

_____

_____

65. _____

_____

_____

66. _____

_____

_____

67. _____

_____

_____

68. _____

_____

_____

69. _____

_____

_____

70. _____

_____

_____

71. _____

72. _____

73. _____

74. _____

75. _____

76. _____

77. _____

78. _____

79. _____

80. _____

Test Key 17, Instructor's Guide

chapter 13
introduction to abbreviations

points: 100 + 5 bonus

_____
name

_____
course or section no.

_____

test

_____

Give abbreviation or terms for the following: (2 points each)

1. Patient is not to have any food or drink   _____

2. Patient may get up to go to the bathroom only   _____

3. Patient is to be given compassionate nursing care   _____

4. Patient is to sit at edge of bed with legs hanging over the side   _____

5. Patient is to be given a large amount of liquid to drink   _____

6. Amount of urine sent to lab for certain test was insufficient   _____

7. All fluids patient drinks and voids are to be measured   _____

8. Patient is to walk twice a day   _____

9. Patient may have aspirin grains ten every four hours as needed   _____

Give the abbreviation for: (2 points each)

10. three times a day   _____   16. grams   _____

11. immediately   _____   17. liters   _____

12. with   _____   18. units   _____

13. without   _____   19. capsules   _____

14. water   _____   20. cubic centimeters   _____

15. oxygen   _____

Identify (spell out):   (2 points each)

21. B. E.   _____   _____

22. IVP   _____   _____

23. GB series   _____

24. upper GI series   _____

25. ECG (EKG)   _____

26. TPR   _____   _____   _____

27. EEG   _____

Write Roman numerals from one to ten: (1 point each)

28. _____   31. _____   34. _____   37. _____

29. _____   32. _____   35. _____

30. _____   33. _____   36. _____

chapter tests, review tests, and final exam

Name *ten* hospital departments: Give abbreviation if there is one. (2 points each)

38. _____ 43. _____

39. _____ 44. _____

40. _____ 45. _____

41. _____ 46. _____

42. _____ 47. _____

48. Orders for hospitalized patients should include (3 points each) _____

_____ _____

Five bonus points: Write an Rx for patient to have 50 milligrams of Demerol every four hours as needed:

_____

Test Key 18, Instructor's Guide

chapter 14
abbreviations: diagnoses and
medical laboratory

points: 100

_____
name

_____
course or section no.

test

1. Define these diagnoses: (2 points each)

   Cardiovascular

   a. CVA _____

   b. MI _____

   c. CHF _____

   Respiratory

   d. URI _____

   e. COPD or COLD _____

   Nervous system

   f. CP _____

   g. MS _____

2. Define these history taking abbreviations: (2 points each)

   a. PH _____

   b. ROS _____

   c. Dx _____

3. Name three divisions of medical laboratory: (2 points each)

   _____   _____   _____

   and one kind of test performed in each, in order: (2 points each)

   _____   _____   _____

4. What is the pap smear or test used for? (2 points) _____

   _____

5. Give the abbreviation for: (2 points each)

   a. hemoglobin _____   b. hematocrit _____   _____

   Spell out the following abbreviations for glucose tests: (2 points each)

   c. FBS _____

   d. GTT _____

6. What is meant by cath spec? Spell out and explain. (2 points) _____

   _____

7. Name three tests performed in routine urinalysis: (2 points each) _____

   _____   _____

Define: (2 points each)

8. erythrocytes _____

9. voided specimen _____

10. WBC and diff. _____

11. culture and sensitivity (C & S) _____

12. type and x-match _____

13. three kinds of leukocytes: (2 points each) _____

_____   _____

True/False: Circle the number of the *true* statements only. Defend your answers. Explain what is "untrue" in the false statements. (2 points each)

14. SMA (SMAC) includes a group of blood chemistry tests.

15. CA is an abbreviation for cancer.

16. Morphology of cells means numbers present.

17. Many kinds of bodily excretions are examined in the laboratory.

18. Serology tests are performed on whole blood.

Spell: (2 points)   **Define first five:** (2 points)

19. _____   _____

     _____

20. _____   _____

     _____

21. _____   _____

     _____

22. _____   _____

     _____

23. _____   _____

     _____

24. _____

Test Key 19, Instructor's Guide

chapter 16
structure of the body

points: 100 + 10 bonus

_____
name

_____
course or section no.

_____

test

_____

Fill in the blank: (3 points each blank)

1. The human body is made up of four structural units. Name them, _in order_, beginning with smallest unit:

   a. _____   b. _____

   c. _____   d. _____

2. Organs that work together are called   _____

3. Name three body systems and one organ in each:

   _____   _____

   _____   _____

   _____   _____

4. Give the other name for the thoracic cavity _____ and the abdominopelvic cavity

   _____ (names derived from the _name of the membrane lining cavity_)

5. The dome-shaped muscle that separates the chest and abdominal cavities is   _____

6. The space between lungs where the heart lies is called   _____

7. The chromosomes in the cell nucleus contain the _____, which pass hereditary characteristics to offspring.

8. Endocrine glands are also called _____ glands.

9. Cells reproduce by a process called   _____

10. GI stands for   _____

11. The main parts of a cell are the   _____ - _____

    _____

True/False: Circle the number of the _true_ statements only. Defend your answers. Explain what is "untrue" in the false statements. (2 points each)

12. The midsagittal plane divides the body into right and left equal sides.

13. The brain and spinal cord lie in the cranial cavity.

14. Metabolism is the sum of all physical and chemical changes that take place in the body.

15. The transverse plane divides the body into "top and bottom" (superior and inferior).

16. The primary tissues (kinds of tissues in the body) are epithelial, smooth, connective and muscular.

17. The coronal plane divides the body into "front and back" (anterior and posterior).

chapter tests, review tests, and final exam

Multiple choice: Circle the correct number (2 points each)

18. Stomatitis is (1) inflammation of the mouth; (2) inflammation of the stomach; or (3) excision of the stomach.

19. A colostomy is (1) excision of the gallbladder; (2) excision of the colon; or (3) a new permanent opening in the colon.

20. Cholecystectomy is (1) opening into colon; (2) colon examination; or (3) excision of the gallbladder.

21. Laparotomy is (1) excision of the stomach; (2) incision into the abdomen; or (3) plastic surgery on the abdominal wall.

Spell: (1 point each)   **Define any five:** (1 point each)

22. _____   _____

_____

23. _____   _____

_____

24. _____   _____

_____

25. _____   _____

_____

26. _____   _____

_____

27. _____   _____

_____

28. _____   _____

_____

29. _____   _____

_____

30. _____   _____

_____

Bonus: Write up to ten words not included on this test that you have learned in this course. (1 point each if correctly spelled)

_____   _____

_____   _____

_____   _____

_____   _____

_____   _____

Test Key 20, Instructor's Guide

chapter 16
structure of the body

name _____

points: 100

course or section no. _____

---

alternate test

Fill in the blank: (3 points for each blank)

1. Name, *in order*, the four structural units of the body, starting with the *largest*: _____

    _____   _____   _____

2. Name an organ in the respiratory system: _____ ;

    the cardiovascular system: _____ ;

    the genitourinary system: _____

    Name the system of which this organ is a part: brain _____ ; pituitary gland

    _____ ; skin _____

3. Specialized cells that are similar in structure and function: _____

4. The largest cavities of the body are the thoracic or chest or _____ and the abdomino-

    pelvic or _____

5. The transverse body plane divides the body into _____

    _____

6. Genes are contained in the _____ which are in the nucleus of the cell.

7. The spinal cord lies in the _____ cavity.

8. GU stands for _____

9. The midsagittal plane divides the body into _____

10. Name three of the four kinds of tissues found in the human body: _____

    _____   _____

11. The brain lies in the _____ cavity.

True/False: Circle the number of the *true* statements only. Defend your answers. Explain what is "untrue" in the false statements. (2 points each)

12. The coronal plane divides the body into superior and inferior sections.

13. Metabolism is the sum of all physical and chemical changes that take place in the body.

14. Cells reproduce by mitosis.

15. The diaphragm is a dome-shaped muscle.

16. Organs that work together are called tissues.

17. The mediastinum (space) is between the lungs.

chapter tests, review tests, and final exam

Define: (2 points each)

18. colostomy _____

19. cholecystectomy _____

20. stomatitis _____

21. laparotomy _____

Spell: (1 point each)   **Define any five:** (1 point each)

22. _____   _____

                                     _____

23. _____   _____

                                     _____

24. _____   _____

                                     _____

25. _____   _____

                                     _____

26. _____   _____

                                     _____

27. _____   _____

                                     _____

28. _____   _____

                                     _____

29. _____   _____

                                     _____

30. _____   _____

                                     _____

Test Key 21, Instructor's Guide

chapter 17
integumentary system

points: 100

_____
name

_____
course or section no.

---

test

Fill in the blank: (3 points each blank)

1. The specialist who treats skin disorders is a _____

2. Three functions of the skin are _____   _____

   _____

3. Give three terms used to describe skin lesions and define:

   _____   _____

   _____   _____

   _____   _____

4. Name three skin diseases: _____   _____

   _____

True/False: Circle the number of the _true_ statements only. Defend your answers. Explain what is "untrue" in the false statements. (2 points each)

5. Perspiration serves no useful purpose.

6. Some systemic diseases produce skin symptoms or manifestations.

7. The outer layer of skin is the dermis.

8. Skin cancer should be suspected when a nevus changes in size or appearance, or begins to bleed.

9. Tinea pedis is athlete's foot. One need not be an athlete to get this disease.

10. Sebaceous glands secrete sebum, which keeps the skin pliable.

11. Blood vessels and nerves are present in the epidermal layer.

12. Areola mamma is the halo or ring around the nipple (breast).

13. Contact dermatitis is inflammation of the skin caused by coming in contact with some irritant.

14. Pruritus means inflammation of the breast.

15. The Dick and Schick skin tests may be used to determine susceptibility to scarlet fever and diphtheria respectively.

Write the word that means: (3 points each; only 2 points if misspelled)

16. Process of stretching or opening wider _____

17. A new permanent opening into the colon _____

18. Plastic surgery on the nose _____

19. Surgical puncture of the abdomen to remove fluid _____

20. Surgical repair of a hernia _____

21. Incision into the trachea _____

Define: (2 points each)

22. Mantoux _____

23. nummular _____

24. biopsy _____

25. erythema _____

26. dermatome _____

Spell: (1 point each)   **Define three:** (1 point each)

27. _____   _____

          _____

28. _____   _____

          _____

29. _____   _____

          _____

30. _____   _____

          _____

31. _____   _____

          _____

32. _____   _____

          _____

33. _____   _____

          _____

34. _____   _____

          _____

Test Key 22, Instructor's Guide

chapter 17
integumentary system

points: 100

name

course or section no.

alternate test

True/False: Circle the number of the *true* statements only. Defend your answers. Explain what is "untrue" in the false statements. (2 points each)

1. A dermatologist is a specialist who diagnoses and treats skin disorders.

2. Macules, papules, and vesicles are terms to describe skin lesions.

3. Athlete's foot is an athlete's disease.

4. Oil glands are called sebaceous glands.

5. The breasts are also called the mammae.

6. Some systemic diseases produce skin symptoms.

7. A mole is a nevus; two moles, nevi.

8. A biopsy is an examination of living tissue.

9. Sweat glands are called sudoriferous glands.

Fill in the blank: (2 points each blank)

10. A blister is called a _____; a larger blister is a _____

11. The skin test used to determine susceptibility to diphtheria is the _____

12. The two outermost layers of the skin are the _____ and the _____

13. Herpes simplex is the medical term for _____

14. The halo around the nipple of the breast is called the _____

15. Three functions of the skin are _____ _____

_____

16. Name three parasitic skin infestations: _____ _____

_____

17. White patches of skin due to loss of pigment produces the disorder called _____

18. Name and describe three other skin diseases:

_____ _____

_____ _____

_____ _____

Write a word that means: (3 points each)

19. Excision of tonsils _____

20. Fixation of a kidney _____

21. Incision into the abdomen _____

22. New permanent opening into trachea _____

23. Tapping of chest to remove fluid _____

Define: (2 points each)

24. laceration _____

25. benign _____

26. malignant _____

27. sebaceous _____

28. lactation _____

Spell: (1 point each)   **Define any seven:** (1 point each)

29. _____   _____

                                    _____

30. _____   _____

                                    _____

31. _____   _____

                                    _____

32. _____   _____

                                    _____

33. _____   _____

                                    _____

34. _____   _____

                                    _____

35. _____   _____

                                    _____

36. _____   _____

                                    _____

37. _____   _____

                                    _____

38. _____   _____

                                    _____

Test Key 23, Instructor's Guide

chapter 18
musculoskeletal system

points: 100

name _____

course or section no. _____

test

Fill in the blank: (2 points each)

1. The five sections of the spinal column, *in order*, starting at the neck are _____

   _____   _____

   _____   _____

2. Two functions of the musculoskeletal system are _____

   _____

3. Bones are attached to other bones by fibrous tissue called _____. Muscles are attached

   to bones by _____.

4. Name of fracture: bone broken, protruding through skin _____; bone cracked, not

   separated _____

5. Flexion and extension mean _____ and _____

6. Moving the arm out to the side, away from the midline is called _____

Name the bones: (2 points each)

7. The longest bone in the human body _____

8. The "shoulder blade" _____ collar bone _____

9. An individual bone in spinal column _____

10. Bones of fingers and toes _____

11. Upper arm bone _____ breast bone _____

True/False: Circle the number of the *true* statements only. Defend your answers. Explain what is "untrue" in the false statements. (2 points each)

12. Bursae are small sacs that serve to cushion joints.

13. The extremities are part of the axial skeleton.

14. The muscles between the ribs are intercostals.

15. Rickets is a disease caused by bacteria.

16. Sinuses are cavities or air spaces in the skull.

17. An osteopath is an MD specialist who treats fractures.

18. Skeletal muscle is also called involuntary muscle.

19. Frontal, occipital, temporal, and peritoneal are all names of skull bones.

Fill in the blank: (2 points each)

20. Name two kinds of arthritis and age groups affected:

_____   _____

_____   _____

21. How are muscles named (two ways)?   _____

_____

_____

22. Three terms used to describe (in bones) "hollow places" or indentations, parts that project outward, and

"holes" in bones   _____   _____   _____

23. Tibia and fibula are bones of the   _____

24. Name a ball and socket joint: _____

Hinge joint: _____

Define: (2 points each)

25. atrophy   _____

26. sutures (in skull)   _____

27. orthopedist   _____

Spell: (1 point each)   **Define:**   (1 point each)

28. _____   _____

_____

29. _____   _____

_____

30. _____   _____

_____

31. _____   _____

_____

32. _____   _____

_____

33. _____   _____

_____

34. _____   _____

_____

35. _____   _____

_____

Test Key 24, Instructor's Guide

chapter 18
musculoskeletal system

points: 104

_____

name

_____

course or section no.

alternate test

Fill in the blank: (2 points each)

1. Four bones of the cranium are   _____   _____

   _____   _____

2. Name and describe three fractures:

   _____

   _____

   _____

3. Tendons attach _____ to _____

4. Other terms that mean: bending _____ and straightening _____

5. Name three large bones of upper extremity: _____   _____

   _____

6. Air spaces or cavities in the cranium are called   _____

7. Small sacs that serve to cushion joints are   _____

8. Seams or articulations between cranial bones are   _____

9. Medical specialist who treats bone disorders is an   _____

10. Skeletal muscle is also called _____ or _____ muscle

11. Name two main skeletal divisions: _____   _____

12. Name three kinds of muscle: _____   _____

   _____

13. Name three large bones of lower extremity: _____   _____

   _____

14. Abduction means   _____

15. Foramen is a   _____

16. Rickets is caused by   _____

17. What are the soft spots in an infant skull called?   _____

18. Name five segments of the vertebral column, _in order, starting from the bottom_ (tail):   _____

   _____   _____   _____   _____

Give a word for: (2 points each)

19. "Any disease" of the joints   _____

chapter tests, review tests, and final exam

20. Wasting away or shrinking of muscle _____

21. Softening of the bones _____

22. Pain in a joint _____

23. Plastic surgery on a joint _____

24. Inflammation of a joint _____

Name and describe two kinds of arthritis: (3 points each)

25. _____   _____

26. _____   _____

Name four other bones not mentioned in previous questions: (2 points each)

27. _____   29. _____

28. _____   30. _____

Test Key 25, Instructor's Guide

chapter 19
cardiovascular system

points: 100

name _____

course or section no. _____

_____
test
_____

Identify: Define or explain. (2 points each)

1. essential hypertension _____

2. myocardium _____

3. atria _____

4. oxygenated blood _____

5. arteriosclerosis _____

6. embolus _____

7. coronary arteries _____

Fill in the blank: (2 points each)

8. Red blood cells are called _____

9. White blood cells are called _____

10. In a white blood count and differential, the different kinds of WBCs are counted. Name the five basic kinds:

    _____   _____   _____

    _____   _____

11. What procedures are done in laboratory to determine compatibility before a transfusion is given?

    _____ and _____

12. Most people have Rh neg/pos blood. (circle one)

13. The top number in the B/P reading is the _____ and the bottom number is the

    _____ pressure.

14. The tiniest blood vessels are called _____

15. In these tiny vessels _____ and _____ (gases) are exchanged.

    Nutrients and _____ are also exchanged.

16. The dividing wall that separates the right and left sides of the heart is called the _____

17. In atherosclerosis, build up of deposits in arteries may occlude the opening or _____
    of the vessel (word that means opening in a tube).

True/False: Circle the number of the *true* statements only. Defend your answers. Explain what is "untrue" in the false statements. (2 points each)

18. Other names for heart attack are coronary occlusion, coronary thrombosis, and myocardial infarct (infarction).

19. A stroke is the same as a heart attack.

20. Lymph nodes help filter out injurious particles such as bacteria.

21. Everyone has one of four blood types (A, B, AB, O). Everyone also has the Rh factor.

22. Valves in the heart and in the veins keep blood from backflowing.

23. Anemia literally means "without blood." It actually means low red cell count.

24. The pulmonary arteries carry deoxygenated blood.

25. The left ventricle of the heart has a thicker muscle than the right ventricle because it has to pump blood farther.

26. Platelets help to clot blood.

27. Varicose veins are dilated, tortuous veins that occur when valves "break down."

28. CVA stands for cerebrovascular accident or stroke.

29. Angiography is an X-ray procedure to determine condition of blood vessels.

Identify:　(1 point each)

30. CCU _____

31. ECG _____

32. Specialist who treats CVD _____

33. Specialist who treats blood diseases _____

34. Trace the circulation from the vessels that bring blood back to the heart to the vessels that carry it out to all parts of the body; name all structures—vessels, chambers, valves, and organs through which it passes, *in sequence*. (13 structures, 1 point each)

a. _____　　f. _____　　j. _____

b. _____　　g. _____　　k. _____

c. _____　　h. _____　　l. _____

d. _____　　i. _____　　m. _____

e. _____

Spell:　(1 point each)

35. _____　　40. _____

36. _____　　41. _____

37. _____　　42. _____

38. _____　　43. _____

39. _____

Test Key 26, Instructor's Guide

chapter 19
cardiovascular system

points: 100

_____

name

_____

course or section no.

---

alternate test

Fill in the blank: (2 points each)

1. Give two other names for heart attack: _____

   _____

2. Name the four blood types (Landsteiner): (2 points for all 4)

   _____ _____ _____ _____

3. In a B/P reading, what is the top pressure called? _____ Bottom pressure?

   _____

4. An embolus is a _____ that is floating freely in the blood stream.

5. The receiving chambers of the heart are called _____

6. _Which_ ventricle of the heart has the thicker muscle and _why_? (4 points)

   _____

7. What are the vessels that carry blood _away_ from the heart called? _____ What are

   the vessels that carry blood _toward_ the heart called? _____

8. The smallest blood vessels are the _____

9. Three layers of the heart are _____ (inner) _____ (outer)

   _____ (muscular)

True/False: Circle the number of the _true_ statements only. Defend your answers. Explain what is "untrue" in the false statements. (2 points each)

10. A CVA is a cerebrovascular accident or stroke.

11. Everyone has the Rh factor.

12. Hypertension is high blood pressure.

13. Platelets are white blood cells.

14. A CBC is a coronary blood center.

15. Hemiplegia means paralyzed from the waist down.

16. The wall that divides the right and left sides of the heart is the septum.

17. Tachycardia means a slow heart rate.

18. Give the names of the five basic kinds of leukocytes: (2 points each) _____

   _____ _____ _____ _____

19. Define WBC and diff: (2 points) _____

   _____

chapter tests, review tests, and final exam

20. Trace the circulation through the heart, starting with the vessels that bring blood back to the heart from the upper and lower parts of the body, naming all chambers, valves, vessels, and organs, *in order*, until the blood leaves the heart to go to all parts of the body. (13 structures, 1 point each)

_____

_____

_____

_____

_____

Define or explain: (2 points each)

21. valves in veins _____

22. coronary arteries _____

23. erythrocytes _____

24. type and x-match _____

25. arteriosclerosis _____

26. hemostasis _____

27. When does the Rh factor present a problem? (4 points)

_____

_____

Spell: (1 point each)   **Define any six:** (1 point each)

28. _____   _____

_____

29. _____   _____

_____

30. _____   _____

_____

31. _____   _____

_____

32. _____   _____

_____

33. _____   _____

_____

34. _____   _____

_____

Test Key 27, Instructor's Guide

chapter 20
respiratory system

points: 100

name _____

course or section no. _____

---

test

Matching: Match the terms (A–CC) with the definitions (1–25), writing the correct corresponding letter in the space provided before each number. Not all of the terms will be used. (2 points each)

_____ 1. Air (gas) expired.

_____ 2. Combination of inspiration and expiration.

_____ 3. Passageway that carries food and gases.

_____ 4. Tube from middle ear to pharynx.

_____ 5. Organs of respiration.

_____ 6. Air left in lungs after expiration.

_____ 7. Medical name for croup.

_____ 8. Diagnostic skin test for TB.

_____ 9. A cough that produces sputum.

_____ 10. Drugs used to treat TB.

_____ 11. Excision of part of a lung.

_____ 12. Allergic disorders of respiratory system.

_____ 13. Secretion from respiratory tract, examined for diagnosis in TB.

_____ 14. Inflammation of air spaces in cranium.

_____ 15. Abnormal lung sounds.

_____ 16. Medical name for infection in bronchi.

_____ 17. Excision of glandular structures in pharynx.

_____ 18. Abbreviated term used for standard chest X-ray film.

_____ 19. Flap of tissue that covers larynx when food is swallowed.

_____ 20. Lower (bottom part) of the lungs.

_____ 21. Referring to both lungs.

_____ 22. Mist type of medication that helps dilate air passages and loosens secretions.

_____ 23. Collapse of lung.

_____ 24. Amount of air that can be forcibly expelled after deep inspiration.

_____ 25. Infection in upper respiratory tract (abbreviation).

A. vital capacity
B. aerosol
C. base
D. URI
E. bilateral
F. adenoids
G. isoniazid and PAS
H. asthma, hayfever
I. sputum
J. lobectomy
K. rales
L. bronchitis
M. CO_2
N. pharynx
O. laryngotracheobronchitis
P. eustachian
Q. lungs
R. valley fever
S. atelectasis
T. residual
U. Mantoux
V. sinusitis
W. tonsillectomy
X. epiglottis
Y. IUR
Z. productive
AA. respiration
BB. AP and lat
CC. spirometer

Give a word for: (2 points each; only 1 point if misspelled)

26. Tiny air sacs in which gases exchange in the lungs _____

27. Air (gas) breathed in (and also given as treatment) _____

28. Muscular partition that separates chest and abdominal cavity _____

29. Dividing wall in nose _____

30. Membrane that covers lung and lines chest cavity _____

31. Windpipe leading to bronchi _____

32. Top (narrower part) of lungs _____

33. Instrument for looking into bronchi _____

34. Difficult or labored breathing _____

35. New permanent opening into trachea _____

36. Incision into trachea _____

37. Procedure of looking into larynx with instrument _____

38. Disease in which alveoli are greatly distended (stretched) _____

39. Cancerous tumor of lung _____

40. Infectious lung disease with tubercle formation _____

41. Inflammation of lungs _____

42. Inflammation of membrane that lines chest cavity _____

43. Surgical puncture of chest (to remove fluid) _____

44. Other words for common cold _____

45. Inflammation that causes loss of voice _____

46. Section of vertebral column that forms back wall of chest _____

47. Can only breathe sitting up _____

48. Rapid breathing _____

49. Temporary periods of no breathing _____

50. ENT specialist _____
(spell out in medical terminology)

Test Key 28, Instructor's Guide

chapter 20
respiratory system

points: 100

name _____

course or section no. _____

alternate test

Fill in the blank: (2 points each)

1. The gas inspired in breathing is _____; that expired is _____

2. Name the structure in the throat through which both food and gases pass _____

3. The tubes from the middle ears to the pharynx are called _____

4. Examination of the larynx with an instrument for "looking into" is called _____

5. The cavity in which the lungs lie (chest) is also called _____ or _____

6. The seven organs (including passageways) through which inspired air passes, *in order*, are the _____

   _____

   _____

7. Another word for rapid breathing is _____ Labored breathing may also be called

   _____

8. The dome-shaped muscle that is located below the lungs and contracts during inspiration is the

   _____ A hernia of this muscle (opening) is called a _____ hernia.

9. Name four diseases or disorders of respiratory system (not mentioned in this test) _____

   _____ _____ _____

10. Two tests for TB are the _____ and the _____

11. Slow breathing is called _____, and a period of no breathing is called _____

12. Atelectasis means _____

13. In emphysema the _____ become distended and inelastic.

14. Rales are _____

15. URI is an abbreviation that means (2 points total) _____ _____

    _____

16. Thoracocentesis means _____

17. The plural of alveolus is _____ and of apex _____

18. Expectorants are medications that _____

19. A spirometer is an instrument used to test _____

Define: (2 points each)

20. tonsillectomy _____

21. tracheostomy _____

chapter tests, review tests, and final exam **281**

22. aerosol _____

23. carcinoma (lung) _____

24. radiologist _____

Spell out: (3 points each)

25. COPD _____

26. IPPB _____

27. SOB _____

28. T & A _____

29. ENT (and give technical name for physician who treats ENT conditions) _____

_____

Spell: (1 point each)

30. a. _____

    b. _____

    c. _____

    d. _____

    e. _____

Test Key 29, Instructor's Guide

chapter 21
gastrointestinal system

points: 100

_____
name

_____
course or section no.

test

Fill in the blank: (2 points each)

1. Two names for the body cavity in which most of the organs of the GI system lie are _____
   and _____

2. The stomach lies in the _____ quadrant; the appendix is attached to the
   _____ (part of colon), and lies in the _____ quadrant.

3. Muscular contractions propelling material through GI tract are called _____

4. Bile is important in the digestion of _____ (food). Bile is produced by the liver and
   stored in the _____

5. The small intestine is lined with tiny projections called _____ These increase the surface area of the intestine, which increases the _____ of nutrients.

6. Write a word that means: excision of the stomach _____; gallstones _____;
   inflammation of liver _____

7. Name any two surgical procedures performed on GI organs:

   _____   _____

8. Name three procedures used in diagnosing GI disorders: _____

   _____   _____

True/False: Circle the numbers of the *true* statements only. Defend your answers. Explain what is "untrue" in the false statements. (2 points each)

9. Choledochitis is inflammation of the common bile duct.

10. Carbohydrates and fats supply the body with heat and energy.

11. The stomach and the abdomen are the same.

12. When the parotid glands are inflamed, the condition is called mumps.

13. Almost all absorption of digested foods occurs in small intestines.

14. Proteins are essential for growth and repair of tissue.

15. The right and left hypochondriac regions of the abdomen are directly below the right and left lumbar regions.

16. The cardiac and pyloric are sphincter muscles of the stomach.

17. The hepatic and cystic ducts join to make the common bile duct.

18. Digestion is both a chemical and a mechanical process.

19. Name three sections of the abdomen (not quadrants and not those already mentioned)

   _____ _____ _____

Write a word for: (2 points each)

20. Inflammation of the tongue   _____

21. Inflammation of the colon   _____

22. Inflammation of the stomach   _____

23. Inflammation of the mouth   _____

24. Inflammation of the ileum   _____

25. Name, *in order*, the 14 organs of the GI tract through which food passes—from intake to excretion (1 point each; total 14)   _____

_____

_____

_____

_____

26. Name six accessory digestive organs (1 point each)   _____

_____

_____

27. Using some of the following words, fill in the blanks: (1 point each) (colostomy, NPO, barium enema, diagnosis, prognosis, proctoscopic, enemas, upper GI series, symptoms)

The physician reviewed the patient's _____ and wrote a tentative _____

He told the patient to take _____ after midnight and to take _____

"until clear" in the morning, in preparation for a _____ (colon X-ray procedure). He

also asked him to schedule another appointment for a _____ exam (looking into rectum

with instrument). The physician tried to reassure the patient by telling him the _____

was favorable, but the patient was worried that the outcome might be a _____

(opening into colon).

Test Key 30, Instructor's Guide

chapter 21
gastrointestinal system

points: 100

_____
name

_____
course or section no.

alternate test

Fill in the blank: (2 points each)

1. Two other names for the GI tract are _____ and _____

2. The duodenum, jejunum, and ileum are parts of the   _____

3. Which cavity holds the GI viscera? _____ or _____

4. The stomach lies in the _____ (quadrant); the liver in the _____ (quadrant).

5. The wormlike appendage, attached to the cecum, which serves no known function except to cause trouble, is the _____

6. During digestion foods are changed into soluble form so that they can be readily _____ into the _____ for use by body cells.

7. An X-ray picture of the lower GI tract is called a _____ or _____ It is a diagnostic tool.

8. The liver produces _____, which is important for the digestion of _____ (certain food). This substance that the liver produces is stored in the _____

9. Name the seven large intestine sections (_in order_):   _____
   _____
   _____

10. Name four accessory digestive organs: _____   _____
    _____   _____

11. The mesentery is sometimes called an "apron" because it   _____
    It is actually part of the membrane that lines the entire cavity, called the   _____

12. There are many "scopes" for looking into GI organs. Name three: _____
    _____   _____

13. Name three surgical procedures commonly performed on GI organs: _____
    _____   _____

14. Peristalsis is   _____

15. What is the common bile duct?   _____
    _____

16. _____   _____ and _____ are three
    main food groups. Two other essential elements for proper nutrition are _____ and
    _____

17. Diagram and label the nine sections of the abdomen: (1 point each)

Spell: (1 point each)

18. a. _____

b. _____

c. _____

d. _____

e. _____

Define four: (1 point each)

_____

_____

_____

_____

_____

_____

_____

_____

_____

Test Key 31, Instructor's Guide

chapter 22
genitourinary system

points: 100

name _____

course or section no. _____

test

Spell out and explain meaning **of five of the following:** (3 points each)

1. D & C _____

_____

2. BOW _____

_____

3. EDC _____

_____

4. LMP _____

_____

5. TUR _____

_____

6. I & O _____

_____

Fill in the blank: (1 point each unless otherwise stated)

7. External genitals are called _____ and _____ in men, and

_____ in women.

8. The sex cell is called _____ in men and _____ in women.

9. Three organs of reproduction in women are _____ _____

_____

10. Name three terms used in describing abortions: _____ _____

_____

True/False: Circle the number of *true* statements only. Defend your answers. Explain what is "untrue" in the false statements. (1 point each)

11. An episiotomy is an incision made to facilitate delivery.

12. The hymen is the afterbirth.

13. The clitoris is a sensitive projection in the vulvar area.

14. ROA and LOA are normal presentations of the infant for delivery.

15. An abortion is a miscarriage.

16. The perineum in the female is the area between the vulva and the anus.

Copyright © 1983 by Addison-Wesley Publishing Company, Inc.

chapter tests, review tests, and final exam **287**

17. Breech always means feet first delivery of infant.

18. A good Apgar score is 9 to 10 at one minute.

19. An enlarged prostate will block the flow of urine.

Fill in the blank: (1 point each)

20. The main function of the kidneys (urinary system) is _____

_____

21. Name three tests included in the Ua: _____   _____

_____

22. Frequency and urgency are symptoms of   _____

23. Give the abbreviation for an X-ray procedure used to determine kidney function: _____

24. Meconium stained amniotic fluid usually indicates   _____

_____

25. Foley and French are names for kinds of   _____

26. STS stands for _____ test for _____

Give a word that means: (1 point each)

27. "Fixation" of kidney   _____

28. "Condition" of the kidney   _____

29. Inflammation of the ovaries   _____

30. Hernia of the bladder   _____

31. Excision of the prostate   _____

32. Inflammation of the renal pelvis   _____

Explain or define: (Choose any 7; 2 points each) (33–42)

33. multipara   _____

34. Pap smear   _____

35. UTI   _____

36. fundus of uterus   _____

37. pudendal block   _____

38. vasectomy   _____

39. kidney transplant   _____

40. peristalsis in ureters   _____

41. enuresis   _____

42. PID   _____

Explain this notation on an OB record   (1 point each): para VI, grav VIII, AB I, SB I:

43.   _____

44. **Diagram urinary system** and label at least three parts: (4 points) Use space on following page.

Spell: (1 point each)

Define any 12: (1 point each)

45. _____

46. _____

47. _____

48. _____

49. _____

50. _____

51. _____

52. _____

53. _____

54. _____

55. _____

56. _____

57. _____

58. _____

59. _____

Test Key 32, Instructor's Guide

chapter 22
genitoruinary system

points: 102

name _____

course or section no. _____

alternate test

Fill in the blank: (2 points each)

1. Name the procedure of looking into the bladder with instrument: _____

2. The tube used to drain urine from the bladder is called a _____
    Name two kinds: _____ _____

3. The score used to determine the infant's condition at one and at five minutes after birth is called _____
    _____

4. What is the medication used to increase urinary output (general category of drug)? _____

5. Name the normal vertex presentations of an infant at delivery time (abbreviations): _____
    _____

6. IVP stands for _____
    Why is it done? _____

7. Two symptoms of UTI are _____ and _____

8. The sterilization procedure in men is called _____; that in women is called
    _____

9. Where is the perineum (in women)? _____

10. Why is a Pap smear done? _____

11. Name the external genitals in the male: _____ _____

12. Name the sex gland and sex cell in women: _____ _____

13. What is the incision made to facilitate childbirth called? _____

14. The first bowel movement of the infant is called _____

15. Name and/or describe three tests done in routine Ua: _____
    _____ _____

16. The two main kinds of VD are _____ and _____

Give the term for: (2 points each)

17. Fixation of fallopian tubes _____

18. Excision of ovaries _____

19. Inflammation of prostate _____

20. Any disease of the kidneys _____

21. Pus in the urine _____

chapter tests, review tests, and final exam

22. Tapping to remove amniotic fluid _____

Explain or define: (choose four out of the six; 2 points each)

23. gravid _____

24. multipara _____

25. pudendal block _____

26. therapeutic abortion _____

27. spontaneous abortion _____

28. I & O _____

Fill in the blank: (2 points each)

29. Name the procedure of opening up the cervix and scraping out the uterus (give abbreviation and spell out):

_____   _____

Give two reasons why this is done: _____   _____

30. Where does fertilization occur? _____

31. Give the medical term for:

a. bedwetting _____

b. procedure of using artificial kidney _____

c. excessive urination _____

32. Give two complications of pregnancy: _____ and_____

True/False: Circle the number of the *true* statements only. Defend your answers. Explain what is "untrue" in the false statements. (1 point each)

33. The placenta is the afterbirth.

34. The main function of the kidneys is to filter the blood.

35. A breech delivery is always buttocks first.

36. A person can live with one kidney.

37. When delivery is accomplished by an incision into the uterus, the procedure is called cesarean section.

38. The fundus is the neck of the uterus.

39. Diagram KUB: (three items, 2 points each)

Test Key 33, Instructor's Guide

chapter 23
nervous system

points: 100

_____

name

_____

course or section no.

test

(Unless noted otherwise, all answers on this test are 2 points each.)

Fill in the blank:

1. Name four lobes of the cerebrum: _____ _____

   _____ _____

2. The largest part of the brain is the _____

3. The membranes covering the brain and spinal cord are called the _____;

   _____ (outer); _____ (middle); and _____ (inner).

4. Name two cranial nerves: _____ and _____

5. Name two divisions of the autonomic nervous system: _____ and _____

   The autonomic nervous system is also called the _____ nervous system because we do not control it.

6. Spinal nerves are designated by abbreviations relating to sections of the spinal column in which they occur;

   C-2 means _____; L-3 _____; T-4 _____

7. The brain and spinal cord are protected by the _____ and _____

   (bony structures) and by _____ (liquid) as well as by membranes.

Define:

8. myelogram _____

9. encephalon _____

10. subdural hematoma _____

11. encephalitis _____

12. EEG _____

13. Name three diseases or disorders of the nervous system not mentioned in this test: _____

    _____ _____

14. Halves or sides of the brain are called _____

15. Glioma and meningioma are kinds of nervous system _____

16. Hemiparesis means _____

Write a word that means:

17. inflammation of meninges _____

18. paralysis from the waist down _____

18. paralysis from the waist down _____

19. deep furrows in the brain _____

20. "water on the brain" _____

21. cavities of the brain _____

22. A spinal tap is also called a _____

23. CSF means _____

24. Injury (damage) to the brain and/or spinal cord generally causes _____ (loss of motor function).

True/False: Circle the number of the *true* statements only. Defend your answers. Explain what is "untrue" in the false statements.

25. All of the body's activities are controlled and coordinated by the central nervous system.

26. The occiput is located at the front of the brain.

27. Neurologic diseases are usually disabling, long-term, and require rehabilitative measures.

28. A person who has a "nervous breakdown" has weak nerves.

29. ECG is a record of electrical impulses in the brain.

Matching: (1 point each)

30. ____ ECT

     ____ membranes

     ____ spinal tap

     ____ functional

     ____ hemiplegia

     ____ gyrus

     ____ plexus

     ____ response

     ____ forehead

     ____ paresis

     ____ paraplegia

     ____ caudal

a. LP
b. paralysis on one side
c. convolutions
d. stimulus
e. frontal
f. paralysis waist down
g. "tail"
h. shock
i. without cause
j. meninges
k. network
l. weakness

Test Key 34, Instructor's Guide

Do not write on this page until assigned

chapter 23
nervous system

points: 100 (All answers in this test are 2 points each.)

name _____

course or section no. _____

---

alternate test

True/False: Circle the number of the *true* statements only. Defend your answers. Explain what is "untrue" in the false statements.

1. Nerve cells are called neurons.

2. A lumbar puncture may be done to relieve pressure or to obtain a sample of fluid for laboratory study.

3. The largest part of the brain is the cerebellum.

4. Because nervous tissue is very delicate, it is protected with coverings of bone, tough membranes, and CSF.

5. An ECG is a record of electrical impulses in the brain.

6. People with weak nerves often have a "nervous breakdown."

Identify: Spell these out. Nerves are located by the section of the vertebral column in which they originate.

7. L-2 _____

8. T-7 _____

9. C-5 _____

10. Co-1 _____

Fill in the blank:

11. Name the four lobes of the cerebrum: _____ _____

_____ _____

12. The three membranes that cover the brain and spinal cord are called _____ Name

the external layer: _____; middle layer: _____; and internal

layer: _____

13. Peripheral means _____ The cranial and spinal _____ are
called the peripheral nervous system.

14. Name the two divisions of the autonomic nervous system:

_____ and _____

Which of these aids the body in emergency situations? _____

15. The skeletal structures that protect the brain and spinal cord are the _____ and the

_____

16. EEG means _____

17. Name three diseases or disorders that affect the nervous system _____

_____ _____

Copyright © 1983 by Addison-Wesley Publishing Company, Inc. *chapter tests, review tests, and final exam* **295**

18. The brain is divided into right and left halves; these are called _____

19. The _____ nerve controls vision and the _____ nerve, hearing.

20. The medical specialist who treats diseases of the nervous system is _____

21. Gyri are convolutions of the _____; sulci are deep _____ in the brain.

Define:

22. hemiplegia _____

23. paraplegia _____

24. quadriplegia _____

25. A group of branching and interconnecting nerves is called a _____

26. Inflammation of the brain is called _____

27. Inflammation of the meninges is called _____

28. The encephalon is the _____

Define:

29. paresis _____

30. concussion _____

_____

31. myelomeningocele _____

_____

32. ventricles (in brain) _____

33. cerebral palsy _____

_____

34. In which cavity does the brain lie? _____

The spinal cord? _____

35. What is the term used to describe the anesthesia injected into the lower part of the spine _____

Test Key 35, Instructor's Guide

chapter 24
eyes, ears, and teeth

points: 100

_____
name

_____
course or section no.

---

test

Fill in the blank: (2 points each)

1. Lenses are measured in units called _____

2. The instrument for measuring pressure within the eyeball is a _____

3. Pink eye is inflammation of mucous membrane. It is a kind of _____ (-itis).

4. "Irrigate OD" means _____

5. The corners of the eye (slit between lids) are called _____

6. The instrument for looking into the eye is an _____

7. Inflammation of the middle ear is _____

8. Two other words for eardrum are _____ and _____

9. Ear wax is also called _____

10. The instrument for looking into the ear is an _____

11. Baby teeth are _____ teeth.

12. Inflammation of the gums is called _____

True/False: Circle the number of the _true_ statements only. Defend your answers. Explain what is "untrue" in the false statements. (2 points each)

13. The pupil dilates when one goes into a dark theater.

14. A cataract is a clouded lens.

15. Glaucoma is a disease that may lead to blindness if untreated.

16. A person with good peripheral vision can only see things far away.

17. Tears leave the eye through the lacrimal duct.

18. Refractive errors are treated with eyeglasses or contact lenses.

19. No medication should be instilled into the eye unless it is an "ophthalmic" preparation.

20. The optic and auditory nerves are cranial nerves.

21. Presbyopia is commonly called lazy eye.

22. Astigmatism can be present with either myopia or hyperopia, or without either of these.

23. The orbital ridge is part of the eye socket of the cranium.

24. The cornea can be successfully transplanted.

25. An otologist is a medical specialist who treats ear diseases.

26. The eustachian tubes connect the middle ear with the pharynx.

27. The machine used to test hearing is called an audiometer.

28. The middle ear controls and affects balance and equilibrium.

29. The iris regulates the size of the pupil.

30. Some forms of deafness cannot be aided with a hearing aid.

31. The periodontist treats diseases of the gums.

32. Gum disease is the primary cause of tooth loss.

33. Permanent first molars usually emerge at about age 6 years.

34. Emmetropia is normal vision.

35. Blepharitis is inflammation of the eyelid.

36. Papilledema can be observed with an ophthalmoscope.

Define: (2 points each)

37. myringotomy _____

38. 20/20 vision _____

_____

39. lensometer _____

40. iridectomy _____

41. pinna _____

42. prophylactic dental care _____

43. prosthetic dentistry _____

44. plaque (dental) _____

45. keratitis _____

46. PERLA _____

47. buccal _____

48. Explain the difference between an ophthalmologist and an optometrist: (4 points) _____

_____

_____

_____

Test Key 36, Instructor's Guide

chapter 24
eyes, ears, and teeth

points: 102

name _____

course or section no. _____

alternate test

Fill in the blank: (3 points each)

1. Sound is measured in units called _____

2. The instrument for looking into the ear is an _____

3. Explain: inflammation OS _____

4. Name the MD specialist who treats eye disease: _____

5. Give two medical terms for an incision into the eardrum: _____

   or _____

6. A clouded lens is called a _____

7. _____ is a disease in which intraocular pressure is increased.

8. Refractive errors are treated with prescription _____

9. The nerve to the eye is the _____ nerve.

10. The _____ is the machine used for testing hearing.

True/False: Circle the number of the *true* statements only. Defend your answers. Explain what is "untrue" in the false statements. (3 points each)

11. The pupil contracts when one enters a dark room.

12. Good peripheral vision means good vision out to the sides.

13. The lacrimal gland produces tears for crying.

14. All preparations instilled into the eye must be ophthalmic preparations.

15. Presbyopia means inability of eye to accommodate quickly to near and far vision.

16. The orbit is the bony cavity of the cranium in which the eye rests.

17. The eustachian tubes connect the inner ear with the pharynx.

18. Some forms of hearing loss can be aided with a hearing aid.

19. The periodontist is a dental specialist in treating gum disease.

20. Dental cavities are the major cause of tooth loss.

21. Permanent first molars appear at about age 3 years.

22. Blepharoptosis is drooping of the eyelids.

23. Papilledema means swelling of the optic nerve where it enters the eye.

24. An ophthalmologist and an optometrist both fit glasses but the first is an MD who also treats eye disease.

Define: (choose *any* 9 out of 11; 3 points each)

25. tonometer _____

26. conjunctivitis _____

27. inner canthus of eye _____

28. otitis media _____

29. cerumen _____

30. gingivectomy _____

31. deciduous _____

32. diopters _____

33. 20/20 vision _____

34. myopia _____

35. amblyopia _____

Test Key 37, Instructor's Guide

chapter 25
endocrine system

points: 100

_____

name

_____

course or section no.

_____

test

_____

Fill in the blank: (2 points each)

1. Endocrine glands are also called _____ glands because their secretions go directly into the bloodstream instead of passing through _____

2. All secretions of endocrine glands are called _____

3. The pituitary glands are located deep in the _____ cavity.

4. The endocrine glands located in the neck, around the larynx, are the _____ and the

   _____

5. Estrogen and progesterone are _____ secreted by the _____

6. The endocrine glands located at the top of each kidney are the _____

7. Excision of the pancreas is called _____

8. All of the organs of the endocrine system are called _____

9. The pituitary is called the _____ gland because it regulates all of the other endocrine glands.

10. Hypoglycemia means (three words, 2 points total) _____

11. Diabetes mellitus is a disease caused by dysfunction of the _____ Treatment usually involves special diet and injection of _____ daily.

12. PBI stands for (three words, 2 points total) _____
    It is a test of _____ function.

13. RAI means (2 points) _____

True/False: Circle the number of the _true_ statements only. Defend your answers. Explain what is "untrue" in the false statements. (2 points each)

14. The parotid glands are a part of the endocrine system.

15. Testosterone is a hormone secreted by the testes.

16. A duct never carries hormones.

17. A goiter is an enlarged adrenal gland.

18. FBS and GTT are tests used to detect diabetes mellitus.

19. The pancreas is located in the LUQ.

20. The Islands of Langerhans are cells in the adrenals.

21. Iodine is essential for thyroid function.

22. Acromegaly means enlarged extremities and is caused by pituitary dysfunction.

23. Postprandial means "after a meal."

24. Insulin is a hormone secreted by the pancreas.

25. The pancreas functions in two systems, GI and endocrine.

26. Name three disorders of the endocrine system (excluding diabetes): _____

    _____   _____

27. People who have diabetes are more susceptible to complications; name three: _____

    _____   _____

28. Give the type of onset, symptoms, and emergency treatment for the following: (4 points each; 8 points total)

    Diabetic coma   *Insulin shock*

Spell: (1 point each)   **Define eight:** (1 point each)

29. _____   _____

    _____

30. _____   _____

    _____

31. _____   _____

    _____

32. _____   _____

    _____

33. _____   _____

    _____

34. _____   _____

    _____

35. _____   _____

    _____

36. _____   _____

    _____

37. _____   _____

    _____

38. _____   _____

    _____

39. _____   _____

    _____

40. _____   _____

    _____

Test Key 38, Instructor's Guide

chapter 25
endocrine system

points: 100

_____

name

_____

course or section no.

_____

alternate test

_____

Fill in the blank: (3 points each blank space)

1. Glands of internal secretion are called _____ or _____ glands.

2. The Islands of Langerhans are cells in the _____, which secretes a _____ called _____

3. The hormone testosterone is secreted by the _____ (organ).

4. Describe the location of the following glands:

   a. hypophysis   _____

   b. suprarenals   _____

   c. thyroid   _____

   d. parathyroids   _____

5. Where is the pancreas located?   _____

6. The gonads in the female are the   _____

7. Spell out:

   a. FBS   _____

   b. GTT   _____

   c. What are they used for?   _____

   _____

8. Name two tests for thyroid function: _____

9. The master gland is the   _____

10. Treatment for diabetic coma is primarily   _____

11. Treatment for insulin shock is primarily   _____

12. Which endocrine gland lies in the cranial cavity?   _____

13. Name three kinds of complications diabetics are susceptible to:

   _____   _____   _____

Define: (3 points each)

14. acute   _____

15. hyperfunction   _____

16. edematous   _____

Spell: (1 point each)

Define eight: (1 point each)

17. _____

18. _____

19. _____

20. _____

21. _____

22. _____

23. _____

24. _____

25. _____

26. _____

27. _____

28. _____

29. _____

30. _____

Test Key 39, Instructor's Guide

medical terminology

name _____

course or section no. _____

points: 200 (Each answer in test is 1 point.)

final exam

Name the medical specialist:

1. Children only _____

2. Internal disorders _____

3. Eye diseases _____

4. Mental illness _____

5. Disorders of skeletal system _____

6. Specialist who interprets X-ray films _____

Identify:

7. DO _____

_____

8. podiatrist _____

_____

9. optometrist _____

_____

10. Name the two largest body cavities: (two names for each)

_____ or _____

_____ or _____

Mark with a check the routine immunizations available and recommended for all with few exceptions. Identify where indicated by blanks:

11. ____ DPT _____ _____ _____

12. ____ varicella

13. ____ parotitis _____

14. ____ influenza

15. ____ rubella _____

16. ____ scarlet fever

17. ____ impetigo

18. ____ syphilis

19. ____ poliomyelitis

20. ____ rubeola _____

Write a word that means:

21. Before birth _____

22. Condition of blueness _____

23. Any disease of glands _____

24. Inflammation of kidney _____

25. Excision of ovaries _____

26. Fixation of fallopian tubes _____

27. Enlarged heart _____

28. Malignant tumor _____

29. Fast heart beat _____

30. High B/P _____

31. Wasting away (muscles) _____

32. Between ribs _____

33. Under the skin _____

34. Treatment with water _____

35. Without rhythm (heart) _____

36. Instrument for cutting thin section of skin _____

37. Instrument for looking into ear _____

38. Excision of gallbladder _____

39. Incision into trachea _____

40. New permanent opening into colon _____

41. Repair of hernia _____

True/False: Circle the number of the *true* statements only. Defend your answers. Explain what is "untrue" in the false statements.

42. Three layers of the heart are endocardium, myocardium, and pericardium.

43. Everyone has the Rh factor (in blood).

44. An isotonic solution has the same salt concentration as that of body fluids.

45. "Diff" in WBC means counting the number of each kind of leukocyte.

46. C & S is a lab procedure done on bacteria to isolate the bacteria causing disease and to determine to which antibiotic the organism is sensitive or resistant (S or R).

47. The words cervix and cervical pertain to the uterus only.

48. Ligaments, tendons, and fasciae are all kinds of connective tissue.

49. A proctoscope is used for looking into the vagina.

50. During inspiration the diaphragm moves upward.

51. The midsagittal plane divides the body into equal R & L sides.

52. Oxygen and carbon dioxide are exchanged in the alveoli (lungs).

Define:

53. capillaries _____

54. vertebrae _____

55. intravenous _____

56. dehydrated _____

57. etiology _____

58. postpartum _____

59. sinuses _____

60. hypertrophy _____

61. speculum _____

62. osteotome _____

63. aseptic _____

64. gastroscopy _____

65. lipoma _____

66. pyogenic _____

67. arthroplasty _____

68. bradycardia _____

69. prognosis _____

70. neuralgia _____

71. laparotomy _____

72. hysterectomy _____

73. thoracocentesis _____

74. sclerosis _____

75. cystocele _____

76. stomatitis _____

77. lithotripsy _____

Matching:

78. _____ Schick   88. _____ FBS

79. _____ EEG   89. _____ CO_2

80. _____ Dick   90. _____ septum

81. _____ WBC   91. _____ voice box

82. _____ C-2

83. _____ lungs

84. _____ A, B, O

85. _____ Kahn

86. _____ cranium

87. _____ CBC

a. pulmonary
b. larynx
c. skull
d. blood types
e. electroencephalogram
f. diphtheria
g. hematology
h. serological test
i. second cervical vertebra
j. "sugar" test
k. dividing partition or wall
l. scarlet fever
m. carbon dioxide
n. leukocytes

Fill in the blank:

92. Prone means face _____ Supination of the hand means palm _____

93. The proximal end of the femur is near the (pelvis, knee). (Underline the correct word.)

94. The distal end of the humerus is nearer the (shoulder, elbow). (Underline the correct word.)

95. Psoriasis, eczema, and verrucae are disorders of the _____ system.

96. Name the five sections of the vertebral column (in order): _____ _____

    _____ _____ _____

97. Paralysis on one side of the body is _____

    From the waist down _____

    From the neck down _____

98. Flexion and extension mean (in order) _____ and _____

99. Toward the midline: _____

    Away from the midline: _____

100. Name three of the five basic kinds of leukocytes:

    _____ _____ _____

101. Name any four bones of the extremities: _____ _____

    _____ _____

102. The largest vein in the body is the _____

    The largest artery is the _____

103. Name any two valves of the heart: _____ and _____

104. The two numbers in a blood pressure reading are called _____ (top number) and

    _____ (bottom)

105. Name two important pathogenic bacteria: (cluster form) _____

    _____ (chain) _____

106. Painful urination is _____ Excessive urination is _____ Urina-

    tion during night is _____

107. Difficult or labored breathing is called _____

    Periods of no breathing is called _____

108. Name four signs of inflammation: _____ _____

    _____ _____

109. Rheumatoid arthritis, bursitis, and fractures are disorders of the _____ system.

110. The pulmonary _____ is the vessel that carries deoxygenated blood from the right
    ventricle to the lungs.

111. The _____ ventricle of the heart has a thicker muscular wall than the

    _____ ventricle because it must pump blood farther.

112. Medical term for heart attack _____ for stroke _____

Abbreviations: (give meaning)

113. prn _____   qid _____

114. stat _____   NPO _____

115. URI _____   COPD _____

116. CVA _____   MI _____

Spell:

Define 117–130:

117. _____

_____

118. _____

_____

119. _____

_____

120. _____

_____

121. _____

_____

122. _____

_____

123. _____

_____

124. _____

_____

125. _____

_____

126. _____

_____

127. _____

_____

128. _____

_____

129. _____

_____

130. _____

_____

131. _____

132. _____

133. _____

134. _____

135. _____

136. _____

137. _____

138. _____

139. _____

140. _____

141. _____

142. _____

143. _____

144. _____

145. _____

146. _____

147. _____

148. _____

149. _____

150. _____

151. _____

Test Key 40, Instructor's Guide

medical terminology

name _____

points: 200 (Each answer in test is 1 point.)

course or section no. _____

alternate final exam

Multiple choice: These may have more than one answer – circle the letter of the correct answer or answers.

1. The serous membrane lining the abdominopelvic cavity is called:

   a. perineum   c. pericardium   e. peristaltic

   b. peritoneum   d. peroneal

2. The two sphincters of the stomach are the:

   a. cardiac   c. pyloric   e. duodenal

   b. hepatic   d. splenic

3. Name three sections of the small intestine in order:

   a. _____   b. _____   c. _____

4. The large intestine is called the _____ It is made up of seven sections, which are: (in order)

   a. _____   d. _____   g. _____

   b. _____   e. _____

   c. _____   f. _____

5. Circle the letter of the diagnostic procedures used in diagnosis of GI disorders:

   a. Upper GI   c. cytoscopy   e. Barium enema   g. sigmoidoscopy

   b. gastroscopy   d. IVP   f. cholangiography

Define and give location and/or function:

6. villi _____

   _____

7. hepatic flexure _____

   _____

8. islands (islets) of Langerhans _____

   _____

9. diverticulosis _____

   _____

Give a word that means:

10. Excision of appendix _____

11. Inflammation of the liver _____

chapter tests, review tests, and final exam   **311**

12. Incision into gallbladder _____

13. New permanent opening into ileum _____

14. X-ray examination of the bile ducts _____

15. Fixation of fallopian tube _____

16. Crushing of stone _____

17. Endocrine gland secretions are all:

   a. bile   b. saliva   c. hormones   d. enzymes

True/False: Circle the number of the *true* statements only. Defend your answers. Explain what is "untrue" in the false statements.

18. Protein is essential for growth and repair of tissues.

19. FBS and GTT are laboratory tests to determine pancreatic function.

20. The fundus of the stomach is the smaller distal portion.

21. The esophagus lies in front of the trachea.

22. The lumbar regions of the abdomen are directly right and left of the epigastric region.

23. Peristalsis moves contents along in the GI tract.

24. A hiatal hernia allows part of the stomach to push upwards through diaphragm opening.

25. The "lumen is patent" means the tube is not plugged.

26. The pituitary gland is also called:

   a. hypophysitis   b. hypophysis   c. hypophrenia

27. DPT (immunization) stands for:

   a. diphtheria   c. parotitis   e. typhoid

   b. whooping cough   d. poliomyelitis   f. tetanus

28. A "D and C" is a procedure often done:

   a. following spontaneous abortion

   b. for diagnostic purposes   d. to relieve pain

   c. to sterilize a woman   e. to abort a fetus

29. Pregnancy outside of the uterus may be called:

   a. ectopic   c. hybrid   e. tubal pregnancy

   b. extrauterine   d. pneumoperitoneum

30. White blood cells are called:

   a. leukocytes   c. thrombocytes

   b. erythrocytes   d. polyphages

31. The lobes of the brain and the bones of the cranium have identical names, which are:

   a. frontal   c. parietal   e. occipital   g. obturator

   b. peritoneal   d. oculomotor   f. temporal   h. paraplegic

32. Dorsal recumbent position means:

   a. lying face down   c. knee-chest   e. lying face up

   b. similar to supine   d. same as prone

33. The regions or areas of the abdomen directly right and left of the epigastric region are:

    a. iliac   c. inguinal   e. hypochondriac

    b. suprapubic   d. lumbar   f. umbilical

34. The pituitary gland is an _____ gland that secretes several _____ to stimulate other target glands. One of these substances is TSH, which means _____ _____ _____ (3 words)

35. Trace the circulation through the heart, from superior and inferior venae cavae to aorta, in order (name chambers, valves, vessels, and organs):

    a. _____   e. _____   i. _____

    b. _____   f. _____   j. _____

    c. _____   g. _____   k. _____

    d. _____   h. _____

Define: (spell out or give meaning)

36. stat _____

37. qid _____

38. subq _____

39. pc _____

40. IM _____

41. BE (X-ray procedure) _____

42. PID _____

43. TUR(P) _____

44. IPPB _____

45. 5% glu D/W _____

46. prn _____

47. bid _____

48. hs _____

49. IV _____

50. NPO _____

51. GB series _____

52. Ua _____

53. Name five sections of the spinal column (vertebrae) in order:

    a. _____   c. _____   e. _____

    b. _____   d. _____

54. Three kinds of abortions (inevitable abortion, for example): _____ _____ _____

55. Write plural form of:

    bronchus _____   testis _____

    atrium _____   sulcus _____

Write any medical term (must be complete word) using the root word for the following and define 15 of these terms: *Must be spelled correctly.*

56. bone _____

_____

57. brain _____

_____

58. heart _____

_____

59. cartilage _____

_____

60. lungs _____

_____

61. blood _____

_____

62. gallbladder _____

_____

63. ovaries _____

_____

64. nose _____

_____

65. ankle _____

_____

66. fingernail _____

_____

67. liver _____

_____

68. ureter _____

_____

69. duodenum _____

_____

70. white _____

_____

71. eye _____

_____

72. colon _____

_____

73. eardrum _____

_____

74. trachea _____

_____

75. pharynx _____

_____

76. tonsil _____

77. fallopian tube _____

_____

Write any medical term using these word parts and define six of these terms: *They must be spelled correctly.*
(not same words as in 56–77)

78. a-, an- _____

_____

79. -emia _____

_____

80. -algia _____

_____

81. -iatrist _____

_____

82. -gram _____

_____

83. -orrhaphy _____

_____

84. hemi- _____

_____

85. -uria _____

_____

86. -oscopy _____

_____

87. -cocci _____

_____

88. -centesis _____

_____

89. -opexy _____

_____

90. Which of the following are eye terms:

a. iridectomy   c. myopia   e. pinna   g. glaucoma

b. myringotomy   d. cataract   f. cerumen

91. Inequality in the size of cells is:

   a. anisocytosis   b. poikilocytosis   c. neutrocytosis

92. The Landsteiner system is a method of designating:

   a. total differential   c. blood types A, B, AB, O

   b. Rh and Hr factors   d. genotype

93. A physician using the stethoscope to check heart sounds would be demonstrating one method of:

   a. percussion   c. consultation   e. concussion

   b. auscultation   d. dilatation

94. Gavage means:

   a. to irrigate   c. to suction

   b. to feed by tube   d. to pump out

95. Premature separation of the placenta is:

   a. abruptio placenta   c. placenta previa   e. hysterorrhexis

   b. retained placenta   d. marginalis

Name the medical specialist (MD or DO) who treats the following: *They must be spelled correctly.*

96. Mental illness _____

97. Fractures and bone disorders _____

98. Children only _____

99. Women only _____

100. Patients with urinary tract disease _____

101. Black stools of the newborn are called:

   a. amnion   b. stridor   c. meconium   d. melena

102. Identify all terms pertaining to malignancy:

   a. metastasis   c. adenocarcinoma   e. adenoma

   b. lipoma   d. sarcoma

103. A neoplasm is a _____ It may be either benign or _____ The cervical smear done to detect abnormal cell growth (cancer and precancer) is called the _____ smear or test.

104. Cancer that has not infiltrated or metastasized beyond its original site is called _____

105. Name seven body systems, one organ in each, and one disorder of each (21 points).

   _____   _____   _____

   _____   _____   _____

   _____   _____   _____

   _____   _____   _____

   _____   _____   _____

   _____   _____   _____

   _____   _____   _____

Test Key 41, Instructor's Guide

appendix g
medications

generic name	brand name	major use
acetaminophen	(Tylenol, Datril, Excedrin, Darvocet-N, Phenaphen, Sinutab)	analgesic, antipyretic
acetaminophen with codeine	(Capital with Codeine Tablets, Phenaphen with Codeine)	analgesic
acetohexamide	(Dymelor)	oral antidiabetic
acetylsalicylic acid (aspirin)	(APC, Empirin, Fiorinal)	analgesic, antipyretic
acetylcysteine	(Mucomyst)	mucolytic
acyclovar ointment	(Zovirax)	herpes infections
albuterol	(Ventolin, Proventil)	bronchodilator
allopurinol	(Zyloprim)	reduces uric acid (gout)
amantadine	(Symmetrel)	antiviral
aminophylline	(Aminophylline, Mudrane)	bronchodilator, mucolytic
amitriptyline	(Elavil, Triavil, Etrafon)	antidepressant
amoxapine	(Asendin)	antidepressant
amoxicillin	(Amoxil, Larotid, Polymox, Sumox)	semisynthetic penicillin
amphotericin B	(Fungizone, Mysteclin-F)	antifungal
ampicillin	(Amcill, Omnipen, Penbritin, Supen, Pen-A, Pensyn, Principen)	semisynthetic penicillin
atropine sulfate	(Atropine sulfate)	reduces salivation and secretions
azathioprine	(Imuran)	immunosuppressive
bacampicillin	(Spectrobid)	semisynthetic penicillin
belladonna	(Donnatal)	antispasmodic
benztropine mesylate	(Cogentin)	parkinsonism
bisacodyl	(Dulcolax)	cathartic
bleomycin sulfate	(Blenoxane)	antineoplastic antibiotic
bretylium tosylate	(Bretylol)	ventricular arrhythmias
bromocriptine mesylate	(Parlodel)	prevents lactation
bromodiphenhydramine, codeine, and so on	(Ambenyl Expectorant)	antitussive, expectorant
brompheniramine maleate	(Dimetane, Dimetapp, Puretane, Puretapp, Histatapp)	antihistamine
busulfan	(Myleran)	antineoplastic
butalbital-aspirin-phenacetin-caffeine	(Fiorinal)	analgesic

generic name	(brand name)	major use
butorphanol tartrate	(Stadol)	narcotic analgesic
calcitriol	(Rocaltrol)	synthetic vitamin D
captopril	(Capoten)	antihypertensive
carbamazepine	(Tegretol)	anticonvulsant
carbenicillin	(Geocillin, Geopen)	semisynthetic penicillin
carbidopa/levodopa	(Sinemet)	parkinsonism
cefaclor	(Ceclor)	respiratory/ear infections
cefadroxil monohydrate	(Duricef)	antibiotic
cefamandole nafate	(Mandol)	lower respiratory
cefotaxime sodium	(Claforan)	antibiotic
cefazolin sodium	(Kefzol, Ancef)	antibiotic
cephalexin	(Keflex)	broad-spectrum antibiotic
cephalothin sodium	(Keflin)	broad-spectrum antibiotic
chlorambucil	(Leukeran)	antineoplastic
chlordiazepoxide	(Librium, Libritabs)	tranquilizer
chlorothiazide	(Diuril, Aldoclor, Chlorothiazide)	diuretic
chlorpheniramine maleate	(Chlor-trimeton, Teldrin, Codimal, Colrex, Coricidin, Extendryl, Rhinex, Ornade)	antihistamine
chlorpromazine hydrochloride	(Thorazine, Chlorpromazine)	tranquilizer, antiemetic
chlorthalidone	(Hygroton)	diuretic
chlorzoxazone and acetaminophen	(Parafon Forte)	analgesic, muscle relaxant
cimetidine	(Tagamet)	inhibits gastric acid (ulcers)
clindamycin	(Cleocin)	antibiotic
clocortolone pivalate	(Cloderm)	topical steroid
clofibrate	(Atromid-S)	lowers cholesterol
clonidine hydrochloride	(Catapres)	antihypertensive
clorazepate dipotassium	(Tranxene)	antianxiety
clotrimazole	(Lotrimin)	topical antifungal (tinea)
cloxacillin sodium monohydrate	(Tegopen)	synthetic penicillin
codeine	(Percogesic with Codeine)	narcotic analgesic
conjugated estrogens	(Premarin, Milprem, Formatrix)	estrogen (in menopause)
cyclacillin	(Cyclapen)	semisynthetic penicillin
cyclobenzaprine hydrochloride	(Flexeril)	relieves muscle spasm
cyclophosphamide	(Cytoxan)	antineoplastic
cyproheptadine hydrochloride	(Periactin)	antihistamine
cytarabine	(Cytosar-U)	antineoplastic
danazol	(Danocrine)	suppresses ovarian function
daunorubicin	(Cerubidine)	antibiotic (cancer)
dexamethasone	(Decadron, Hexadrol)	corticosteroid
dexbrompheniramine and pseudoephedrine sulfate	(Drixoral)	antihistamine, vasoconstrictor
dextroamphetamine sulfate	(Dexamyl, Dexedrine)	cerebral stimulation (narcolepsy, obesity)

generic name	(brand name)	major use
diazepam	(Valium)	tranquilizer
dicyclomine hydrochloride	(Bentyl)	GI muscle spasm
diethylpropion hydrochloride	(Tenuate)	anorectic
digoxin	(Lanoxin, Digoxin)	increases strength and force of heart beat
dihydroergotamine mesylate	(D.H.E. 45)	aborts vascular headache
diphenhydramine and alcohol	(Benylin)	antihistaminic, antitussive
diphenhydramine hydrochloride	(Benadryl, Ambenyl)	antihistamine
diphenoxylate hydrochloride	(Lomotil)	antispasmodic (diarrhea)
disopyramide phosphate	(Norpace)	antiarrhythmic
dobutamine hydrochloride	(Dobutrex)	strengthens heart muscle
docusate sodium	(Colace, Comfolax, Dilax, Disonate, Modane Soft)	stool softener
doxepin hydrochloride	(Adapin, Sinequan)	treatment of depression or anxiety
doxorubicin hydrochloride	(Adriamycin)	antineoplastic antibiotic
doxycycline monohydrate	(Vibramycin)	bacteriostatic
doxylamine succinate	(Bendectin)	antiemetic
ephedrine sulfate	(Isuprel, Marax, Efed)	relaxes bronchioles
epinephrine	(Adrenalin)	respiratory distress and hypersensitivity reactions
ergot alkaloids	(Hydergine, Deapril-ST, Circanol, Hydergot)	mental deterioration in elderly
ergotamine tartrate	(Cafergot, Ergomar, Migral, Gynergen, Wigraine)	migraine
erythromycin	(Ethril, Erythrocin, Bristamycin, Ilotycin)	antibiotic
ethosuximide	(Zarontin)	anticonvulsant
fenoprofen calcium	(Nalfon)	nonsteroid anti-inflammatory
ferrous sulfate	(Feosol, Iberet, Mol-Iron, Fero-Folic-500, Obron-6)	iron deficiency
fluocinolone acetonide	(Synalar)	topical steroid
fluocinonide	(Lidex, Topsyn)	anti-inflammatory antipruritic
5-fluorouracil	(Fluorouracil)	antineoplastic
fluphenazine hydrochloride	(Permitil, Prolixin)	psychoses
flurandrenolide	(Cordran, Cordran SP)	anti-inflammatory, antipruritic corticosteroid (topical)
flurazepam hydrochloride	(Dalmane)	vasoconstriction, hypnotic
furosemide	(Lasix)	diuretic
gentamicin sulfate	(Garamycin)	antibiotic
glutethimide	(Doriden)	hypnotic
guaifenesin	(Actifed-C, Dimetane, Robitussin, Triaminic)	expectorant
guanethidine sulfate	(Ismelin)	antihypertensive

generic name	(brand name)	major use
heparin sodium	(Lipo-Hepin, Panheprin, Heparin)	anticoagulant
hepatitis B vaccine	(Heptavax-B)	prevention of hepatitis B in high-risk population
hydralazine hydrochloride	(Apresoline, Ser-Ap-Es)	antihypertensive
hydrochlorothiazide	(Esidrex, HydroDIURIL, Hydro-Z-50, Oretic)	diuretic
hydrocortisone	(Cortef, Cort-Dome)	steroid
hydromorphone hydrochloride	(Dilaudid)	narcotic
hydroxyzine hydrochloride	(Atarax, Vistaril)	tranquilizer, muscle relaxant
hyoscyamine sulfate, atropine sulfate, phenobarbital, hyoscine hydrobromide	(Donnatal, Acro-Lase, Anaspaz, Cystospaz)	relaxant (GI spasm)
ibuprofen	(Motrin)	nonsteroid anti-inflammatory
imipramine hydrochloride	(Tofranil, SK-Pramine, Presamine)	antidepressant
indomethacin	(Indocin)	nonsteroid anti-inflammatory
insulin	(NPH Iletin, Lente, Protamine Zinc, Semi-lente, Ultralente)	injectable in diabetes
ipecac		emetic
iron dextran	(Imferon)	iron deficiency
isocarboxazid	(Marplan)	monoamine oxidase inhibitor (MAO) in depression
isoetharine and phenylephrine	(Bronkosol)	bronchodilator
isoniazid	(INH, Nydrazid)	anti-infective (tuberculosis)
isoproterenol solution	(Isuprel Mistometer)	bronchodilator
isosorbide dinitrate	(Isordil, Sorbide, Sorbitrate)	vasodilator
isoxsuprine hydrochloride	(Vasodilan)	vasodilator
kanamycin sulfate	(Kantrex)	antibiotic
kaolin	(Donnagel)	antispasmodic (GI)
ketoconazole	(Nizoral)	antifungal
lactulose	(Cephulac)	acidifies colon (hepatic coma)
levodopa	(Larodopa, Sinemet)	parkinsonism
lidocaine	(Xylocaine)	antiarrhythmic, anesthetic
lincomycin hydrochloride monohydrate	(Lincocin)	antibiotic
lindane (gamma benzene hexachloride)	(Kwell)	scabies and lice
liotrix	(Euthroid, Thyrolar)	thyroid hormones
lomustine	(CeeNU)	antineoplastic
loperamide hydrochloride	(Imodium)	inhibits peristalsis (acute diarrhea)
maprotiline hydrochloride	(Ludiomil)	tetracyclic antidepressant
measles virus vaccine	(Attenuvax)	measles vaccine
mechlorethamine hydrochloride	(Mustargen)	antineoplastic

generic name	(brand name)	major use
meclizine hydrochloride	(Antivert)	antihistamine (nausea, vomiting)
meclocycline sulfosalicylate	(Meclan)	antibiotic cream
meclofenamate sodium	(Meclomen)	nonsteroid anti-inflammatory
melphalan	(Alkeran)	antineoplastic
meperidine	(Demerol)	narcotic analgesic
mephenytoin	(Mesantoin)	anticonvulsant
meprobamate	(Deprol, Equagesic, Equanil, Meprobamate, Milpath, Miltown)	tranquilizer
mercaptopurine	(Purinethol)	antimetabolite (leukemias)
methenamine mandelate	(Mandelamine, Uroqid)	antibacterial (UTI)
methocarbamol	(Robaxin)	musculoskeletal pain
methotrexate	(Methotrexate)	antimetabolite
methyclothiazide	(Aquatensen, Enduron, Diutensen, Eutron)	diuretic, antihypertensive
methyldopa	(Aldomet)	antihypertensive
methylphenidate hydrochloride	(Ritalin)	CNS stimulation
methylprednisolone	(Depo-Medrol, Solu-Medrol)	steroid, anti-inflammatory immunosuppressive
methysergide maleate	(Sansert)	vascular headache
metoclopramide hydrochloride	(Reglan)	stimulates upper GI motility
metolazone	(Diulo, Zaroxolyn)	diuretic
metoprolol tartrate	(Lopressor)	hypertension
metronidazole	(Flagyl)	trichomonal and amebicidal action; anaerobic bacterial infections
metyrosine	(Demser)	pheochromocytoma
miconazole	(Monistat)	fungicidal (moniliasis)
minoxidil	(Loniten)	peripheral vasodilator (antihypertensive)
mumps virus vaccine	(Mumpsvax)	mumps vaccine
nadolol	(Corgard)	angina, hypertension
nulbuphine hydrochloride	(Nubain)	analgesic (synthetic narcotic)
nalidixic acid	(NegGram)	UTI (gram negative)
naloxone hydrochloride	(Narcan)	narcotic antagonist
naproxen	(Naprosyn)	nonsteroid anti-inflammatory
nitrofurantoin	(Furadantin, Macrodantin, Nitrex)	bactericidal (UTI)
nitroglycerin	(Nitro-Bid, Nitrostat, Nitrol, Nitrospan)	vasodilator (in angina)
norepinephrine bitartrate	(Levophed)	peripheral vasoconstrictor
nylidrin	(Arlidin)	vasodilator
nystatin	(Achrostatin, Declostatin, Mycolog Cream)	antibiotic (fungal)
orphenadrine citrate-aspirin-phenacetin-caffeine	(Norgesic)	analgesic (musculoskeletal)

generic name	(brand name)	major use
oxamniquine	(Vansil)	*Schistosoma mansoni* infection
oxazepam	(Serax)	anticonvulsant, antianxiety
oxtriphylline	(Choledyl)	bronchodilator
oxycodone	(Percodan)	narcotic analgesic
oxytocin	(Pitocin)	uterine stimulant
pancuronium bromide	(Pavulon)	muscle relaxant
papaverine hydrochloride	(Papaverine Hydrochloride)	relieves arterial spasm
pentazocine hydrochloride	(Talwin)	analgesic
pentobarbital sodium	(Nembutal)	barbiturate (short acting)
phenazopyridine hydrochloride	(Azo-Gantanol, Pyridium, Azo-Gantrisin, Urobiotic)	relief of pain in UTI
phenelzine sulfate	(Nardil)	MAO inhibitor (in depression)
phenobarbital	(Belap, Bentyl, Luminal, Peritrate, Valpin)	sedative, antispasmodic
phenoxybenzamine hydrochloride	(Dibenzyline)	vasospastic disorders (Raynaud's)
phentermine resin	(Ionamin)	anorexic
phenylbutazone	(Butazolidin, Azolid, Sterazolidin)	nonsteroid, anti-inflammatory
phenylpropanolamine-chlorpheniramine-codeine and alcohol	(Novahistine DH)	antitussive, decongestant, antihistamine
phenylpropanolamine-phenylephrine-phenyltoloxamine-chlorpheniramine	(Naldecon)	antihistamine vasoconstrictor
phenytoin sodium	(Dilantin)	anticonvulsant
phytonadione	(AquaMEPHYTON, Konakion)	synthetic vitamin K
pilocarpine	(Ocusert)	antiglaucoma
polymyxin B-bacitracin-neomycin-gramicidin	(Neosporin)	topical antibiotic
plus hydrocortisone	(Cortisporin)	topical antibiotic
potassium chloride	K-Lor, K-Lyte, Kaon-Cl)	potassium depletion
povidone-iodine	(Betadine)	germicide
prazosin hydrochloride	(Minipress)	antihypertensive
prednisone	(Orasone, Meticorten, Deltasone, Prednisone)	steroid, anti-inflammatory immunosuppressive
primidone	(Mysoline)	anticonvulsant
procarbazine hydrochloride	(Matulane)	antineoplastic (Hodgkin's)
prochlorperazine	(Compazine, Combid)	tranquilizer, antinauseant
promethazine	(Phenergan, Quadnite, Zipan)	antihistamine, antiemetic, tranquilizer
propantheline bromide	(Pro-Banthine)	inhibits GI motility (in ulcers)
propoxyphene hydrochloride	(Darvon, Dolene, SK-65, Wygesic)	analgesic

generic name	(brand name)	major use
propranolol hydrochloride	(Inderal)	antihypertensive, angina, migraine
protamine sulfate		for overdose of heparin
quinestrol	(Estrovis)	synthetic estrogen
quinidine sulfate	(Quinidine, Quinora)	cardiac depressant (in arrhythmias)
rabies vaccine		pre- and post-exposure vaccine
rauwolfia serpentina	(Raudixin)	diuretic, antihypertensive
reserpine	(Hydropres, Renese-R, Serpasil)	hypertension
ritodrine hydrochloride	(Yutopar)	prolongs gestation
secobarbital sodium (with amobarbital)	(Seconal Sodium) (Tuinal)	barbiturate
sodium levothyroxine	(Levothroid, Synthroid)	thyroid hormone
sodium warfarin	(Coumadin, Panwarfin)	anticoagulant
spectinomycin hydrochloride	(Trobicin)	antibiotic (penicillin-resistant GC)
spironolactone	(Aldactone)	diuretic
sulfasalazine	(Azulfidine)	sulfonamide (ulcerative colitis)
sulfisoxazole	(Gantrisin, SK-Soxazole, Soxomide)	sulfonamide (UTI)
sulindac	(Clinoril)	nonsteroid anti-inflammatory
tetracycline hydrochloride	(Achromycin, Retet 250, Robitet, Sumycin, Tetracycline, Achrostatin)	antibiotic
theophylline	(Tedral, Bronkodyl, Isuprel, Marax)	bronchodilator
thioridazine	(Mellaril)	major tranquilizer
thyroglobulin	(Proloid)	thyroid
ticarcillin disodium	(Ticar)	antibiotic
ticrynafen	(Selacryn)	antihypertensive, diuretic
timolol maleate	(Timoptic)	reduces intraocular pressure (glaucoma)
tobramycin sulfate	(Nebcin)	antibiotic (gram negative)
tolazamide	(Tolinase)	oral hypoglycemic
tolbutamide	(Orinase)	oral hypoglycemic
tolmetin sodium	(Tolectin)	nonsteroid anti-inflammatory
tranylcypromine sulfate	(Parnate)	MAO inhibitor (depression)
trifluridine	(Viroptic)	antiviral (eye)
trihexyphenidyl hydrochloride	(Artane, Tremin)	smooth muscle relaxant (Parkinson's)
trimethobenzamide hydrochloride	(Tigan)	antiemetic
triprolidine hydrochloride and pseudoephedrine hydrochloride	(Actifed)	antihistamine, decongestant
vincristine sulfate	(Oncovin)	antineoplastic

generic name	(brand name)	major use
zinc undecylenate and undecylenic acid (powder)	(Desenex)	topical antifungal
zomepirac sodium	(Zomax)	anti-inflammatory, analgesic, antipyretic

appendix h
abbreviations

General hints regarding abbreviations: Periods are generally omitted. Some abbreviations are shown in capital letters; some will be seen in either capitals or lower case letters.

A   American, association

AP   anterior/posterior

D   disease

F   Fellow

L/R   left/right

N   national

P   physicians

S   surgeons, syndrome

U/L   upper/lower

GENERAL ABBREVIATIONS

A   anterior, accommodation, atrium, artery

AA   Alcoholics Anonymous, Associate of Arts (degree)

$\overline{\text{aa}}$ of each (pharmacy)

AAA   abdominal aortic aneurysm

AAE   active assistive exercise (physical therapy)

ab   abortion (if spontaneous, same as miscarriage)

ABO   Landsteiner blood groups

ABS   acute brain syndrome

ac   before meals

ACP   American College of Physicians

ACS   American College of Surgeons

ACTA   type of scanner

ACTH   adrenocorticotropin hormone

A & D   admission and discharge (hospital department)

A & P (or P & A)   auscultation and percussion (listening and tapping)

A & P repair   anterior/posterior repair of perineum

A & W   alive and well

AD   right ear (auris dextra)

ADA   American Dietetic (Diabetic, Dental) Association

ADC   Aid to Dependent Children (also AFDC, "families")

ADL   activities of daily living

ad lib   as desired, at will

ADR   Adriamycin (antineoplastic drug)

AE   above elbow (amputation)

AFB   acid-fast bacillus (TB and related organisms)

AGA   approximate gestational age (length of pregnancy)

AgNO₃   silver nitrate (instilled in newborn's eyes to prevent GC)

AHA   American Heart (Hospital) Association

AI   artificial insemination

AJ   ankle jerk (reflex)

AK   above knee (amputation)

AL   axillary line (right or left)

ALL   acute lymphocytic leukemia

ALP   alkaline phosphatase (high in Ca of prostate)

ALS   amyotrophic lateral sclerosis (Lou Gehrig's disease)

AMA   American Medical Association, against medical advice

AMD   actinomycin D (antineoplastic drug)

AMI   acute myocardial infarction

AML   acute myeloblastic (myelocytic, myelogenous) leukemia

ANA   antinuclear antibodies (lab test; presence may indicate autoimmune disease), American Nurses' Association

ANS autonomic nervous system

AP anterior/posterior

APC aspirin, phenacetin, caffeine (analgesic medication)

APGAR score of newborn's condition (Dr. Apgar)

APL anterior/posterior/lateral

Aq aqueous (water)

ARA C (Ara C) cytosine arabinoside (antineoplastic drug)

ARDS acute (adult) respiratory distress syndrome

ARE active resistive exercise

AS left ear (auris sinistra), aortic stenosis

ASA acetylsalicylic acid (aspirin)

ASAP as soon as possible

ASCP American Society of Clinical Pathologists (medical lab)

ASCVD arteriosclerotic and cardiovascular (or cerebrovascular) disease

ASD atrial septal defect (congenital heart defect)

ASHD arteriosclerotic heart disease, atrial septal heart defect

as tol as tolerated (diet, and so on)

Au gold (metallic element; salts used in treatment; radioactive gold used in certain Ca cases and liver scan)

AV arteriovenous (shunt), atrioventricular

AVR aortic valve replacement

AZT Aschheim-Zondek test (for pregnancy)

B bacillus, buccal

B₆ pyridoxine vitamin

Ba barium (opaque substance used in X-ray procedures)

B/A backache

Bab Babinski reflex (neurologic test; normal in infant but abnormal after 6 months)

baso basophil (white blood cell type)

BBB bundle branch block (heart); blood-brain barrier

BCG Calmette-Guerin (TB bacillus), used as vaccine

BD birthdate

BE barium enema, below elbow (amputation)

BEAM brain electrical activity mapping in diagnosis of tumors, epilepsy

BHA bilateral (or benign) hilar adenopathy

BM bowel movement

BMR basal metabolic rate

BOW bag of waters (amniotic sac)

BP (B/P) blood pressure

BPH benign prostatic hypertrophy

BRP bathroom privileges

BS bowel sounds, breath sounds, blood sugar

BSA body surface area (important measurement in burn patients)

BSP bromosulphthalein (lab)

BT bleeding time, brain tumor, body temperature

BU Bodansky units (lab term)

BUN blood urea nitrogen (lab test of kidney function)

BVR Bureau of Vocational Rehabilitation

BW birth weight, body weight

Bx biopsy

C centigrade, celsius, costal (rib), cervical, carbon, cesarean

c cubic, centimeter

c̄ with

C & S culture and sensitivity (bacteriology lab)

C-1, C-2, and so on cervical first, second, and so on vertebra or spinal nerve

CA cancer, carcinoma, chronologic age

Ca calcium, cancer

CABG "cabbage" (coronary artery by-pass graft)

cal calorie

caps capsules

CAT computerized axial tomography (also CT) (scan); multiple X-rays fed into computer provide cross sections of multiple planes

cath catheterized

Cauc caucasian (white race)

CBC complete blood count

CBD common bile duct, closed bladder drainage

CBS chronic brain syndrome

CC chief or current complaint, crippled children, compensation case

cc cubic centimeter (also written cm³)

CCI chronic coronary insufficiency

CCU coronary care unit

CD communicable disease

CDC communicable disease center

CF Christmas factor (in blood, bleeding disorder), cystic fibrosis, complement fixation

C/F colored female

CHD coronary heart disease, congenital heart disease

CHF congestive heart failure

CHO carbohydrate

CLL chronic lymphocytic leukemia

cm centimeter (cm^3 = cubic centimeter)

C/M colored male

cm costal margin (left or right)

CML chronic myelocytic leukemia

CN cranial nerve (also written Cr_I, Cr_{II}, and so on)

CNS central nervous system

Co cobalt (chemical element, used in CA treatment)

CO carbon monoxide

CO₂ carbon dioxide

comp compensation

COPD chronic obstructive pulmonary disease (also COLD, chronic obstructive lung disease)

CP cerebral palsy

CPD cephalopelvic disproportion (in birth canal, head too large)

CPK creatinine phosphokinase (enzyme released when heart or muscle is damaged)

CPM cyclophosphamide (antineoplastic drug)

CPR cardiopulmonary resuscitation

CPZ chlorpromazine (drug)

CRF chronic renal failure, corticotropin releasing factor

crit hematocrit (blood test)

CRP (A) C-reactive protein (antiserum)

C section cesarean section (caesarean)

CS central service (supply), coronary sinus

CSF cerebrospinal fluid

Cu copper (metal); small quantities used by body

cu cubic

cu cm cubic centimeter (cm^3)

cu mm cubic millimeter (mm^3)

CV cardiovascular, cerebrovascular

CVA cerebrovascular accident (stroke); cardiovascular accident

cva costovertebral angle (area over the kidney)

CVD cardiovascular (cerebrovascular) disease

CVP central venous pressure; Cytoxan, vincristine, prednisone (combination of drugs used in cancer treatment)

CW crutch walking

cysto cystoscopy

CXR chest X-ray (procedure)

D dorsal, diopter, disease, divorced

d deceased, dead, distal, dorsal

D-1, D-2, and so on dorsal (thoracic) vertebra, spinal, nerve, or rib

DAT diet as tolerated

DC (D/C) discontinue, discharged, Doctor of Chiropractic

D & C dilatation and curettage (uterus)

db decibel (unit of sound)

DD differential diagnosis, dry dressing

DDS Doctor of Dental Surgery

DES diethylstilbestrol (hormone)

DIC disseminated intravascular clotting

DIP distal interphalangeal (joint) – joint near tip of finger

diff differential (count of each type of WBC)

DJD degenerative joint disease

DK diet kitchen

DLE disseminated lupus erythematosus

DM diastolic murmur, diabetes mellitus

DMD Doctor of Medical Dentistry

DMSO dimethyl sulfoxide (controversial drug)

DNA deoxyribonucleic acid (present in chromosomes of nuclei of cells, carries genetic information)

DNR dorsal nerve root

DNS did not show (for appointment)

D/ns (D/s) dextrose in normal saline (IV solution)

DO Doctor of Osteopathy or Optometry

DOA dead on arrival

DOB date of birth

dorsi dorsiflexion (of foot, turned to posterior aspect of body as in "pointing toes")

DOU definitive observation unit (just below intensive care)

DPT diphtheria, tetanus, pertussis (immunization); also DTP, DT

DR dorsal root, doctor, dressing

DSD dry sterile dressing

DTs delirium tremens (in alcoholism)

DTR deep tendon reflex

DVR Department of Vocational Rehabilitation

DVT deep vein thrombosis

D/W dextrose in water (DW = distilled water)

Dx diagnosis

E enema, eye, extremity

E & H environment and heredity

EA educational age

ED emergency department

ECF extended care facility

ECG electrocardiogram

echo sound

ECHO virus (enterocytopathogenic human orphan virus)

E. coli *Escherichia coli* (bacterium)

ECT electroconvulsive therapy (shock treatment)

EDC estimated date of confinement (due date for delivery)

EEG electroencephalogram (brain wave recording)

EFP (R) effective filtration pressure (rate)

EGD esophagogastroduodenoscopy

EKG electrocardiogram

EM electron microscope

EMG electromyogram (muscle)

EMI type of scanner

EMT emergency medical technician

ENG electronystagmography (to test vestibular function by assessing eye motion)

ENT ear, nose, and throat

EOM extraocular movements

eos, eosin eosinophil (type of white blood cell)

ER emergency room, external rotation

ERV expiratory residual volume (pulmonary function test)

ES emergency service

ESP extrasensory perception

ESR erythrocyte sedimentation rate (blood test)

EST electroshock therapy (same as ECT)

EUA examination under anesthesia

ext external

F Fahrenheit, female, Fellow, frequency

FACP, FACS Fellow of American College of Physicians, Surgeons

FANA fluorescent antinuclear antibodies

FB, Fb fingerbreadth, foreign body

FBS fasting blood sugar

FDA Food and Drug Administration

Fe iron

FeSO₄ ferrous sulfate

FEV forced expiratory volume

FH family history

FHT fetal heart tones

F-N finger to nose (coordination)

FOB fiberoptic bronchoscopy, foot of bed

FP flat plate (X-ray procedure)

Fr French (size of catheter)

FROM full range of motion (of joint)

FSH follicle-stimulating hormone

FTA fluorescent treponemal antibody (syphilis test)

FTND full-term normal delivery

FU, 5-FU fluorouracil (cancer drug)

FUO fever of undetermined origin

Fx fracture

G glucose, gingival, specific gravity

g (Gm, gm) gram (unit of weight); 29 g in 1 oz

Ga gallium (rare metal, used in scans)

GA gestational age, gastric analysis

GAS general adaptation syndrome

GB gallbladder

GBS gallbladder series (X-ray film)

GC gonorrhea (venereal disease)

GE gastroenteritis

GFR glomerular filtration rate (kidney test)

GG gamma globulin (protein in blood, used therapeutically for passive temporary immunity)

GH growth hormone

GI, GIS gastrointestinal, series (X-ray film)

GP general practitioner, gram positive

gr grain, gravida, gravity

gram cystogram (X-ray film of bladder)

Grav I, II, and so on   gravida I, II, and so on (number of pregnancies)

gtt drop

GT, GTT glucose tolerance (test)

GU genitourinary

GV gentian violet (dye used in lab and as topical medication)

gyn gynecology

H hydrogen, hypo

H⁺ hydrogen ion

h hour

H₂O water

Hb, Hgb hemoglobin (iron-containing pigment in RBCs, carries oxygen to tissues)

HBO   hyperbaric oxygen therapy

HBP   high blood pressure (hypertension)

HCl   hydrochloric acid (normal in the stomach)

HCO₃   bicarbonate

Hct   hematocrit (blood test, low in anemias)

HD   Hodgkin's disease (type of cancer), Hansen's disease (leprosy), hip disarticulation

HDL   high-density lipoprotein

HEENT   head, eyes, ears, nose, throat

HEW   Health, Education, and Welfare

HF   high frequency (sounds)

Hg   mercury (metallic element)

Hgb   hemoglobin

HGH   human growth hormone

HH   hard of hearing

HID   headache, insomnia, depression (syndrome)

HLA   homologous (human) leukocytic antibodies

HMD   hyaline membrane disease (of newborn babies)

HMO   Health Maintenance Organization

HNP   herniated nucleus pulposus (hernia of intervertebral disc)

h/o   history of

HP   high-power field (microscope)

hs   bedtime

HS   heart sounds, head sling

HSG   hysterosalpingography (gram)

HSO   hysterosalpingoooophorectomy

HSV   herpes simplex virus (causes cold sores, genital herpes)

HVD   hypertensive vascular disease

hypo   injection, hypoglycemic diet

Hx   history

I   iodine (nonmetallic element, used as medication and in diagnosis of thyroid disorders)

¹³¹I   radioactive isotope of iodine

I & D   incision and drainage

I & O   intake and output

IC   intensive care, intercostal

ICA   internal carotid artery

ICM   intercostal margin

ICN   intensive care nursery

ICS   intercostal space

ICT   insulin coma therapy

ICU   intensive care unit

IgA   immunoglobulin A

IH   infectious hepatitis

IHD   ischemic heart disease

IM   intramuscular (injection)

INH   isoniazid (TB drug)

in situ   in position or original place (not metastasized)

IPPB   intermittent positive pressure breathing (treatment)

IQ   intelligence quotient

IU   international units

IUD   intrauterine device (for contraception)

IV   intravenous (into vein)

IVC   intravenous cholangiogram, inferior vena cava

IVD   intervertebral disk (between vertebrae)

IVP   intravenous pyelogram (X-ray film of kidney)

J   joint, journal, Jewish

JAMA   Journal of the American Medical Association

K   potassium (mineral) — essential in diet

KCl   potassium chloride (one of the ingredients in Ringer's solution for IV)

kg   kilogram

KJ   knee jerk (reflex)

KMnO₄   potassium permanganate (antiseptic)

KRP   Kolmer Reiter protein (syphilis test)

KUB   kidneys, ureters, bladder

KVO   keep vein open (do not allow IV to run dry)

L   liter, left, lower, lumbar

L-1, L-2, and so on   first, second, and so on lumbar vertebra or spinal nerve

LI, LII, LIII   primary, secondary, tertiary lues (syphilis)

L & A   light and accommodation (eye)

L & D   labor and delivery

L & W   living and well

LA   left atrium or auricle (of heart)

LASER   light amplification by stimulated emission of radiation (has some uses in surgery)

lat   lateral

LATS   long-acting thyroid stimulator

LCM   left costal margin

LDH   lactic dehydrogenase (enzyme, lab test)

LDL   low-density lipoproteins

LE   lupus erythematosus, lower extremity, left eye

LGI   lower gastrointestinal (series), same as barium enema

LH luteinizing hormone

LKS/np liver, kidney, spleen (also LSK – liver, spleen, kidney) nonpalpable

LLB lower leg brace

LLL lower left lobe, lower left lid

LLQ lower left quadrant

LMP last menstrual period (to calculate due date)

LN lymph node

LOA, LOP left occiput anterior, posterior (presentation at delivery)

LOM limitation of motion

LP lumbar puncture, low power (microscope)

LPN licensed practical nurse (LVN = licensed vocational nurse)

LRQ lower right quadrant

LRS lactated Ringer's solution (for IV)

LS lumbosacral

LTB laryngotracheobronchitis (croup)

LSD d-lysergic acid (hallucinogenic drug)

LTH luteotropic hormone (pituitary hormone, prolactin)

LUL left upper lobe

LV left ventricle

LVH left ventricular hypertrophy

lymph lymphocyte (type of blood cell)

M mean, medium, male, married, medical, morphine, murmur, mortality, morbidity

M₁ first mitral sound, heart sound at apex

m murmur, minim, monocyte, meter

MA mental age, menstrual age, Master of Arts, mentum anterior (presentation at delivery)

MAO monoamine oxidase (inhibitor) (type of medication)

MCH mean corpuscular hemoglobin (blood test), maternal and child health

MCHC mean corpuscular hemoglobin concentration (Hgb in each RBC or per unit of blood)

MCV mean corpuscular volume (measurement of size of individual red cell)

MD Doctor of Medicine, muscular dystrophy

mEq/L milliequivalent per liter (measurement of concentration of a solution)

MF meat free (diet)

MFD minimal fatal dose

MG myasthenia gravis

mg (mgm) milligram

MH mental health, marital history

MI myocardial infarction, mitral insufficiency

mL (ml) milliliter (same as cc)

MM mucous membrane

mm millimeter

mm³ cubic millimeter

mm HG millimeters of mercury

MMPI Minnesota Multiphasic Personality Inventory (test)

MMR measles, mumps, rubella (combined immunization)

MO mineral oil

MOM Milk of Magnesia

mono mononucleosis, monocyte (white blood cell)

MOPP nitrogen mustard, Oncovin, prednisone, procarbazine (drugs used in combination for some cancers)

MOR minor operating room

MR may repeat, metabolic rate, mentally retarded, medical records

MRL medical records librarian

MS multiple sclerosis, mitral stenosis, morphine sulfate, muscle strength, musculoskeletal

MT medical technologist (lab)

MT (ASCP) medical technologist (American Society of Clinical Pathologists)

MTX methotrexate (cancer drug)

MVP mitral valve prolapse (heart valve)

MVR mitral valve replacement

N nitrogen, Negro, negative, normal, national

n normal (saline), nasal, nerve

NI, NII, and so on nerves by number

N₂O nitrous oxide (anesthetic gas)

n & t nose and throat

n & v nausea and vomiting

Na sodium

NaCl sodium chloride (salt)

NAD no acute distress

NaHCO₃ sodium bicarbonate

NB newborn

NBM nothing by mouth

NED no evidence of disease

NER no evidence of recurrence

n/f Negro female

NFTD normal full-term delivery

NG nasogastric (tube)

NH₃ ammonia

NIH National Institute of Health

n/m Negro male

nm neuromuscular

NMR nuclear magnetic resonance (gives chemistry of an organ)

NP neuropsychiatric, nasopharygeal

NPH neutral protein Hagedorn (insulin)

NPN nonprotein nitrogen (lab test)

NPO nothing by mouth

nr no repeat (no refill of Rx)

ns normal saline (salt solution equal in concentration to that of body fluids)

NYD not yet diagnosed

O occiput, oculus, oral, aught, oxygen

O & C onset and course

O$_2$ oxygen

OA occiput anterior, old age, osteoarthritis

OAA old age assistance

OASI old age and survivor's insurance

OB obstetrics

OB-GYN obstetrics-gynecology

OBS organic brain syndrome

OCG oral cholangiogram (bile ducts X-ray film)

od every day

OD right eye, overdosed, Doctor of Optometry, occupational disease

OJ orange juice

OOB out of bed

OPD outpatient department

OR operating room

ORT operating room technician

OS left eye

OT occupational therapy

OTC over the counter (medications)

OTR occupational therapist registered

OU both eyes, each eye

OV office visit

P phosphorus, pulse, passive, proximal, pupil, para (live births)

p post, pupil (of eye), para, p wave (ECG)

P & A percussion and auscultation (tapping and listening)

PA posterior/anterior, pulmonary artery, pernicious anemia

PABA para-aminobenzoic acid (sunscreen preparation)

PAN periarteritis nodosa

PaO$_2$ arterial oxygen pressure

PAP primary atypical pneumonia

Pap Papanicolaou (smear for cancer detection)

Para I, II, and so on number of live births, full term

PAT paroxysmal atrial tachycardia

PBI protein-bound iodine (thyroid test)

PBZ pyribenzamine (antihistamine medication)

pc after meals

pCO$_2$ pressure or tension of carbon dioxide

PD Doctor of Pharmacy

PDA patent ductus arteriosus (open duct between pulmonary artery and aorta)

PDR Physician's Desk Reference (listing of prescription drugs)

PE physical examination

Peds pediatrics

PEG pneumoencephalogram

PEEP positive end respiratory pressure

PERRLA pupils equal, round, react to light and accommodation (eye)

PF push fluids

pg pregnant

pH hydrogen ion concentration (measure of acidity/alkalinity)

PH past history, public health

PICA posterior inferior cerebellar artery

PID pelvic inflammatory disease

PIP proximal interphalangeal joint

PIIS posterior inferior iliac spine

PKU phenylketonuria (causes retardation)

PM physical medicine, postmortem, afternoon

PMI point of maximum intensity

PMN polymorphonuclear (leukocyte)

PN peripheral nerve, practical nurse

PND paroxysmal noctural dyspnea, postnasal drip

PNS peripheral nervous system

PO phone order, postoperative

PO$_4$ phosphate (important in acid-base balance of blood)

PO$_2$, pO$_2$ pressure of oxygen

POD postoperative day

POMP prednisone, Oncovin, methotrexate, 6-mercaptopurine (combination of cancer drugs)

PP postprandial (after a meal)

PPD purified protein derivative (TB test), permanent partial disability

PRE progressive resistive exercise

prn as needed

PROM premature rupture of membranes

PSP phenolsulfonphthalein (renal excretion test)

PSRO professional standards review organization

PT physical therapy, prothrombin time

pt patient

PTD permanent total disability

PTA prior to admission

PTCA percutaneous transluminal coronary angioplasty (compression of atherosclerotic plaque to increase diameter of lumen)

PVC/B premature ventricular contractions/beats

PVD peripheral vascular disease

pvO$_2$ venous oxygen pressure

Px prognosis

PZI protamine zinc insulin

q every

qd every day

qh, q2h every hour, every 2 hours

qid four times a day

qm every morning

qn every night

qns quantity not sufficient (for test ordered)

qod every other day

QRS complex (ventricular complex in ECG)

R, r right, rectally, resistant, roentgen

Ra radium

RA rheumatoid arthritis, right atrium, residual air

RAD, rad radiation absorbed dose (unit of measure for X-rays)

RAI radioactive iodine

RAIU radioactive iodine uptake

RBC red blood cell, red blood count

RBD right border dullness

RBF renal blood flow

RC Red Cross, respiratory center, red cell, Roman catheter

RCD relative cardiac dullness

RCM right costal margin

RD retinal detachment (eye), respiratory disease

RDS respiratory distress syndrome

RE right eye, readmission

REM rapid eye movements (during dreams)

rep repeat

RF respiratory failure, rheumatic fever, rheumatoid factor

Rh factor in blood (Rh+ have the factor)

RHD rheumatic heart disease

RhoGAM injection given to Rh-negative women after delivery to prevent antibody formation against Rh factor

RLF retrolental fibroplasia (eye condition that causes blindness)

RLL right lower lobe

RLQ right lower quadrant

RML right middle lobe, right mediolateral (episiotomy)

RNA ribonucleic acid

R/O rule out

ROA right occiput anterior (presentation at delivery)

ROAD reversible obstructive airway disease

ROM range of motion, rupture of membranes

Rom Romberg (neurologic test for balance)

ROP right occiput posterior (presentation)

ROS review of systems

RP retrograde pyelogram

RPR rapid plasma reagent (syphilis test)

RPT registered physical therapist

RSB right sternal border

RT radiotherapy, recreational therapy, radiologic technologist

RTC return to clinic

RUE right upper extremity

RUL right upper lobe

RUQ right upper quadrant

RV right ventricle, residual volume, rubella virus

RVH right ventricle hypertrophy

RVHD rheumatic valvular heart disease

Rx prescription, recipe, treatment, therapy

rx reaction

S, s sacral, stimulus, sulfur, sinister (left), saline, sensitive, section

s̄ without

S-1 first sacral spinal nerve or vertebra

SA sinoatrial node (pacemaker in heart), sarcoma

SAH subarachnoid hemorrhage

SB stillborn, sternal border (right/left, upper/lower)

SBE   subacute bacterial endocarditis

Sc   subcutaneously

SC   sickle cell

SCUBA   self-contained underwater breathing apparatus

SD   shoulder disarticulation

sed   sedimentation rate (rate at which blood settles)

seg   segmented white blood cells (mature forms with segmented nuclei)

SF   salt free

sg, sp gr   specific gravity (weight as compared to water)

SGOT   serum glutamic oxaloacetic transaminase (enzyme, lab test)

SGPT   serum glutamic pyruvic transaminase (enzyme, lab test)

SH   serum hepatitis (hepatitis B), social history

SHS   Sayre head sling

SIADH   syndrome of inappropriate antidiuretic hormone

S/ICU   surgery/intensive care unit

SIDS   sudden infant death syndrome

sig   let it be labeled (label on prescription)

SIJ   sacroiliac joint

SLB   short leg brace

SLC   short leg cast

SLE   systematic lupus erythematosus

SMA, SMAC 6, 12, or 18   sequential multiple analysis (series of blood chemistry tests)

SMR   submucous resection (nasal surgery)

SNAFU   situation normal, all fouled up

SNDO   standard nomenclature of diseases and operations

SO₄   sulfate

SOB   short of breath

SOL   space-occupying lesion

soln   solution

SOPM   stitches out in afternoon

sp gr   specific gravity

sq, subq   subcutaneously

Sr   strontium (metallic element)

SR   sedimentation rate, systems review, sinus rhythm, stimulus/response

SS   social service, Social Security, soap solution, sterile solution, saline soak, supersaturated, signs and symptoms

s̄s̄   one half

SSE   soapsuds enema

SSKI   saturated solution potassium iodide (medication)

stabs   nonsegmented white blood cells (immature forms)

staph   *Staphylococcus* (bacterium)

stat   immediately

STD   sexually transmitted disease, skin test dose

STH   somatotropin (growth hormone)

strep   *Streptococcus* (bacterium)

STS   serologic test for syphilis

subq, subcu   subcutaneously

SV   stroke volume

SVC   superior vena cava

SW   short wave (diathermy)

Sx   signs, symptoms

T, t   temperature, thoracic, total, tetanus, tablespoon

T-1, T-2, and so on   first, second, and so on thoracic vertebra or spinal nerve

T + 1, T + 2   increased intraocular tension

T − 1, T − 2   decreased intraocular tension

T₃, T₄   thyroid function tests

T & A   tonsillectomy and adenoidectomy, tonsils and adenoids

T & C   turn and cough

TAB   typhoid, paratyphoid A and B (vaccine), therapeutic abortion

tab   tablet

TAH   total abdominal hysterectomy

TAT   toxin antitoxin, toxoid antitoxin, tetanus antitoxin, Thematic Apperception Test

Tb, Tbc   tubercle bacillus, tuberculosis

TBW   total body weight

TC   tissue culture

TCNS   transcutaneous electrical nerve stimulation (also TENS, TNS)

TED   thromboembolus (support hose to prevent emboli)

temp   temperature, temporal

TF   tuning fork

TH   thyroid hormone

THI   thiamine

TIA   transient ischemic attack

tid   three times a day

tinc, tr   tincture (alcohol preparation)

tiw   three times a week

TKO   to keep open (vein)

TL   tubal ligation (sterilization)

TLA   translumbar aortogram

TLC   total lung capacity, tender loving care

TLCA   transluminal coronary angioplasty

TM   tympanic membrane, temporomandibular

TMJ   temporomandibular joint (jaw)

TNC   too numerous to count (lab)

TNM   tumor, nodes, metastasis (cancer staging system)

TNS   transcutaneous nerve stimulation

TO   telephone order

TOF   tetralogy of Fallot (congenital heart defect)

TP   total protein, testosterone proprionate, *Treponema pallidum*

TPC   *Treponema pallidum* complement test (syphilis test)

TPI   *Treponema pallidum* immobilization test

TPN   total parenteral nutrition

TPR   temperature, pulse, and respirations

Tr   trace, tincture, traction

trach   trachea, tracheotomy, tracheostomy

TSB   total serum bilirubin (lab test)

TSH   thyroid-stimulating hormone

TT   tilt table, transfer to

TTD   temporary total disability, transverse thoracic diameter

TTH   thyrotropic hormone

TUR, TURP   transurethral resection of prostate gland

TV   tidal volume, total volume, television

TVC   timed vital capacity (pulmonary function test)

TW   tap water

Tx   traction, treatment

U   unit, upper, uranium

U & C   urethral and cervical

Ua   urinalysis

UCG   ultrasound cardiogram

UE   upper extremity (arm)

UG   urogenital

UGI   upper GI series (X-ray film)

UN   urea nitrogen (lab test); same as BUN

ung   ointment

U/O   under observation

URI   upper respiratory infection

USP   US Pharmacopoeia (list of medications)

USPHS   US Public Health Service

UTI   urinary tract infection

U/S   ultrasound

UV   ultraviolet

V   ventricle, volt, volume, virulence, valve, vein, Roman numeral for number 5

VA   Veterans Administration

VC   vital capacity, vocal cord

VCG   vector cardiogram

VCR   vincristine (cancer drug)

VCU   voiding cystourethrogram

VD   venereal disease

VDRL   Venereal Disease Research Laboratories

Vf   ventricular fibrillation, visual field

VR   vocational rehabilitation, venous return, ventral root

VS   vital signs

VSD   ventricular septal defect

W   water, week, west, widow, with, watt, weight, width, wife

WAIS   Wechsler Adult Intelligence Scale

WB   whole blood

WBC   white blood count, white blood cell

WBC & diff   white blood count and differential (count of each type WBC)

WC   wheelchair

WD   well developed, wet dressing

WDWN   well developed, well nourished

W/F, wf   white female

WHO   World Health Organization

WISC   Wechsler Intelligence Scale for Children

W/M, wm   white male

WN   well nourished

WNL   within normal limits

WP   wet pack, whirlpool

WPW   Wolff-Parkinson-White syndrome (disturbance in conduction in Purkinje fibers of heart)

X   cross (match), cross section, Roman numeral for 10

X ray   roentgen ray

XU   excretory urogram

XX   female chromosome

XY   male chromosome

Y/O   year old

Z zero

Zn zinc

symbols

♂ male

♀ female

> greater than

< less than

℥ ounce

ℨ dram

± plus or minus

↑ increased, elevated

↓ decreased, lowered

PHYSICAL THERAPY ABBREVIATIONS
kinds of treatment

E. stim electrical stimulation

fluido fluidotherapy

FT$_x$ Fontaine traction

HP hot pack

HT Hubbard tank

IC T$_x$ intermittent cervical traction

IP T$_x$ intermittent pelvic traction

MWD microwave diathermy

parr paraffin (wax)

PT physical therapy

ST$_x$ Sayre traction

SWD shortwave diathermy

TENS transcutaneous electrical nerve stimulation

US ultrasound

WP whirlpool

WT wading tank

movement

AAROM active assistive range of motion

abd abduction

add adduction

AROM active range of motion

elev elevation

ER external rotation

ext or / extension

flex or √ flexion

IR internal rotation

lat flex lateral flexion

PROM passive range of motion

ROM range of motion

SAQ short arc quad

SLR straight leg raise

general

act active

act assist active assistive

ADL activities of daily living

AE amp above elbow amputee

a g antigravity

AK amp above knee amputee

amp amputation

BE amp below elbow amputee

BIW twice a week

BK amp below knee amputation

FOB foot of bed

ft foot or feet

FWB full weight bearing

LLE left lower extremity

LUE left upper extremity

MED minimal erythemal dosage

NWb non-weight bearing

pass passive

‖ bars parallel bars

PRE progressive resistive exercise

pt patient

PWB partial weight bearing

reed reeducation

rehab rehabilitation

RLE right lower extremity

RUE right upper extremity

Rx treatment or therapy

SB side bending

TIW three times a week

TO telephone order

x times or repetitions

T$_x$ traction

WC wheelchair

W/cm² watts per centimeter squared

WFL within functional limits

wt weight

PULMONARY FUNCTION ABBREVIATIONS

CaO$_2$ concentration of oxygen in arterial blood

CcO$_2$ concentration of oxygen in end capillary blood

C$\bar{v}$O$_2$ concentration of oxygen in mixed venous blood

DL$_{CO}$ diffusing capacity of the lung for carbon monoxide

DL$_{O_2}$ diffusing capacity of the lung for oxygen

ERV expiratory reserve volume

FE$_{CO_2}$ fraction of carbon dioxide in expired air

FEF$_{25\%-75\%}$ forced midexpiratory flow (between 25% and 75% of FVC)

FE N$_2$ fraction of nitrogen in expired air

FEV$_1$ forced expiratory volume in 1 second

FEV$_3$ forced expiratory volume in first 3 seconds

FEO$_2$ fraction of oxygen in expired air

FIN$_2$ fraction of nitrogen in inspired air

FIO$_2$ fraction of oxygen in inspired air

FRC functional residual capacity

FVC forced vital capacity

IC inspiratory capacity

IRV inspiratory reserve volume

MVV maximum voluntary ventilation

P$\bar{A}_{CO}$ mean partial pressure of carbon monoxide in alveolar gas

PA$_{CO_2}$ partial pressure of carbon dioxide in alveolar gas

P$\bar{A}_{CO_2}$ mean partial pressure of carbon dioxide in alveolar gas

Pa$_{CO_2}$ partial pressure of carbon dioxide in arterial blood

P$_{alv}$ alveolar pressure

PA$_{H_2O}$ partial pressure of water in alveolar gas

Pao pressure at airway opening

Pa$_{O_2}$ partial pressure of oxygen in arterial blood

PA$_{O_2}$ partial pressure of oxygen in alveolar gas

P$\bar{A}_{O_2}$ mean partial pressure of oxygen in alveolar gas

PB atmospheric pressure

Pbs pressure at external surface of chest

P$_{CO_2}$ partial pressure of carbon dioxide

P$\bar{c}_{O_2}$ mean partial pressure of oxygen in capillary blood

P$\bar{E}_{CO_2}$ mean partial pressure of carbon dioxide in mixed expired air

P$_L$ recoil pressure of lung

pN$_2$ partial pressure of nitrogen

PO$_2$ partial pressure of oxygen

Ppl pleural pressure

PRS recoil pressure of total respiratory system

PW recoil pressure of chest wall

$\dot{Q}$x shunt flow

$\dot{Q}$t total cardiac output

R respiratory exchange ratio

Raw resistance of tracheobronchial tree to flow of air into lung

Re Reynolds number

RQ respiratory quotient

RUS resistance of upstream segment of tracheobronchial tree

RV residual volume

SO$_2$ percentage saturation of hemoglobin with oxygen

Sa$_{O_2}$ percentage saturation of hemoglobin with oxygen in arterial blood

TLC total lung capacity

$\dot{V}$ gas volume per minute

V$_1$ inspiratory volume of ventilation per minute

VA volume of alveolar gas

$\dot{V}$A/$\dot{Q}$c ratio of alveolar ventilation to pulmonary blood flow

Vc volume of blood in pulmonary capillary bed

VC vital capacity

$\dot{V}_{CO}$ rate of carbon monoxide uptake per minute

$\dot{V}_{CO_2}$ amount of carbon dioxide eliminated per minute

VD volume of dead space gas

$\dot{V}$E expiratory volume of ventilation per minute

$\dot{V}_{max}$ maximal rate of airflow during forced expiration

$\dot{V}_{max\ 50}$ rate of airflow at 50% of vital capacity

$\dot{V}_{O_2}$ rate of oxygen uptake per minute (oxygen consumption)

V$_T$ tidal volume (also TV)

CANCER ABBREVIATIONS*

This form is presented to acquaint the student with some abbreviations used in cancer cases. The breast is used as an example for the anatomic site of cancer; however, definitions are for all time periods.

primary tumor (T)

____ **TX** tumor cannot be assessed

____ **TO** no evidence of primary tumor

____ **TIS** Paget's disease of the nipple with no demonstrable tumor

* Adapted from Data Form for Cancer Staging. Permission by The American Joint Committee for Cancer Staging and J. B. Lippincott Co., Philadelphia.

___ **T1** tumor 2 cm or less in greatest dimension

___ **T1a** no fixation to underlying pectoral fascia or muscle

___ **T1b** fixation to underlying pectoral fascia and/or muscle

    I tumor – 0.5 cm or less
    II tumor – more than 0.5–1.0 cm or less
    III tumor – more than 1.0–2.0 cm or less

___ **T2** tumor more than 2 cm but not more than 5 cm in greatest dimension

___ **T2a** no fixation to underlying pectoral fascia or muscle

___ **T2b** fixation to underlying pectoral fascia and/or muscle

___ **T3** tumor more than 5 cm in its greatest dimension

___ **T3a** no fixation to underlying pectoral fascia or muscle

___ **T3b** fixation to underlying pectoral fascia and/or muscle

___ **T4** tumor of any size with direct extension to chest wall or skin (chest wall includes ribs, intercostal muscles, and serratus anterior muscle, but not pectoral muscle)

___ **T4a** fixation to chest wall

___ **T4b** edema (including peau d'orange), ulceration of the skin of the breast, or satellite skin nodules confined to the same breast

___ **T4c** both of the above

lymph nodes (N)   (definitions for clinical–diagnostic stage)

___ **NX** regional lymph nodes cannot be assessed clinically

___ **N0** homolateral axillary lymph nodes not considered to contain growth

___ **N1** movable homolateral axillary nodes considered to contain growth

___ **N2** homolateral axillary nodes considered to contain growth and fixed to one another or to other structures

___ **N3** homolateral supraclavicular or infraclavicular nodes considered to contain growth, or edema of the arm (edema of the arm may be caused by lymphatic obstruction, and lymph nodes may not then be palpable)

lymph nodes (N)   (definitions for surgical evaluative and postsurgical treatment – pathologic)

___ **NX** regional lymph nodes cannot be assessed (not removed for study, or previously removed)

___ **N0** no evidence of homolateral axillary lymph node metastasis

___ **N1** metastasis to movable homolateral axillary nodes not fixed to one another or to other structure; further classified as to number of metastases and size

___ **N2** metastasis to homolateral axillary lymph nodes that are fixed to one another or to other structures

___ **N3** metastasis to homolateral supraclavicular or infraclavicular lymph node(s)

distant metastases (M)   (all time periods)

___ **MX** not assessed

___ **M0** no (known) distant metastasis

___ **M1** distant metastasis present

    specify: _____

tumor size

_____ × _____ × _____ cm

Predominant lesion measured on:

___ patient

___ mammogram

___ pathologic specimen

location   (multiple when necessary)

___ OUQ*

___ OLQ*

___ IUQ*

___ ILQ*

___ nipple/areola

performance status of host (H)

Several systems for recording a patient's activity and symptoms are used and are more or less equivalent as follows:

H0   normal activity

H1   symptomatic but ambulatory – cares for self

H2   ambulatory more than 50% of time – occasionally needs assistance

---

* Quadrants: outer upper, outer lower, inner upper, inner lower.

H3   ambulatory 50% or less of time — nursing care needed

H4   bedridden — may need hospitalization

stage

_____ clinical–diagnostic

_____ surgical evaluative

_____ postsurgical treatment – pathologic

_____ stage TIS: in situ

_____ stage X: cannot stage (unstageable)

_____ stages I–IV (further broken down; too detailed for this text)

histologic type of cancer   (check predominant type)

  ductal

_____ intraductal (in situ)

_____ invasive with predominant intraductal component

_____ invasive, NOS*

---

* Not otherwise specified.

_____ comedo

_____ inflammatory

_____ medullary with lymphocytic infiltrate

_____ mucinous (colloid)

_____ papillary

_____ scirrhous

_____ tubular

_____ other (specify)

lobular

_____ in situ

_____ invasive with predominant in situ component

_____ invasive

nipple

_____ Paget's disease, NOS

_____ Paget's disease with intraductal carcinoma

_____ Paget's disease with invasive ductal carcinoma

_____ other (specify)

histologic grade

_____ G1: well-differentiated

_____ G2: moderately well-differentiated

_____ G3–G4: poorly to very poorly differentiated

glossary/index

All abbreviations are listed separately in Appendix h, as are drug names in Appendix g. Words in case reports are not included here unless they appear elsewhere in the text. Foreign word definitions are on the back inside cover.

Systems, root words, suffixes and prefixes are not listed. Check table of contents. Only reference page number is given for words that require a long definition. Italicized number indicates illustration.

ankylosis condition of stiffening or fusion.

anomaly any abnormality.

anorexia (nervosa) the state of being without appetite (aversion to food) 154, 193

anoxia without oxygen 146

anteflexion bending forward.

anterior (ventral) toward the front, or in front of 67

antibiotic "against life"; medication effective in treatment of bacterial infections 101

anticoagulant medication to delay clotting of blood 137

anticonvulsive medication to prevent convulsions.

antineoplastic medication used in cancer treatment.

antiseptic against sepsis, used to prevent infection.

anuria no urinary output.

anus (anal) body outlet for solid waste at the end of the colon (pertaining to) 151

aorta largest artery in the body, arises from the left ventricle 132

aperture an opening.

apex (apices) the peaked portion or narrower part of an organ 131, 143

Apgar (score) system of evaluating condition of newborn 168

aphagia a state of not eating or being without appetite.

aphasia a condition of being unable to speak 178

apnea periods of no breathing 146

aponeurosis flattened tendon, resembles a membrane 118

appendectomy excision 157

appendicitis inflammation 154

appendix (appendices) useless appendage attached to cecum 151

apyrexia afebrile; without fever.

arachnoid "resembling a web"; middle meninx 173

arrhythmia without rhythm; erratic heart beat 136

arteriosclerosis (atherosclerosis) hardening of arteries (with build-up of fatty plaque) 136

artery (arteritis) vessel that carries blood away from the heart (inflammation).

arthritis inflammation of the joints 122

arthrocentesis joint puncture to remove fluid.

arthroplasty plastic surgery on a joint.

arthroscope (arthroscopy) lighted instrument for looking into a joint (procedure) 125

arthrotomy incision into a joint 125

articulation a joint; bones coming together 118

ascites the presence of excessive serous fluid in peritoneal cavity 157

asepsis, aseptic without contamination; sterile.

asphyxiation suffocation due to interference with breathing 145

asthma respiratory disorder with wheezing 145

astigmatism irregularity of curvature of the eye 182

astrocytoma malignant brain tumor.

asymptomatic without symptoms.

asystole cardiac standstill 136

ataxia lack of muscle coordination 178

atelectasis incomplete dilatation of lungs, which are collapsed 145

atraumatic not causing trauma, as in atraumatic needles.

atresia abnormal closing of a structure that should be open. esophageal 156

atrioventricular node impulse-conducting fibers in heart septum (Purkinje fibers) 132

atrium (atria) upper receiving chambers of the heart 131

atrophy without growth; wasting 122

atypical not typical or usual.

audiometer device for testing hearing 187

auditory pertaining to hearing 187 nerve 173

auscultation listening, as with a stethoscope or while tapping with fingers.

autism complete withdrawal from reality 179

autoclave sterilizer using pressurized steam.

autoimmune produces antibodies against self (own tissues) 126

autonomic (nervous system) self-controlling 173–5

avascular without blood vessels.

axilla, axillary the armpit.

azotemia uremia; the state of having nitrogenous waste in the blood 64

Babinski reflex big toe turns up when sole of foot is stroked 177

bacillus rod-shaped bacterium 57

bacteriology the study of bacteria 57

bacterium (bacteria) microscopic organism 57

bands immature forms of white blood cells 135

bariatrician (bariatrics) physician specialist who treats obesity (specialty).

basophil type of white blood cell 135

Bell's palsy paralysis of one side of the face 176

benign innocent, not deadly 53

Beta streptococcus hemolytic type (blood destroying).

bicuspid having two cusps (as a tooth or heart valve).

bifurcation division into two 146

bilateral both sides 67

bile (biliary) substance produced by the liver, important in digestion of fats 153, 154

bioavailability amount of drug actually assimilated by the body.

biochemistry chemistry of living things 96–7, 156

biofeedback type of training given to control some autonomic functions 175, 178

biology the study of living things.

biomed technician one trained in medical electronics.

biopsy examination of living tissue 110, 156

biweekly once every 2 weeks; twice a week 71

bladder a sac that usually holds fluid. distention 164 gallbladder 153, 154 urinary 162, 163

blepharitis inflammation of eyelids 182

blepharoptosis drooping of upper eyelid 182

blindness loss of sight, 20/200 or less. color inability to distinguish colors 182

blood vital fluid that circulates through the body 135 cells 135 chemistry 96–97, 156 gases 146 pressure 139 tests 88, 91 types 135

bloody show bloody mucus passed during late labor 168

"blue baby" infant not receiving adequate oxygen (any cause).

botulism severe food poisoning 154

bougie a dilating instrument (male urethra).

bradycardia slow heart beat 137

Braille raised alphabet for blind 185

brain mass of nerve tissue in cranium; encephalon 173 stem pons and medulla, upper portion of cord.

tumor new growth causing pressure on brain 177

bronchiectasis chronic lung disease 145

bronchitis inflammation of bronchi 145

bronchodilators medications to dilate bronchi.

bronchogenic arising from the bronchi 145

bronchopneumonia inflammation of bronchi and lungs 146

bronchoscope (bronchoscopy) lighted instrument to view bronchi (procedure) 146

bronchospasm contraction of bronchial tubes 146

bronchus (bronchi) large airway tubes to lungs 143

buccal pertaining to the cheek or mouth 157

bulla (bullae) large blister, as seen in burns 110

bundle of His part of impulse-conducting system of the heart 132

burns first, second and third degree 113

burr holes openings made with a trephine in the skull to permit access 177

bursa (bursae) pad-like structure in joints 118, *121*

bursitis inflammation of a bursa 122

by-pass surgery (coronary) grafting of new vessels to by-pass blocked artery (may be double or triple) *137*, 137
  GI for treatment of severe obesity 157

cachexia state of severe malnutrition, wasting 157, 194

calcaneus (os calcis) the heel bone.

calculus stone.
  renal (in kidney) 162

callus localized hyperplasia, thickening, caused by friction 113

calorie unit of heat 157

canthus (canthi) inner and outer corners of the eye 185

capillaries venous and arterial, the smallest blood vessels *132*

carbohydrates members of one of the basic food groups 154

carbon dioxide gas expired when breathing out 146

carbuncle pustular lesion; boil 112

carcinoma (carcinomata) cancerous or malignant tumor of epithelial or "surface" type tissue 53, 112, 145, 154

cardiac arrest heart action ceased 136

cardiac technician (biomed) a technician who takes electro-cardiograms, works with pacemakers, and so on.

cardiologist (cardiology) physician specialist in concerns of the heart (specialty) 30

cardiopulmonary resuscitation method of restoring circulation and breathing.

caries cavities in teeth 188

carpals bones of the wrist.

cataract clouding of lens of the eye 182, 194
  extraction surgical removal of lens 184

catatonic rigid, without speech or movement 179

catgut type of suture material.

catheter tube used for insertion into body.
  Swan-Ganz tube for insertion into vein in arm or groin to allow pressure in right heart and pulmonary artery to be read and pressure in LA to be approximated.

catheterization introduction of a catheter.
  cardiac into heart to detect abnormal flow 137
  urinary into bladder to drain urine 164

cauda equina "horse's tail"; group of nerves at the end of the spinal cord 178

caudal pertaining to the tail or end of spine 67
  anesthesia anesthesia injected into epidural space (regional).

cautery electrical machine for destruction of tissue 110

cavity a hollow space.
  cranial 106
  dental 188
  nasal 143
  peritoneal 106
  pleural 106
  spinal 106

cecum pouch at the beginning of the large intestine 151

celiotomy incision into abdomen; laparotomy.

cell the basic unit of all living things 106

cellulitis inflammation of the skin and subcutaneous tissue 112
  See case history 115

cephalic pertaining to the head 67

cerebellum part of the brain 173

cerebral palsy paralysis resulting from brain defect or trauma 176

cerebrospinal fluid (CSF) fluid that circulates around the brain and cord, in the subarachnoid space 173, *174*

cerebrum (cerebral) (pertains) to largest part of the brain 173

cerumen the wax in ear canal 186
  impacted 187

cervicectomy excision of the cervix of the uterus.

cervix (cervices) outlet of the uterus (the neck) that extends into vagina.

cesarean (C section) delivery by way of incision into abdomen and uterus 168

chalazion meibomian cyst; small hard tumor on eyelid 182

chancre primary lesion of syphilis, on genitals.

cheiloplasty plastic surgery of the lip 157

chemonucleolysis injection of a substance to destroy a herniated nucleus pulposus (disk).

chemotherapy treatment with chemicals, especially drugs used in treatment of cancer.

Cheyne Stokes irregular breathing 146

chiropractor (DC) one who treats disease with manipulation only 31

cholangiogram (cholangiography) X-ray picture of bile ducts (procedure) 156

cholecystectomy excision of the gallbladder 157

choledochoduodenostomy creation of a new permanent opening between the CBD and the duodenum 157

choledochostomy creation of a new permanent opening in the CBD through the abdominal wall.

cholelithiasis gall stones 154

cholesterol a chemical component of oils and fats produced by the body; in the diet considered to be a risk factor in blocking arteries 157

cholinergic nerve endings that release acetylcholine (para-sympathetic) 175

chondrectomy excision of cartilage.

chondritis inflammation of cartilage.

choroid dark brown layer between sclera and retina in the eye 182

chromic type of catgut suture material.

chromosomes "colored bodies" in the nucleus of cells, carry genetic material 106

chronic of long duration, usually not curable.

cicatrix, cicatricial a scar 113

ciliary muscle muscle that changes the shape of the eye lens 182

circulation process by which oxygen and nutrients are carried to tissues and wastes are carried away 132, *134*

  collateral expanded vessels 137

  portal from abdominal organs to liver 132

  pulmonary from right side of heart to lungs 132

  systemic from left side of heart to all parts of the body 132

circumcision the cutting around foreskin of penis 166

cirrhosis *cirrh* means orange yellow and describes the color of the liver with this disease 154

clavicle the collar bone 117

cleft lip/palate congenital defect; split lip/palate 154

Clinitest simple method of testing urine 164

coarctation narrowing of vessel walls 136

coccidioidin (cocci) test for valley fever (skin test) 114

coccidioidomycosis lung infection caused by a fungus; valley fever 145

coccus (cocci) round-shaped bacterium 57

coccyx, coccygeal tail bone, end of spine 117, *120*

colectomy excision of the colon or part of it.

colitis inflammation of the colon 154

collagen connective tissue (body protein) 122

colon the large intestine 151

colonoscope (colonoscopy) lighted instrument, flexible, for viewing colon (procedure).

colostomy a procedure creating a new permanent opening into colon 157

colpitis inflammation of the vagina; vaginitis.

colporrhaphy surgical repair of vagina; A & P repair 167

colposcope (colposcopy) magnifying instrument for viewing cervix (procedure) 167

coma (comatose) unconscious, unresponsive state 178

  diabetic complication of diabetes 194

combining form root word plus "o" as used when combining two root words: gastro/intestinal 4

commissurotomy cutting of the heart valve to improve circulation (mitral valve) 137

commode bedside portable toilet.

common bile duct (CBD) union of hepatic and cystic ducts, carries bile to the duodenum *153*, 157

communicable disease one that spreads from person to person.

concussion brain trauma, usually with loss of consciousness 176

congenital defect defect present at birth.

  atresias 156

  heart 136

congestive heart failure (CHF) failure to maintain circulation 136

conjunctiva (e) mucous membrane covering of the eye 182

conjunctivitis inflammation of membrane of eye (pink eye) 184

consolidation lung tissue being dense and solid 146

constriction narrowing (vasoconstriction) 44

contact dermatitis skin irritation due to contact with irritant 112

continent able to control voiding and defecation 164

contracture permanent contraction of a muscle, producing a stiffened joint 122

contraindicated not indicated (should not be used), especially medications in certain cases.

contrecoup occurring on the opposite side; injury to the brain on the side opposite to the blow 178

convulsion seizure (uncontrolled spasms) as in epilepsy, stroke, high fever in children 176, 194

Coomb's (test) blood test used to diagnose hemolytic anemias for presence of antibodies 168

cor pulmonale heart failure due to pulmonary disease 145

cordotomy cutting nerve fibers to relieve severe pain 177

coronary pertaining to the heart.

  arteries first branches from the aorta, supply blood to heart muscle 132, *133*

  occlusion blockage of coronary artery 136

  thrombosis clot in coronary artery 136

cortex outer layer of an organ 162

coryza the common cold, viral caused 145

costal pertaining to a rib.

craniotomy incision into the cranium 177

cranium (cranial) the skull.

  bones 117

  cavity 106

cretinism congenital hypothyroid condition 193

crisis (crises) in medicine, the time of greatest danger.

cryoextraction use of cold to extract lens of eye 184

cryoprobe cold probe, surgical instrument 185

cryoretinopexy fixation of detached retina with use of cold 184

cryosurgery use of cold in surgery.

cryptitis inflammation of crypts at opening of anus and penis 154

cryptorchidism "hidden testes"; undescended 58, 166

curettage using a curette to scrape inner surface of uterus; D & C 167

curvature a curve or bending.

  greater curved portion of the stomach on larger side 122

  lesser curved portion of stomach on smaller side (top).

  of the spine lordosis, kyphosis, scoliosis 151

cyanosis condition of blueness; skin, nailbeds and gums are pale, blue-tinged 146

cyst type of nodule or lump 110

  Bartholin 167

  pilonidal "hair nest" at base of spine (coccygeal area).

cystectomy excision of the bladder; excision of a cyst.

cystic fibrosis disorder of mucous glands leading to pancreatic insufficiency; mucoviscidosis 145

cystitis inflammation of the urinary bladder 162

cystocele hernia of the bladder 167

cystoscope (cystoscopy) lighted instrument for viewing interior of bladder (procedure) 164

cystostomy new permanent opening from bladder to surface.

cystotome instrument for cutting into bladder or anterior lens capsule of the eye; may be spelled cystitome (for eye incision) 185

cystotomy incision into the bladder.

cytometer instrument used to count cells.

cytoplasm the material of a cell outside of the nucleus 106

dacryoadenitis inflammation of lacrimal (tear) gland 184

dacryocystitis inflammation and obstruction of lacrimal sac 184

dacryocystotomy incision of the lacrimal sac 185

dacryolith a stone in the lacrimal duct 184

dangle to hang legs over side of bed.

datum (data) collection of factual material.

deafness hearing impairment, partial or total 187

debridement removal of dead tissue around a wound with cutting instrument or medication 110

decibel unit used in measuring sound 187

deciduous (teeth) "falling away," baby teeth 188

decongestant medication to relieve congestion 101

decubitus lying down.
  ulcers bed sores from lying down 67

defibrillate stopping fibrillation; a procedure to restore rhythm with electrical device that applies shock to heart.

deglutition swallowing 157

dehydrate remove water.

delirium mental confusion or excitement 179

delivery explusion of infant.
  forceps with instruments.

deltoid large triangular muscle that covers the shoulder prominence *121*

delusion a false belief 179

dental assistant a person who works chairside, handing materials to dentist 35

dental hygienist a graduate of a 2- or 4-year program, who does prophylactic dental care and takes X-ray pictures 35

dentalgia (dentodynia) tooth ache.

dentist (DDS or DMD) Doctor of Dental Surgery, Doctor of Medical Dentistry 35

depression a condition characterized by a lack of hope or despondency with all bodily functions slowed down 179

dermabrasion abrasion of the skin, used in plastic surgery 110

dermatitis inflammation of the skin 112

dermatologist (dermatology) physician specialist for skin disorders (specialty) 30

dermatome skin area innervated by various spinal cord segments; instrument for cutting thin section of skin 110

dermatosis any abnormal condition of the skin.

dermis (corium) the deeper layer of skin, under the epidermis 109

detail man (or woman) representative of a drug company 101

dextro to the right, or the right 67

diabetes mellitus a major disease of endocrine system 193–94

diagnosis (diagnoses) the identification of a disease; may be tentative, differential, presumptive.

dialysis the procedure of filtering blood with a machine 162
  peritoneal the process of using peritoneal membrane instead of a machine (fluid introduced and removed).

diaphoresis excessive perspiring 194

diaphragm a dome-shaped muscle 143

diarrhea running through of watery stools.

diastole, diastolic the least amount of force on vessel walls; lower number in B/P reading 139

diathermy therapeutic application of heat.

diet, low salt lowers B/P by reducing blood volume 82, 139

differential (diff) count a procedure to determine the percentage of each type of white blood cell in the blood 135

digital (exam) use of gloved finger (hand) to palpate for irregularities, especially of the rectum and prostate gland 156

digitalized, digitalization subjection of patient to digitalis drug at proper level to maintain heart contraction force without side effects 137

dilatation a process of stretching, opening 44

dilator instrument to stretch an opening.

diopter unit of measure for lenses 185

diphtheria acute infectious disease, bacterial 145

diplococcus round bacterium, in pairs 57

diplopia double vision.

disease disturbance in structure or function of an organ.
  Addison's 193
  Alzheimer's 176
  autoimmune 126
  Buerger's chronic inflammatory disease of arteries and veins in lower extremities.
  collagen 122
  Cushing's 193
  Hodgkin's 113, 136
  hyaline membrane 145
  Legg Calve Perthe's 122
  Meniere's 187
  Osgood-Schlatter's 125
  Parkinson's 177
  Raynaud's severe pain in toes and fingers with redness,

blueness, and coldness.
  rheumatic heart 136
  sexually transmitted 167
  Simmond's 193

distal farthest, from center or point of origin 67

diuresis (diuretic) increased output of urine (drug to produce this) 137, 164

diverticulosis, diverticulitis presence of diverticula (out-pouchings), inflammation of diverticula, especially in colon 154

dogs (guide and hearing) specially trained animals 187

Doppler ultrasonic probe that checks blood flow in the artery under it 137

dorsal referring to the back 67

dorsiflexion position with toe not pointed, but turned upward 68

duct a tube or channel.
  cystic *153*, 154
  hepatic *153*, 154
  common bile *153*, 154
  Wirsung pancreatic duct *153*

duodenum (duodenectomy) first section of small intestine (excision) 151

dura mater outer tough layer of the meninges 173

dyscrasia (blood) any abnormal condition 137

dysentery severe diarrhea 156

dysmenorrhea painful menstruation.

dysphagia difficulty eating or swallowing.

dysphonia a condition of impaired voice 146

dysphoria exaggerated feeling of depression.

dyspnea a condition of difficult breathing 146

dystocia difficult labor 168

dystrophy poor development 122

dysuria painful urination 164

ear organ of hearing 186, *186*

ecchymosis bruise or black and blue mark due to bleeding under the skin 113

echocardiogram (echocardiography) photograph of echo produced from sound waves emanating from heart (procedure).

echolalia repetition of anything that is said 179

ectopic out of place 168

eczema red, itching skin usually due to allergy 112

edema a condition of excessive fluid in body tissues.

EEG technician person who administers electroencephalography.

effusion "flowing out" of liquid, especially into pleural cavity 145

ejaculatory (duct) carries semen to urethra 165

electrocardiogram (electrocardiography) recording of electrical impulses of the heart (procedure) 137

electrocardiograph machine used in electrocardiography.

electrodesiccation destroying and drying out with electricity 110

electroencephalogram (electroencephalography) picture or recording of brain waves (procedure) 177

electroencephalograph machine used in electroencephalography.

electrolytes substances that, in solution, conduct an electric current (acids, bases, salts).

electronystagmography method of testing inner ear function 187

emaciation severe wasting with loss of body tissue 194

embolus, embolism a thrombus or clot (air, fat) that is moving through the circulatory system until it blocks a vessel 136

emesis vomiting.

emmetropia normal vision 185

emphysema condition characterized by distended or ruptured alveoli in lungs 145

empyema the presence of pus in the pleural cavity 145

encephalitis inflammation of the brain 176

encephalon (encephalopathy) the brain (disease of) 178

endarterectomy "boring out" the inner lining of an artery to increase flow 137

endocardium (endocarditis) membrane lining inside of heart chambers (inflammation) 136

endocrine (glands) glands which secrete hormones directly into blood stream instead of through a duct 191
system 191

endocrinology (endocrinologist) the study of endocrine glands (specialty, specialist) 30

endodontist dental specialist who works inside the tooth 35

endogenous arising from within.

endometriosis condition arising when cells of inner lining of uterus spread into pelvis 167

endoscope lighted instrument for looking into an orifice of the body.

enema (enemata) introduction of fluid into the rectum 157

enemas until clear until solution

comes back with no sign of fecal material 157

Fleet's prepared, disposable type of enema.

enterostomy the creation of a new permanent opening into the small intestine.

enucleation removal of eye 185

enuresis bedwetting 164

enzymes complex proteins manufactured by living tissues (necessary for digestion) 158

eosinophil (eos) type of white blood cell 135

epidermis (cuticle) outermost layer of skin (epithelial tissue) 109

epididymis (epididymitis) small body on top of testis; first part of excretory duct in male (inflammation) 165–66

epigastric over the stomach area 154

epiglottis flap of tissue that covers entrance to trachea to prevent aspiration of food 143

epilepsy seizure disorder 176

epinephrine (adrenaline) hormone secreted by medulla of adrenal glands.

episiotomy incision of perineum to facilitate delivery and avoid laceration 168

epithelium, epithelial protective type of tissue on surface areas (skin and lining of organs) 106

erosion "eating away" as an early ulcer 110

eruption any rash or "breaking out" 113

erysipelas an acute febrile disease with fiery red skin (streptococcal) 113

erythema redness 113

erythrocyte red blood cell 135

eschar (escharotomy) hard crust over a burn (cutting) 110

esophagogastroduodenoscopy (EGD) a procedure using scope to examine esophagus, stomach, duodenum 156

esophagus (esophagitis) food tube to the stomach (inflammation) 151, 156

essential (hypertension) high blood pressure without apparent organic cause 139

estrogen female hormone secreted by ovaries 191

euphoria exaggerated feeling of well-being.

eustachian (tubes) tubes from pharynx to middle ear to equalize pressure 143, 186

euthanasia "good death."

euthyroid normal thyroid.

eutocia easy labor (childbirth).

eversion turning outward, or inside out.

eviscerate viscera extruding from wound.

exacerbation an acute flare-up of symptoms, usually following period of remission.

exanthem rose-colored eruption 113

excise, excision to cut out.

excoriation severe abrasion 113

excrete, excretion elimination of waste products.

exfoliation the condition of scaling, flaking.

exocrine type of gland that externally secretes through a duct (salivary or sweat glands and so on).

exogenous, ectogenous arising from outside the body.

exophthalmic pertaining to protrusion of eyeballs 193

expectorant medication to loosen secretions in airways 146

extension straightening 122, *123*

external outside.
fixation devices used to reduce fractures in place of casting 125

extrauterine outside of the uterus; ectopic.

extremities arms (upper) and legs (lower).

eye organ of sight 182, *183*

fallopian tubes female ducts for egg traveling from ovary 166

family practice specialist (specialty) physician specialist who treats all types of patients 30

fascia (ae) fibrous covering, supporting and separating muscles; unites skin with underlying tissue 118

fats member of one of the basic food groups 154

febrile feverish; having an elevated temperature.

femur (femora) thigh bone; largest bone of the body 117

fenestration artificial opening to by-pass damaged middle ear 187

fibrillation quivering of individual muscle fibers causing ineffectual contraction of the heart and circulatory failure 136

fibroid resembling fiber; fibrous tumors 167

fibroma fibrous tumor.

fibrosis abnormal formation of fibrous tissue usually due to previous infections; often idiopathic (cause unknown) 145

fibula one of the lower leg bones (outer side) 117

fissure crack in skin surface, especially anal 110; deep furrow in the brain 178

fistula any abnormal passageway that occurs between organs or to outside surface of body 158, 167

flaccid floppy, lacking muscle tone 178

flail chest erratic movement of chest due to multiple injuries of ribs, sternum 145

flat plate term used in X-ray picture of abdomen.

Fleet's (enema) prepared, disposable enema 158

flexion bending 122

flexure a curve 156

  hepatic curve in the colon near the liver 151

  splenic curve in the colon near the spleen 151

floaters particles in the vitreous humor of the eye 184

"flu" influenza originally; now means almost any viral infection 145

focus (foci) the main or chief place involved in a morbid process (illness).

foramen (foramina) hole in a bone for vessels and nerves to pass through 118

  magnum opening in base of skull for spinal cord 178

forceps delivery involves use of instruments to deliver infant 168

forensic medicine medicine in relation to the law.

fossa (ae) a depression or hollow; indentation in a bone 118

fracture a break in a bone 122, *124*

  reduction 125

  skull 176

fulguration destruction of tissue with electric sparks 110

functional without organic cause (cause unknown) 179

funduscope, funduscopy examining instrument for the eye (procedure) 185

fungus (fungi) type of microorganism.

furuncle (furunculosis) pustular lesion 187

gallbladder an organ that lies behind the liver; stores and concentrates bile *153*, 154

  series X-ray procedure 157

gamma globulin substance containing antibodies formed by the blood; given as medication to people who need passive immunity (especially hepatitis contacts) 157

ganglion a knot of many nerve cell bodies outside the cord and brain 178

gangrene the presence of necrotic (dead) tissue 113, 194

gastrectasis dilatation of the stomach.

gastrectomy excision of the stomach (or part of it) 157

gastritis inflammation of the stomach 156

gastroduodenostomy the creation of a new permanent opening between the stomach and duodenum.

gastroenterology (gastroenterologist) specialty dealing with GI disorders (specialist) 30

gastrointestinal pertaining to the stomach and intestines 151

  series (upper, lower) X-ray procedures 157

gastroscope (gastroscopy) lighted instrument for looking into the stomach (procedure) 157

gastrostomy the creation of a new permanent opening into stomach (for feeding).

gastrotomy incision into the stomach.

gavage to feed by introducing a tube into the stomach (through nose) 158

generic drug the nontrade name of a pharmaceutical preparation 101

genetics branch of biology that deals with heredity 52

genitals, genitalia organs of reproduction 52, 165–66

  external (male) scrotum and penis 165

  external (female) vulva 166

geriatrics science of aging.

gestation period of pregnancy (280 days in human) 168

gigantism (giantism) abnormal overdevelopment of the body due to excessive production of growth hormone (pituitary gland) 191

gingivectomy excision of gum tissue (dental).

gingivitis inflammation of the gums 188

gland an organ that secretes (lymph nodes are often referred to as glands) 194

  prostate 165

  Bartholin 166

  sebaceous (oil) 109

  sudoriferous (sweat) 109

  salivary 151

  Also see endocrine

glaucoma increased intraocular pressure due to flow blockage of aqueous humor (eye) 184

glioma tumor of glia cells in brain or cord 177

glomerulonephritis form of nephritis involving glomeruli 162

glossitis inflammation of the tongue 156

glossopharyngeal relating to tongue and pharynx; ninth cranial nerve; sense of taste 173

gnathodynia pain in the jaw.

goiter enlarged thyroid gland 193

gonads sex glands (ovaries, testes) 191

gonioscopy procedure used in diagnosis of closed angle glaucoma 185

Gonococcus causative organism in gonorrhea 57

gonorrhea one of the major venereal diseases 57

gout one type of acute arthritis, due to uric acid crystals accumulating in joints 122

graft, by-pass any surgical procedure to create an alternate route for blood flow by detouring around obstructed vessel; coronary and aortoiliac are examples.

graft, skin tissue taken from one place to replace a defect elsewhere 110

grand mal (seizure) severe seizure in epilepsy with loss of consciousness.

granulocytes white blood cells with granules in the cytoplasm 135

granuloma granular tumor, usually of lymphoid and epitheloid cells.

gravida, gravid a pregnant woman; pregnant 168

groove shallow linear depression in a bone or tooth 118

guaiac (test) for blood in stool.

gynecology (gynecologist) specialty combined with obstetrics, concerned with diseases of women (specialist) 30

gyrus (gyri) convolutions of the brain (cerebrum) 178

hallucination hearing or seeing things not present 179

hayfever allergic coryza, pollinosis 145

heart hollow muscular organ that functions as a pump *131*, 132

  attack myocardial infarction; blockage of a coronary artery 136

  block disturbance in regular rhythm 136

failure (congestive)   failure of heart to maintain circulation 136

murmur   soft, blowing sound indicating heart valve may be incompetent 136

hemangioma   benign tumor of dilated vessels 64

hemarthrosis   condition of having blood in the joints (often seen in hemophilia) 64

hematemesis   vomiting blood (from GI tract).

hematology (hematologist)   the study of the blood (specialist) 30

hematoma   swelling due to blood clot 176

hematuria   blood in the urine, gross or microscopic 164

hemiparesis   weakness on one side.

hemiplegia   paralysis on one side (as seen in stroke victims).

hemisphere   either lateral half of the brain 178

hemoglobin   pigment in red blood cells that contains iron; its function is to transport oxygen 137

hemolysis   destruction of blood.

hemophilia   congenital lack of clotting factor 136

hemoptysis   spitting up blood from respiratory tract 64, 146

hemorrhage   uncontrolled bleeding.

hemorrhoids (hemorrhoidectomy)   dilated veins in rectum (excision).

hemostasis   control of bleeding during surgery, using hemostat clamps, cautery and so on.

hemothorax   blood in the thoracic cavity 145

Hemovac   closed system for wound drainage.

heparin   an anticoagulant drug 137

lock   system of maintaining an open vein for intermittent frequent intravenous use (using heparin).

hepatitis   inflammation of the liver 156

hepatoma   tumor of the liver.

hernia   projection of a part out of its normal place 156
  inguinal (direct, indirect) *155*
  umbilical 156
  hiatal 145

herniated nucleus pulposus   intervertebral disk rupture 122, 127, *128*

herniorrhaphy   surgical repair of a hernia 157

herpes   viral-caused blister type lesions 112

genitalis 167
simplex 112
zoster 112, 176
ophthalmic 184

hiatus, hiatal   an opening, especially in the diaphragm 145–46

hiccough, hiccup   spasm of diaphragm; singultus 145

high risk   more likely to succumb to certain morbid conditions; factors include heredity, age, use of tobacco and alcohol, degree of stress, lack of exercise, and so on.

hilus   root of lung where vessels, nerves and bronchi enter 146

hirsutism   excessive body hair 113

histoplasmosis   a fungal respiratory disease
  skin test 145

holistic (wholistic)   philosophy of treating the whole person instead of only the disease.

Holter monitor   portable ECG 137

homeostasis   state of equilibrium (sameness) that the body strives to maintain 107

homogenous, homogeneous   derived from like sources; uniform, same throughout 52

homosexual   one who is attracted to own sex.

hordeolum (stye)   inflammation of sebaceous gland, eyelid 184

hospital departments 85

humerus   bone of the upper arm 119

humor   fluid or semifluid substance.
  aqueous   in front of lens of eye 182
  vitreous   inside eyeball 182

Huntington's chorea   hereditary disease, purposeless movement, uncontrolled, and leading to dementia 176

hydrocele   fluid "hernia" in testes 165

hydrocephalus   cerebrospinal fluid not circulating properly in ventricles of brain, causing large head, mental retardation 176

hydronephrosis   collection of urine in pelvis of kidney due to obstruction of outflow 162

hydrophobia   fear of water; rabies.

hydrosalpinx   fluid collection in fallopian tubes 167

hydrotherapy   treatment with water.

Hyfrecator   commercial name for type of machine for destroying tissue (acronym for High Frequency Eradicator).

hyperactive   excessively active.

hyperalimentation   method of supplying body with nutrients

with a subclavian catheter 158

hypercapnia   increased CO_2 in the blood 146

hyperopia   far sightedness 184

hypertension   high blood pressure 136, 139

hyperthermia   unusually high temperature, induced in some cases to treat disease.

hypertrophy   excessive growth or development 122

hyperventilation   increased rate and/or depth of breathing 146

hypoactive   with less than normal activity.

hypochondria   "under the cartilage," of ribs (area of the abdomen); also, one who thinks he or she is sick without the presence of pathology 154, 179

hypodermic   under the dermis (skin); a method of giving an injection or the syringe used.

hypoglossal   under the tongue; twelfth cranial nerve, muscles of the tongue 174

hypoglycemia   low blood sugar.

hypophysectomy   excision of pituitary 194

hypophysis   the pituitary gland 191

hyposensitization   treatment in which increasing doses of an offending substance are given to build up tolerance (in allergic states) 146

hypotension   low blood pressure.
  orthostatic   occurring after suddenly rising to upright position, or from standing still.

hysterectomy   excision of the uterus 167

hysteria   extremely emotional state 179

hysteropathy   "any disease" of the uterus.

hysterorrhexis   breaking open of the uterus (rupture).

hysterosalpingogram   picture of uterus and tubes to determine patency 167

hysterosalpingo-oophorectomy   excision of uterus, tubes, ovaries.

iatrogenic   any condition arising from treatment by a physician 29

icterus   jaundice (bile pigment coloring tissues of the body a yellowish color).

idiopathic   arising from unknown cause.

ileocecal   pertaining to the ileum and cecum (a valve) 151

ileostomy   the creation of a new permanent opening into the

ileum (last portion of small intestine) 157

ileum last portion of small intestine 151

ilium bones of the upper half of the pelvis.

immunity; immunization the response of the body to an antigen (production of antibodies); preventive measure with use of various vaccines to stimulate production of antibodies 78

impaction tightly wedged.
fecal 156
wisdom tooth 188

impetigo skin disease, crusted lesions 112

in situ in position; said of cancer that has not metastasized 53

incision a cut into.

incontinent, incontinence inability to control urination and/or bowels 164
stress incontinence occurs only with hard coughing, sudden sneeze.

induction starting labor by use of medication or by rupturing membranes 168

infarct, infarction area of necrotic tissue.

inferior (sub, infra) below.

inflammation reaction of tissues to injury, characterized by the presence of redness, heat, swelling and pain.

influenza acute, infectious viral disease 145

infrasternal below the sternum.

inguinal pertaining to the groin 154

insemination impregnating with sperm from mate or donor, without intercourse 168

insulin injected medication used in treatment of diabetes mellitus; antidiabetic hormone 151, 194
dependent diabetic who requires insulin 194
pump method of giving insulin 195

integument, integumentary the skin (covering) 109

intercostal (muscles) between the ribs 143

intern physician (student) getting practical experience 31

internal inside.

internal medicine (internist) specialty that treats various types of patients (specialist) 30

interphalangeal (joints) joints between finger and toe bones (DIP distal) (PIP proximal) 118

intervertebral disks cartilage substance between the vertebrae; the center is the nucleus pulposus 118

intestine alimentary canal from pylorus to anus 151
small duodenum, jejunum, ileum; function is absorption of nutrients.
large the colon (about 5 feet long), from the cecum to the anus.

intramuscular (IM) within the muscle; injection method.

intrathecal within the spinal canal; method of introducing spinal anesthetic.

intravenous (IV) within the vein; using a needle to supply fluids, blood, medications.

introitus vaginal cavity 44

intubate to insert a tube.

intussusception telescoping of intestine into itself 156

involutional melancholia mental illness in menopause 179

ipsilateral on the same side 178

iridectomy, iridencleisis surgery in treatment of glaucoma, excision of part of the iris 185

iris (iritis) colored band of choroid surrounding the pupil of the eye (inflammation) 182, 184

ischemia insufficient supply of blood to any part 136

isocytosis condition of equal cells (all the same).

isothermal containing equal amounts of heat.

isotonic having the same salt concentration as body fluids; normal saline.

jaundice yellow coloring to body tissues due to bile pigment; symptom of liver disease, bile duct obstruction, carcinoma, hemolytic disease.

jejunostomy the creation of a new permanent opening into jejunum (small intestine).

jejunum that part of the small intestine following the duodenum and preceding the ileum 151

juvs immature forms of white blood cells 135

keloid overgrowth of scar tissue 113

keratitis inflammation of the cornea (eye).

keratoconus cone-shaped cornea; causes myopia 184

keratoplasty plastic surgery on cornea; transplant 185

keratosis hard, horny skin 112
actinic due to sun exposure.

seborrheic benign skin tumor (wart) especially in elderly.

ketosis accumulation of ketone bodies due to incomplete metabolism of fatty acids 194

kidneys lie behind the abdominal organs against muscles of the back (two) 162, *163*
floating displaced and moveable 162

Kussmaul (breathing) deep, gasping type of breathing 146

kyphosis the presence of hunch or hump back; spine deformity 122

labial (labia) pertaining to lips.

laboratory 88–97

labyrinthitis inflammation of inner ear 187

laceration a cut.

lacrimal, lacrimation pertaining to tears 185
glands secrete tears (superior to eyeball) 182
ducts passageway for tears.

lamina (laminae) the thinnest part of a vertebra on either side of the arch 118

laminectomy surgical excision to gain access to ruptured intervertebral disk 125, 177

Landsteiner (types) ABO blood groups.

laparoscope, laparoscopy lighted instrument for looking inside the abdomen (procedure); laparoscopic sterilization of female 167

laparotomy incision into abdomen.
exploratory in cases of acute abdomen when cause is not known 157

laryngectomy excision of the larynx (voice box) 146

laryngitis inflammation of the larynx 145

laryngospasm spasm of larynx, interferes with breathing.

laryngotrachobronchitis croup, with air hunger 145

larynx the voice box, first part of the airways 143

laser acronym for Light Amplification by Stimulated Emission of Radiation; produces intense heat, used in surgery 185

lateral side.

lavage to wash out 146, 158

leiomyoma tumor of smooth muscle.

lens transparent colorless structure in the eye 182

lensometer device that reads prescription of eyeglasses 185

lesion any kind of "sore"; a change in tissue structure *111*, 113

leukemia "white blood"; many types of malignant disease of the bone marrow 136

leukocyte (leucocyte) white blood cell 135

leukocytosis increase in white blood cell count.

licensed practical nurse (or vocational nurse) 34

lien the spleen.

ligament type of connective tissue, connecting bone to bone 118

limbic system part of the brain having to do with emotional behavior 178

lingual (sublingual) pertaining to the tongue (under the tongue) 158

lipoma tumor of fat; benign.

lithotomy "to cut out a stone" but refers to a position, lying on back with legs in stirrups 68

lithotripsy crushing a stone or calculus.

liver largest organ in the body 151

lividity skin discoloration due to venous congestion.

lobectomy excision of a lobe (lung) 146

lobotomy incision into a lobe of the brain (surgery sometimes used to treat certain mental illnesses).

lochia vaginal discharge following delivery 168

lordosis convex curvature of spine; swayback 122

lumbar that portion of the back at the waist.
  puncture (LP) insertion of needle into subarachnoid space of spinal canal for various reasons (spinal tap) 177

lumen (lumina) opening within a tubular structure (vessel, catheter and so on) 44, 138

lumpectomy excision of a lump (breast).

lungs organs of respiration 143

lupus erythematosus (LE) classified with rheumatoid diseases (autoimmune) 113, 122
  discoid 113
  systemic 122

lymph (lymphatic) alkaline fluid in lymphatic vessels; formed in tissue spaces all over the body and gathered into small vessels which carry it into bloodstream *132*
  nodes 133
  system *132*, 133

lymphocyte type of white blood cell 135

lymphoma tumor of lymphatic system.

lymphosarcoma malignant disease of lymphatic system.

macule spot on skin 110

malaise general feeling of being ill; nonspecific term for vague symptoms.

malignant deadly 53

malingering pretending, making believe 179

malleolus protuberance on either side of the ankle 118

malocclusion poor occlusion; teeth coming together improperly 188

mammary the breast.
  gland lobe of glandular tissue drained by ducts.

mammogram (mammography) X-ray picture of breasts to detect nonpalpable lesions (procedure).

mammoplasty plastic surgery on the breast.

mandible lower jaw bone 117, *118*

manic depressive one who suffers from a major psychosis 179

manometer apparatus to measure pressure 178

Mantoux (PPD) TB skin test (purified protein derivative) 146

Marshall Marchetti surgical repair of cystocele for stress incontinence 167

mastectomy removal of a breast
  radical with underlying muscle removed.

mastitis inflammation of the breast.

mastoid (mastoiditis) bony process of the temporal bone of the skull (inflammation); mastoidectomy is excision 187

maxilla upper jaw bone 117, *118*

meatus passage or opening, especially urinary meatus (urethra) 44, 162
  acoustic 187

meconium black tarry substance; first bowel movement of newborn 168

medial (mesial) middle.

mediastinum cavity between two principal portions of an organ 131

medical technologist (MT) laboratory technician 30

medium (media) in medicine refers to substance used to grow cells, organisms.

medulla inner or central portion of an organ 162

megacolon extremely dilated colon (congenital).

megalocardia, cardiomegaly enlarged heart.

megalomania mental state of having delusions of grandeur 179

meibomian cyst chalazion 182

melanoma "black tumor," a highly malignant tumor of the skin that metastasizes.

menarche onset of menses.

meninges (meninx) three membranes that cover the brain and spinal cord 173

meningitis inflammation of the meninges 177

meningocele hernia of the spinal cord meninges 177

meniscectomy excision of a meniscus 125

meniscus the saucer-like cartilage on the superior aspect of the tibia (knee) 118

menopause cessation of menses.

menorrhagia hemorrhage during menses.

menstruation monthly period if fertilization does not take place (menses).

mesentery peritoneal fold 158

mesopexy surgical fixation of the mesentery.

mesosternum in the middle of the sternum.

metabolism all physical and chemical changes that take place within the body; change of foodstuff to energy or heat 107, 154

metacarpals "beyond wrist"; bones of the hand.

metastasis, metastasize to spread to other parts of the body, as cancer cells do.

metatarsals "beyond ankle"; bones of the foot.

metrorrhagia hemorrhage between menstrual periods.

microbiology the study of small life (bacteriology) 57

microscope a magnifying instrument for looking at small objects.

microtome instrument for cutting something small (in laboratory, to make frozen sections).

micturate to void, pass urine 164

minerals inorganic elements, essential in small amounts for good health 54

miotic (myotic) drug that contracts pupil of eye 185

miscarriage spontaneous abortion; see abortion 167

mitosis cell multiplication by division 106

mitral (bicuspid) pertaining to valve in the heart (left side) 131

Monilia, moniliasis yeast-like fungus infection, vagina and tongue (thrush) 167

monocyte type of white blood cell 135

mucoid resembling mucus.

mucosa mucous membrane.

mucus a thick, sticky fluid secreted by mucous membranes and glands.

multipara woman who has borne more than one term infant 168

multiple sclerosis (MS) degeneration of myelin 177

myalgia pain in a muscle.

myasthenia gravis debilitating disease characterized by lack of muscle strength 122

mydriatic drug that dilates pupil of eye 185

myelin white fatty substance surrounding certain nerve fibers 178

myelogram (myelography) X-ray picture of spinal cord after dye injection 125, 178

myeloma (multiple) tumor originating in cells of bone marrow; malignancy.

myelomeningocele hernia of spinal cord and meninges 177

myelosuppression suppression of bone marrow function; produced by drugs used in treatment of cancer (leukemias).

myocarditis inflammation of the heart muscle 136

myogram, myograph, myography recording of muscular contractions, the machine used and the procedure (same as electromyography) 24, 125

myoma tumor of muscle tissue.

myopia nearsightedness 63

myositis inflammation of muscle 125

myringitis (tympanitis) inflammation of eardrum 187

myringotomy incision into the eardrum 187

myxedema condition due to hyposecretion of thyroid 193

nares the nostrils 143

naturopath, naturopathy one who uses natural forces to treat patients 31

nausea inclination to vomit.

necrosis, necrotic condition of having dead tissue.

neonatal (period) first 4 weeks of life following birth 168

neoplasm a new growth; tumor 53

nephrectomy excision of a kidney.

nephrolithiasis kidney stones 162

nephron kidney cell and capillaries 162

nephropexy suturing of the kidney.

nephroptosis prolapse of the kidney.

nephrorrhaphy surgical repair of the kidney 162

nerve structure that transmits impulses.
    auditory 173
    block 178
    cranial 173
    parasympathetic 175
    spinal 174
    sympathetic 175

neuralgia pain in a nerve.

neurasthenia ill-defined weakness, not relieved by rest 179

neurectomy excision of a nerve.

neurilemma membrane around peripheral nerves (sheath of Schwann) 178

neuritis inflammation of a nerve.

neurodermatitis skin condition for which no external or obvious reason exists (psychologic) 113

neurodynia pain in a nerve.

neurologic examination 176

neurology (neurologist) the study or science of the nervous system (specialist) 30

neuron nerve cell; functional unit of the nervous system 176

neuropathy "any disease" of the nerves 177, 194

neurosis "condition of the nerves" literally; a form of mental disturbance 179

neurospasm spasm or twitching of a nerve.

neurotripsy surgical crushing of a nerve.

neutrophil type of white blood cell (polymorphonuclear leukocyte); phagocytic 135

nevus (nevi) mole; flat or fleshy growth 112

nocturia, nycturia getting up to void during the night 164

nodule large raised lesion; a cyst 110

noninvasive (procedure) diagnostic procedure that does not require inserting needles, tubes and so on.

  tumor one that does not spread.

nonstriated muscle that does not have striped appearance 118

nosocomial (infection) one that results from a hospital stay.

nuclear medicine the branch concerned with diagnostic, therapeutic and investigative use of radionuclides.

nucleus (nuclei) the center, main portion of a cell 106

nucleus pulposus the relatively soft inner part of an intervertebral disk 122, 127, *128*

nummular having the shape of a coin 113

nurse midwife a nurse who delivers uncomplicated births 34

nurse practitioner performs routine examinations 34

nurse's aid, assistant one who performs bedside nursing care, simple office procedures.

nystagmography (electronystagmography) method of testing vestibular (inner ear) function (procedure) 187

nystagmus rapid, side-to-side movement of eyeballs 184

obese, obesity extremely fat, 20–30% over average weight.

oblique at an angle 67

obstetrics (obstetrician) specialty combined with gynecology, the care of pregnant women (specialist) 30

occult hidden, producing no symptoms.

occupational therapist (OTR) 34

oculomotor pertaining to eye movement 173

Oedipus complex intense love of child for parent of opposite sex, especially son for mother.

olecranon bony process on ulnar bone, elbow 118

olfactory pertaining to sense of smell 173

oliguria scanty output of urine 164

oncology (oncologist) study of tumors, especially malignant ones (specialist) 31

onychia (paronychia) inflammation around fingernail.

oophorectomy excision of an ovary 167

ophthalmology (ophthalmologist) the study of the eye (specialist) 30

ophthalmoscope instrument for looking into the eye 185

optic pertaining to vision. nerve 173

optometrist (OD) one who fits eyeglasses 31

oral surgeon dental specialist 35

orchidoplasty surgical repair of testes.

orchiectomy castration; excision of testes 166

orchiopexy, orchidoplasty surgery to place undescended testes into scrotum 166

orchitis inflammation of testes 166

organomegaly the condition of having enlarged organs.

orifice any opening 44

orthodontist dental specialist 35

orthopedics, orthopedist specialty, specialist for musculoskeletal disorders 30

orthopnea a condition in which the subject can breathe only while sitting upright 147

os mouth, opening 44

osteochondritis (osteochondrosis) inflammation of bone and cartilage (condition) 125

osteogenic originating in the bone.

osteolysis destruction of bone.

osteomalacia softening of the bone.

osteomyelitis inflammation of the bone and marrow 125

osteopath, osteopathy 30

osteoporosis porous condition of bones in old age 125

osteotome instrument for cutting bone.

otitis inflammation of the ear; media, externa, interna 187

otalgia pain in the ear.

otolaryngologist or otorhinolaryngologist ENT specialist 30

otology (otologist) study of the ear (specialist) 30

otoplasty plastic surgery on outer ear 187

otosclerosis stiffening of middle ear bones 187

otoscope (otoscopy) lighted instrument for looking into ear (procedure) 187

ovary one of the sex glands in the female; gonad 166

ovum (ova) female sex cell; egg.

oxygen gas inhaled and carried by hemoglobin; used in medical treatments 147

pacemaker battery-powered device implanted under skin to regulate heart rate 138

palliative used to relieve pain.

palpable, palpation able to be felt; to feel 167

pancreas, pancreatectomy excretes pancreatic juice and secretes insulin; excision 151 function tests 193

pancreatitis inflammation of the pancreas 156

pandemic large scale epidemic.

Papanicolaou (Pap) smear for cancer detection; sloughed off cells taken from cervical area 167

papilla (papillae) any nipple-like elevation or projection. of Vater 151

papilledema swelling of the optic nerve; choked disk 184, 186

papule raised spot on skin 110

paracentesis surgical puncture to remove fluid.

paralyzed, paralysis inability to move a part 122, 178

paramedical, paramedics allied health workers 34

paranoid, paranoia a condition of feeling persecuted 177

paraplegia paralysis from the waist down.

parasympathetic 175

parathyroids four endocrine glands 191

paratyphoid similar to typhoid.

parenchyma the functional part of any organ 147

paresis weakness 122, 178

paresthesia abnormal sensation 178

parietal pertaining to or forming the wall of a cavity; parietal bones of the skull and parietal lobes of the brain. membrane 132, 143

paronychia inflammation around fingernail 113

parotid (parotitis) "near the ear," salivary glands; inflammation (mumps).

paroxysm sudden unexpected attack.

patella the knee cap.

patent open, not plugged 44
  ductus arteriosus open duct between the pulmonary artery and the aorta in the fetus that should close after birth but remains open.

pathogen, pathogenic disease-producing 52

pathology (pathologist) the study of disease (specialist) 107

pediatrics (pediatrician) specialty that deals with children (specialist) 30

pedicle (graft) attaching skin to injured area from another part of the body, but leaving the graft attached to its source of blood supply until union takes place.

pediculosis lice infestation.
  capitis 112
  corporis 112
  pubis 112

pedodontist dental specialist who treats children 35

pelvimeter, pelvimetry instrument for measuring pelvis; procedure using instrument, X-ray, or ultrasound 168

pelvis any basin shaped structure; support for vertebral column and articulation with lower limbs *119*

renal the expanded proximal end of the ureter 162

percussion tapping, as with fingers during examination to ascertain presence of fluid or gas in underlying structures.

perforation a hole, caused by ulcer or injury 44

perfusion supplying organ with oxygen and nutrients 147

pericardium, pericarditis double membrane covering outside of heart 132; inflammation 136

perineum, perineal area between vulva and anus in female, between penis and anus in male.

periodontist dental specialist for gum diseases.

peripheral at the outer edges; farthest (from beginning) 67, 186

peristalsis rhythmic contraction of smooth muscle 154

peritoneum, peritoneal membranes that line abdominopelvic cavity and hold viscera 106, 158

peritonitis inflammation of the peritoneum 156

peritonsillar, paratonsillar around the tonsils.

pertussis whooping cough 145

petechia (petechiae) tiny pinpoint hemorrhages; evidence of bleeding disorder.

petit mal type of mild seizure characterized by brief periods of unconsciousness 177

phagocyte, phagocytosis "eating cell"; process of white cells ingesting foreign material 135

phalanges (phalanx) finger and toe bones.

pharmacology, pharmacist study of drugs; druggist 34

pharynx, pharyngitis the visible part of the throat; inflammation 143, 151

pheochromocytoma tumor of the adrenal medulla 193

phlebitis inflammation of a vein.

phlebotomist one trained to draw blood.

phlebotomy incision into a vein; cut down 138

phobia exaggerated fear 179

phthisis wasting; tuberculosis.

physiatry (physiatrist) specialty dealing with physical medicine and rehabilitation (specialist) 30

physician one who has successfully completed the requisites to practice medicine, either MD or DO 29–30

assistant usually, one who has academic and practical apprenticeship with a physician 34

physiology study of the function of the body and its components.

pia mater internal layer of meninges, directly covering the brain and cord 173

pituitary master endocrine gland (hypophysis) 191

placenta the afterbirth 168

previa low-lying placenta, near or covering the cervix so it would deliver first; *also see* abruptio.

plane imaginary line that divides 107

coronal 107

midsaggital 107

transverse 107

plantar flexion position of foot with toe pointed *123*

plaque silvery scales of psoriasis; material that builds up in arteries.

dental 188

platelets clotting particles in blood; thrombocytes 135

pleura, pleurisy the membrane covering the lungs and lining chest cavity 143; inflammation with effusion causing severe pain and dyspnea 145

plexus network of nerves or blood vessels.

pneumoconiosis any of the pulmonary disorders caused by an irritant such as asbestiosis, silicosis 145

pneumoencephalogram (PEG) "picture" of the brain after injection of air or gas into ventricles; pneumoencephal-ography is the procedure 178

pneumogastric pertaining to lungs and stomach; vagus nerve 173

pneumonia, pneumonitis inflammation of the lung, may be bacterial, viral; may involve lobes, bronchi 145

pneumothorax introduction of air into thoracic cavity either to collapse lung, or as a result of injury 147

podiatry, podiatrist (DPM) treatment of foot disorders; the practitioner 31

poliomyelitis inflammation of the gray matter of the spinal cord; acute, infectious viral disease 177

polycystic containing many cysts; polycystic kidneys, ovaries.

polymorphonuclear many shaped nuclei (pertaining to leukocytes) 135

polyp, polypoid type of tumor attached by a pedicle; resembles a polyp.

polyposis condition of having polyps, especially in the intestine 156

polyuria large volume of urine output.

porta cava shunt shunting of portal vein to inferior vena cava to by-pass obstructed liver 157

positions 68

Fowler's 68

knee chest 68

lithotomy 68

Sims' 68

Trendelenburg 68

post-operative following surgery.

posterior (dorsal) toward the back, or in back of 67

postmortem after death; refers to autopsy, examination of a body with family permission or, in unusual circumstances, required by law.

postpartum period following childbirth 168

postural drainage by the patient's position, loosening secretions to improve ventilation 147

practitioner one who practices; a physician, a nurse, or therapist.

prefix group of letters at the beginning of a word that alters the word's meaning.

premature not mature, especially an infant.

prenatal care care of a pregnant woman.

pre-operative before surgery.

presbycusis nerve deafness in older people 187

presbyopia loss of accommodation (vision) in older people 184

presentation position of infant for delivery 168

breech with buttocks or footling emerging first.

vertex with head emerging first.

primigravida a woman in her first pregnancy.

primipara a woman bearing her first child 168

proctology (proctologist) specialty dealing with diseases of the lower digestive tract (specialist) 30

proctoscope (proctoscopy) lighted instrument inserted into the rectum (procedure) 157

prodromal running before; early (symptoms).

progesterone female hormone secreted by ovaries *192*

prognosis (prognoses) prediction of the outcome of a disease.

prolapse drooping down 167

prone, pronation face down, palm down 122, *123*

prophylaxis, prophylactic any preventive measure such as immunization, regular dental care 188

prostate; prostatectomy accessory gland in the male 165; excision 166

prosthodontist dental specialist who designs and fits dentures 35

protein member of one of the basic food groups 154

protoplasm thick substance of a cell (cytoplasm).

proximal nearest to the center or point of origin 122, *123*

pruritus itching 113

pseudocyesis false pregnancy.

psoriasis chronic, hereditary dermatosis 113

psychiatric (tests) 179

psychiatry (psychiatrist) specialty that deals with mental illness (specialist) 30

psychology the study of the mind 31

psychosis mental illness 179

psychosomatic relating mind and body; bodily ill due to or aggravated by mental processes.

pterygium a growth of the conjunctiva over inner portion of eye 185

ptosis drooping.

public health (nurse, officer) that branch of medicine which deals with control of disease to prevent epidemics; PHN nurse usually makes home visits and operates clinics; PH officer is the physician in charge of public health operations.

pulmonary pertaining to the lungs.

function tests various diagnostic procedures 147

pupil an opening in the iris, which regulates the size of the pupil 182

purulent producing pus.

pustule lesion containing pus 110

pyelitis inflammation of the pelvis of the kidney 163

pyelogram, pyelography X-ray picture of the kidney, procedure; can be done intravenously (IVP) or retrograde (introducing dye from below).

pylorus, pyloric the outlet at the distal end of the stomach 151

stenosis obstruction of the pylorus, so food does not pass through 156

spasm spasmodic contractions of the pylorus.

pyorrhea "flow of pus," refers to gums that are inflamed and exuding pus 188

quadrant quarter, especially of the abdomen 154

quadriplegia paralysis of all four extremities; tetraplegia.

radiograph, radiography X-ray picture; procedure of taking X-ray pictures 24

radiologic technologist (RT) X-ray technician who prepares patients and takes pictures 34

radiology, radiologist specialty that deals with diagnosis and treatment with radiant energy; specialist 31

radionuclide atom that disintegrates by emission of electromagnetic radiation; radioactive isotope used in diagnostic procedures.

radius one of the bones of the forearm, thumb side *119*

rales sounds in the chest 147

rarefaction decreased density in an area on X-ray film 147

reaction (of a substance) the acidity or alkalinity; the pH, with 1–7 as acidic, 7–14 as alkaline.

rectocele hernia of the rectum.

rectum, rectal last section of the colon before anus 151

recumbent lying down; dorsal recumbent, lying on back 67

reduction (of fracture) bringing fractured parts into alignment; may be closed or open reduction.

reflex involuntary response to a stimulus 178

refractive errors vision disorders that are correctable with lenses 186

registered nurse (RN) a graduate nurse who has passed State Board examinations 34

registered physical therapist (RPT) a graduate physical therapist who has passed State Board examinations 34

rehydrate replace water or fluids.

remission period in which symptoms subside and which is often followed by an exacerbation; characteristic of some diseases.

renal pertaining to the kidney 162
failure 163
transplant 163

replantation reconstructing of a severed body part 125

resident physician who has completed his or her internship

and is working toward a specialty.

respiration the act of breathing 143

respirator a machine for prolonged artificial respiration; intermittent or continuous positive pressure 147

respiratory therapist (ARRT) graduate respiratory therapist who has passed State Board examinations 34

reticulocytes immature red blood cells, in bone marrow 135

retina innermost layer of the eye.
detached separated *183*, 184

retinitis inflammation of the retina 184

retinoblastoma malignant tumor of the retina 184

retinopathy any disorder of the retina 184

retrograde (flow) introduction of fluid from opposite direction in which it normally flows.
pyelogram kidney X-ray procedure where dye is introduced through the urethra 164

retroperitoneal behind the peritoneum.

retroversion turned or tipped backward.

Rh factor a factor in blood of those we call Rh positive 135

rhachialgia pain in the spine.

rhegma a rupture or tear.

rheumatic, rheumatism pertaining to general feelings of muscle and joint stiffness 125
heart disease a form of myocarditis with mitral valve insufficiency; a sequela to rheumatic fever 136
fever a systemic, febrile disease occurring usually in childhood; its onset usually follows a streptococcal infection.

rhinitis inflammation of the nose 145

rhinoplasty plastic surgery on the nose 147

rhizotomy the procedure of cutting roots of spinal nerves to relieve pain 178

RhoGAM vaccine given to Rh-negative mother after delivery of first Rh-positive fetus to prevent antibodies from forming 135

rhonchi sounds in the chest and throat 147

rhytidectomy excision of wrinkles (plastic surgery).

rib one of a series of 12 pairs of curved bones that form the thorax; connected to the sternum by cartilage, except two

lower floating ribs, and to the spinal column *119*

rickets juvenile osteomalacia, due to vitamin D deficiency 125

roentgenology, roentgenologist *see* radiology

root word the base part of a word.

rotation (version) turn.

rubella German or 3-day measles 113

rubeola regular/hard/red measles 113

sacroiliac pertaining to the sacrum and ilium (lower part of the spine).

salivary pertaining to saliva.
glands three pairs: parotid, sublingual, submandibular; send saliva into the mouth 151

salpingectomy, salpingitis excision of fallopian tube; inflammation 167; salpingitis can also refer to inflammation of the eustachian tubes 187

salpingopexy suturing of the fallopian tube 167

sarcoma malignant or cancerous tumor of underlying tissue, such as bone, muscle, connective tissue, bladder, kidneys, liver, lungs, and spleen 53, 125

scabies skin infestation by a small parasite called a mite 112

scan any of a number of procedures used in diagnosis, some employing radioactive substances to produce a contrast that can be detected 82–83, 147, 157, 164, 177

scapula the shoulder blade 117

schizophrenia (schizoid) literally means "split mind" but is a major psychosis affecting usually young people 179

Schlemm (canal of) opening through which aqueous humor flows (eye) 185

Schwannoma tumor of nerve fiber's sheath (neurilemma) 178

sciatica inflammation of sciatic nerve 177

sclera outer covering of eye 182

sclerosis condition of hardening.

scoliosis lateral curvature of the spine 125

sebaceous pertaining to the oil glands (sebum).

sedative drug that produces a relaxing effect or sleep 101

segs segmented nuclei in white blood cells (*see* footnote) 135

semicomatose unconscious, with some response to voice or touch at times.

seminal pertaining to semen.
duct 165

septal defect opening in the atrium or ventricle wall allowing deoxygenated blood to return to systemic circulation; congenital.

septum a dividing wall.
heart 132
nasal, deviated 145

sequela (sequelae) a result or after-effect.

series procedures for taking X-ray pictures 157
gallbladder 157
gastrointestinal (upper and lower) 157

serum (sera) (serous) blood plasma minus fibrinogen, the clotting factor; fluid from serous membranes 135

sesamoid resembling a seed.

shock disruption of circulation, characterized by drop in B/P, rapid, weak pulse; moist, clammy skin; anxiety.
anaphylactic reaction to penicillin or bee sting, for example; a type of neurogenic shock.
cardiogenic heart unable to adequately circulate blood.
hypovolemic loss of blood volume and body fluids.
neurogenic blood pools in peripheral veins and tissues as a result of severe cord injury, anesthesia.
septic toxins in blood impede pumping action of heart.

shunt any device used to divert or bypass; an artifically created passage or detour 177

sialolithiasis stone in a salivary duct 156

sigmoid S-shaped part of colon before the rectum 151

singultus hiccups.

sinistro to the left, or the left 67

sinoatrial node SA node; the pacemaker of the heart in the right atrium 132

sinus hollow space in cranium 118, 143; also refers to a dilated channel for venous blood.
rhythm regular heart rhythm.

skeleton bony framework of the body 117, *119*
appendicular 117
axial 117

slit lamp special narrow beam lamp of high intensity for examining the eye 185

slough dead tissue separation.

Snellen chart for screening vision for myopia 186

spastic having forceful uncontrollable contractions 178

specialties, specialists 30–31

speculum a type of dilating instrument, used especially for vagina or nose 167

spermatozoon (spermatozoa) male sex cell; sperm 165

sphincter a circular muscle.
anal closes the anus 151
cardiac, pyloric proximal and distal stomach openings.
of Oddi at entrance in duodenum from common bile duct.

sphygmomanometer blood pressure apparatus 139

spina bifida congenital defect in spine; *see* meningocele 125

spinal cord column of nervous tissue enclosed in the spinal canal; nerves to the trunk and limbs issue from it, and it is the center of reflex action to and from the brain 173
injuries 177

spirometer, spirometry instrument and procedure used in pulmonary function testing 147

spleen (splenectomy) vascular organ in left upper quadrant; forms white blood cells and acts as a filter (excision) 133

spondylitis (ankylosing) inflammation of vertebrae with spontaneous fusing, causing deformity 125

spondylolisthesis dislocation by forward displacement of a vertebra 122

spondylosyndesis surgical type of ankylosis; spinal fusion 125

sputum secretions from bronchial tree 147

stabs immature forms of white blood cells 135

stapedectomy excision of stapes (middle ear bone) 187

Staphylococcus **(cocci)** type of bacterium (round, growing in clusters) 57

stapling a method of suturing.
of stomach drastic method of controlling morbid obesity by placing staples across most of the stomach 157

steatoma fatty tumor 112

stenosis a narrowing.
pyloric congenital narrowing of stomach outlet so that food does not pass through.

sterilization process of rendering barren.
female tubal ligation or laparoscopic (Band-aid surgery) 167
male vasectomy 166

sterilized made free of organic matter.

sternum breast bone (manubrium, gladiolus, and xiphoid process) 119

stethoscope instrument for listening to sounds in the body.

stillborn (SB) infant dead before birth 168

stimulus any environmental element that brings about a response 178

stoma opening established in abdominal wall by colostomy 44, 158

stomach organ in which food processing begins 151

stomatitis inflammation of the mouth.

stool feces; bowel movement.
specimen feces sent to laboratory for analysis 157

strabismus any deviation of the eyes 184

Streptococcus **(cocci)** type of bacterium, round, growing in chain formation 57

striated striped; skeletal or voluntary muscle 106

stroke cerebrovascular accident; clot or hemorrhage in the brain 136

stye (hordeolum) lesion on eyelid 184

subcutaneous under the skin; layer under dermis 109

subluxation partial dislocation 122

subnormal below normal.

sudden infant death (SID) cessation of breathing during sleep, cause unknown, usually within first 3 months of life.

sudoriferous pertaining to the sweat glands 109

suffix group of letters at the end of a word that alters the word's meaning.

sulcus (sulci) grooves or furrows in the brain 178

superfluous (hair) unnecessary (especially on women's faces).

supine, supination face up or palm up 122, *123*

suprapubic above the pubic area.

surgeon specialist who performs surgery, general or specialized 31, 35

surgical technologist operating room technician, "scrub nurse."

suture various types of material used to stitch wounds; also the immovable joints of the cranium.

sympathectomy cutting fibers of sympathetic nerve 177

sympathetic nervous system 175

syncope fainting 178

cord/brain 177
Wilms' 164

tuning fork steel instrument used in testing hearing 187

turbinates cone-shaped nasal bones.

20/20 vision ability to see at distance of 20 feet what most people see at 20 feet; term used in screening vision 186

tympanectomy excision of the eardrum.

tympanic membrane, tympanum eardrum; separates middle and external ear; same as myringa 186

tympanoplasty plastic surgery on eardrum 187

type and crossmatch test to determine compatibility of bloods before transfusion 135

typhoid, paratyphoid acute, infectious bacterial diseases transmitted through food and water.

ulcer tissue destruction; a deep lesion 110
  decubitus 110
  gastric 156
  corneal 184
  varicose 110

ultrasound, ultrasonography procedure of using high frequency sound to produce an image of an organ or tissue 83, 157, 164

umbilicus (umbilical) the navel or belly button 154

universal donor one whose blood can allegedly be given to a person of any other blood type; type O 135

universal recipient one who can allegedly receive blood from a donor of any other type; type AB 135

upright standing.

uremia urine components in the blood instead of being excreted 163

ureter (ureterectomy) narrow tube that drains the urine from the kidney to the bladder (two) (excision) 162

ureterostomy the formation of a new permanent opening into a ureter 162

urethra the outlet for urine to leave the body; in the male also carries seminal fluid 162, 165

urethritis inflammation 164

urinalysis (urinalyses) (Ua) testing the urine 91, 164

urogenital pertaining to the urinary and reproductive systems.

urology (urologist) specialty dealing with urinary tract disorders (specialist) 31

urticaria hives; raised itchy welts 113

uterus womb; female organ in which fetus develops 166

uvea (uveitis) vascular coat of the eye beneath the sclera (inflammation) 184

uvula muscle tissue that hangs down from the soft palate 143

vagina birth canal, from cervix to vulva 166

vaginitis inflammation (*see Monilia, Trichomonas*) 167

vagus nerve, vagotomy tenth cranial nerve 173; incision 157, 178

valley fever coccidioidomycosis 145

valves (heart) structures in veins, lymph vessels, and in the heart, to keep blood from backflowing.
  aortic 131
  mitral 131
  pulmonary 131
  tricuspid 131

varicella chickenpox; vesicles that itch and scab 113

varices (varix) dilated, varicose veins; varicosities 136
  esophageal 156

varicocele varicose veins near the testes 166

varicose veins enlarged, twisted superficial veins, due to incompetent valves 136

variola smallpox; an acute, infectious viral disease now considered to be extinct.

vas deferens continuation of duct from epididymis; excretory duct 165

vasectomy excision of all or a segment of the vas deferens; sterilization procedure 166

vasoconstriction narrowing of vessels.

vasodilator medication that causes dilatation or widening of vessels 138

vasopressor agent that stimulates contraction 138

vein vessel that carries blood toward the heart 132

vena(e) cava(e) largest veins in the body, superior and inferior 132

venereal disease (VD) sexually transmitted disease (STD); *see* syphilis, gonorrhea, herpes 167

venipuncture puncture of a vein for any purpose 138

venogram (phlebogram) X-ray picture of the veins.

ventilator device that provides mechanical assistance to ventilate the lungs.

ventricle either of two lower chambers of the heart 131; cavity in the brain *174*

ventriculography injection of air into ventricles of the brain for X-ray purposes 178

vernix caseosa cheesy white substance on skin of newborn 169

verruca(e) wart; epithelial tumor 112

vertebra(e) individual bone of spinal column *120*

vertebral column the spine 117, *120*

vertigo sensation of whirling motion 187

vesicle lesion containing fluid; blister 110

vesico-vaginal pertaining to the bladder and vagina 164

villus (villi) tiny, fingerlike projections in the small intestines 154

virus pathogenic agent, much smaller than bacteria, that depends on nutrients inside cells for existence and reproduction.

viscera, visceral (viscus) internal organs, especially the abdominal organs 158

viscosity, viscous thickness; sticky, gummy.

vital capacity volume of air that can be expelled after full inspiration 147

vitamins substances needed for normal function and maintenance of health 154

vitiligo loss of pigment in skin 113

vitrectomy aspiration of vitreous fluid in eye 185

void to empty; pass urine 164

vomiting, vomit ejecting stomach contents through the mouth.
  projectile with great force.

wheal an individual hive or elevated area on skin 110

"whiplash" hyperextension of neck; injury caused by sudden jerking 177

whooping cough pertussis 145

X-ray (roentgen ray) rays which can penetrate solid matter and act on photographic film; used in diagnosis and treatment.
  chest 147
  flat plate 156
  routine X-ray picture of chest taken on admission to hospital, AP and lat.

xanthoma benign yellow tumor.

xiphoid (process) pointed bottom portion of sternum (breastbone).